1 Rod
, Laurie
Hikes within 60 miles :
Houston, including
Huntsville, Beaumont, and
$17.95
ocn707256049
ed.   11/29/2011
WITHDRAWN

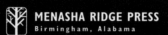

MENASHA RIDGE PRESS
Birmingham, Alabama

60 HIKES WITHIN 60 MILES

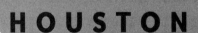

HOUSTON

INCLUDING
HUNTSVILLE, GALVESTON, AND BEAUMONT

SECOND EDITION

LAURIE RODDY

60 HIKES WITHIN 60 MILES: HOUSTON

Copyright © 2012 by Laurie Roddy
All rights reserved
Printed in the United States of America
Published by Menasha Ridge Press
Distributed by Publishers Group West
Second edition, first printing

Library of Congress Cataloging-in-Publication Data
  Roddy, Laurie, 1958–
    60 hikes within 60 miles : Houston, including Huntsville, Beaumont,
    and Galveston / Laurie Roddy. — 2nd ed.
      p. cm.
    Includes index.
    ISBN-13: 978-0-89732-931-6
    ISBN-10: 0-89732-931-7
    1. Hiking Texas—Houston Region—Guidebooks. 2. Houston Region
    (Tex.)—Guidebooks. I. Title. II. Title: Sixty hikes within sixty miles.
    GV199.42.T492H687 2011
    796.5109764141'1—dc23
                        2011037364

Cover and text design by Steveco International
Cover photo © Chad Ehlers / Alamy
Author photo by Jim Roddy
Cartography and elevation profiles by Laurie Roddy, Scott McGrew, and Chris Erichson

Menasha Ridge Press
P.O. Box 43673
Birmingham, AL 35243
menasharidge.com

DISCLAIMER
This book is meant only as a guide to select trails in the Houston area and does not guarantee hiker safety in any way—you hike at your own risk. Neither Menasha Ridge Press nor Laurie Roddy is liable for property loss or damage, personal injury, or death that result in any way from accessing or hiking the trails described in the following pages. Please be aware that hikers have been injured in the Houston area. Be especially cautious when walking on or near boulders, steep inclines, and drop-offs, and do not attempt to explore terrain that may be beyond your abilities. To help ensure an uneventful hike, please read carefully the introduction to this book, and perhaps get further safety information and guidance from other sources. Familiarize yourself thoroughly with the areas you intend to visit before venturing out. Ask questions, and prepare for the unforeseen. Familiarize yourself with current weather reports, maps of the area you intend to visit, and any relevant park regulations.

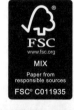
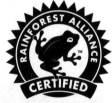

**FOR JIM AND MITCH,
THE TWO MEN IN MY LIFE WHOM I ADORE**

— LAURIE RODDY

TABLE OF
CONTENTS

ACKNOWLEDGMENTS

I am most thankful for the support my husband, Jim, and son, Mitch, gave me during the hiking and writing of this book. While completing 60 hikes in nine months took me away many weekends and even some holidays, neither of them complained and oftentimes they had dinner ready or the restaurant picked out when I got home. Mitch was with me on my first hike and then again on the only other hike I completed during the summer. What a trooper to hike in Houston during July.

I also want to thank my hiking, golfing, shopping, and just hanging-out buddy, Pam. She was there when I needed her most, even through her sore knee, knee surgery, and knee-surgery recovery. Her moral and emotional support were invaluable in keeping me focused and on schedule. I love her dearly.

My family and friends encouraged me along the way with enthusiasm for the project. To a person they expressed excitement about a hiking book in Houston. I also want to thank the Lone Star Hiking Trail Club, and in particular Carol, who sent me copious amounts of information on trails that the club had mapped out and recommended. The club's website is a great resource for information on hiking in this area.

Thank you to my Menasha Ridge Press editor, Russell Helms, who helped me throughout the project and particularly in the beginning, when I was just learning about GPS use and map creation. His knowledge, patience, and guidance were sorely needed at times. Also, I want to thank Molly Merkle, who took all my files and actually made a book. Amazing!

The volunteers and employees of state, city, and county agencies that support all the parks must also be recognized. Without them there would be no parks, no hiking trails, and a very dreary world. Thanks for your time and support.

And last I want to thank my mom, Shirley Cook, for instilling in me the love of the outdoors and the belief that I can do anything to which I put my mind. I think of her every day and miss her in my life.

—LAURIE RODDY

FOREWORD

Welcome to Menasha Ridge Press's *60 Hikes within 60 Miles*. Our strategy was simple: First, find a hiker who knows the area and loves to hike. Second, ask that person to spend a year researching the most popular and very best trails around. And third, have that person describe each trail in terms of difficulty, scenery, condition, elevation change, and all other categories of information that are important to hikers. "Pretend you've just completed a hike and met up with other hikers at the trailhead," we told each author. "Imagine their questions, and be clear in your answers." An experienced hiker and writer, author Laurie Roddy has selected 60 of the best hikes in and around the Houston metropolitan area. From the greenways and urban hikes that make use of parklands to flora- and fauna-rich treks along the ravines and hills in the hinterlands, Roddy provides hikers (and walkers) with a great variety of hikes—and all within roughly 60 miles of Houston.

You'll get more out of this book if you take a moment to read the Introduction explaining how to read the trail listings. The "Topographic Maps" section will help you understand how useful topos will be on a hike, and will also tell you where to get them. And though this is a "where-to" rather than a "how-to" guide, those of you who have hiked extensively will find the Introduction of particular value. As much for the opportunity to free the spirit as well as to free the body, let these hikes elevate you above the urban hurry.

All the best,
The Editors at Menasha Ridge Press

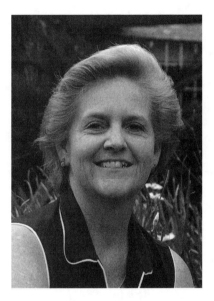

A native of Houston, **Laurie Roddy** has been writing for almost 30 years on everything from computers to sports. She started her own company, Roddy Communications, Inc. in 1997 after working as a technical writer for Compaq Computer Corporation for ten years. Her main interests and current writing career include hiking, golf, and traveling. She has hiked the Rocky Mountains, Mt. Olympia, Mt. Rainier, the Davis Mountains, Big Bend, the Smokey Mountains, St. Johns in the U.S. Virgin Islands, and all around the Houston area. She is a contributing writer for *Cy-Fair* magazine, *Community Impact News,* **Trails.com,** **Livestrong.com,** and a freelance writer.

PREFACE

The most frequent question I was asked was, "Where are you going to find 60 hikes around Houston?" Not only did I find 60 hikes, but I could have added another 10 to 15 hikes if the book were called 75 Hikes within 75 Miles: Houston. And, with the number of trails being added in the next few years, I expect that number to increase. Another comment I got was, "Since we don't have mountains, where are you going to hike?" Again, not a problem. The Houston area has the Gulf Coast in the south, Texas coastal prairies in the south and west, marshes along the coast, East Texas forests north and east, rolling hills north, and riparian landscapes along rivers, creeks, and bayous all around the city. To my surprise some of the hikes in the Sam Houston National Forest had elevation changes of 200 to 300 feet, and while that doesn't seem like much to people in other parts of the country, I think it's more than what most people would expect around here.

Houston, the Bayou City, has in the last few years decided to capitalize on the waterways that meander through most of the area. Once thought of only as flood-control channels, many of the bayous were reconstructed with concrete in the 1960s and 1970s. That has all changed as the City of Houston is now embracing the bayous as important assets to the aesthetics and environmental viability of the city. With the work of the Buffalo Bayou Partnership and other environmentally minded groups, Buffalo Bayou has become the focal point of the recent downtown revitalization. Its rich and diverse plant and animal life are important to the urban ecosystem of Houston. What this change in attitude means to hikers is a boon in hiking and biking trails throughout the city. Sims Bayou, Buffalo Bayou, White Oak Bayou, Armand Bayou, and Brays Bayou all have trails, and in many cases, paved and lighted trails that run parallel to each waterway. More and more parks are planned, with most containing some form of hiking trails.

From easy hikes in county parks to long, demanding hikes in the Sam Houston National Forest, there is a hike for everyone. And, while Houston has subtropical weather in the summer, it also has that same subtropical weather in the winter, making the area ideal for winter hiking. There is nothing like getting out on a trail in January under a cloudless, deep blue sky in 45-degree weather. The air is clear, the humidity is low, the temperature is just cold enough to need a jacket, and the sun is just warm enough to make the hike perfect. Golf is not the only 12-month activity in this area—hiking, biking, canoeing, and kayaking can all be enjoyed year-round.

ABOUT THE HIKES

While I could have added more long hikes from the Sam Houston National Forest and the Lone Star Hiking Trail, I felt that the urban hikes are just as important because they are more accessible to a greater number of people and a more diverse group of hikers (for example, children, the disabled, and beginning hikers). These hikes are not only easier to get to, but they tend to be shorter and on paved, level ground. Because Houston is only 50 miles from the coast, only 16 hikes are south and east of the city, with the other 44 hikes located in Houston and north and west of the city limits.

URBAN HOUSTON

Hikes in Houston are generally on paved paths that run parallel to the bayous. They are heavily used on weekends and in the evenings during the week, but you should see very few people on most mornings Monday through Friday. The paths are used by cyclists, so stay to the right at all times and be aware of your surroundings. The hikes in Memorial Park (while only minutes from downtown Houston) are all located in a wooded, secluded area. These trails were originally created by Houston cyclists, so you may want to hike them during the week to avoid the cycling crowd on the weekends. The Memorial Park Conservancy is working on a master plan to build more trails and enhance the existing trails for use by hikers, cyclists, and equestrian riders. Many new trails within the 610 Loop area have been added by the City of Houston over the last few years, including the West White Oak Bayou Trail, Halls Bayou Trail, and Heights Hike and Bike Trail. Check out the Houston Parks and Recreation website for a listing of all the new trails.

SOUTH

Due to the proximity of the Gulf of Mexico to Houston, there is not much land south of Houston before you reach the water, limiting the number of hikes in this area. However, the three hikes in this region were some of my favorites because they offer incredible bird-watching opportunities in the winter and early spring before the northward migration. I saw more wildlife at San Bernard and Brazoria National Wildlife Refuge than on any hike north of the city. You can expect to see herons, ducks, geese (by the thousands), alligators, snakes, deer, and wild pigs on most days.

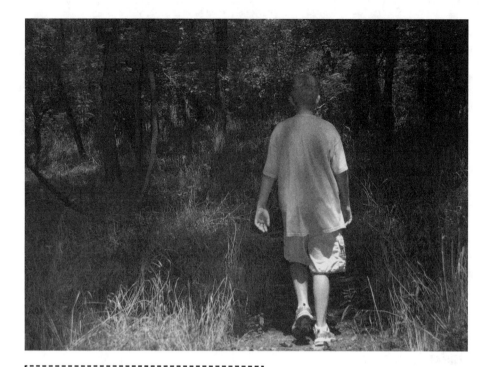

My son, Mitch, hiking in Stephen F. Austin State Park.

SOUTHWEST

There's only one hiking park southwest of Houston and that is Brazos Bend State Park, one of the best parks in Texas. Included on The Brazos River Trail, this park offers some of the best camping and nature-watching in the state. Besides the trails described in this book, there are numerous other short, backcountry, and camp hikes. Again, as with the hikes south of Houston, the wildlife is abundant here, with alligators, snakes, and deer.

WEST

As you head west out of Houston, the terrain changes to open grasslands and prairie.Included in this section are hikes in Terry Hershey Park and George Bush Park that run parallel to Interstate 10 from Beltway 8 to Fry Road. You can hike or bike the entire 10 miles one way without having to get off the trail or cross a major road. Also included in this section are Stephen F. Austin State Park and the Attwater Prairie Chicken National Wildlife Refuge, both worth visiting due to the uniqueness of the landscape as compared with the rest of the Houston area.

NORTHWEST

The hikes in this section are all what I would call children-friendly hikes. They are all relatively short and in parks where there are learning centers, playgrounds, and fishing lakes. You can learn local history at Kleb Woods Nature Preserve and the Jesse H. Jones Park, both favorite parks for Cub Scout trips. While these hikes are close to the city, they all offer very wooded environments with abundant flora and fauna to observe. As part of the newly dedicated Spring Creek Greenway (a 12,000-acre greenway that runs along Spring Creek), many new trails have been added to the area, including trails in George Mitchell Nature Preserve and Pundt Park.

NORTH (including Huntsville)

The Lone Star Hiking Trail is a 128-mile National Recreation Trail that stretches from the eastern edge of the forest near Montague Church on FM 1725 close to Cleveland to the extreme western edge near Richards, Texas. A large part of the trail is maintained and mapped by the Lone Star Hiking Trail Club, which you can find at **lshtclub.com**. Affiliated with the American Hiking Society, this club works year-round to ensure trails are maintained and cleared. These trails are all located in heavily wooded areas that can be dark and difficult to hike, so make sure you have the proper gear and experience before you tackle these trails. The trails in Huntsville State Park offer the most elevation change in the area. While the park is well maintained, it is heavily used on spring and fall weekends.

NORTHEAST

"Deep East Texas piney woods" best describes the hikes in this region. Lake Houston Park is now a city and county park that was turned over by the State of Texas in August 2006. Although the Big Thicket National Preserve is a bit out of the 60-mile range, I thought it important to add at least one hike to bring attention to the area. The Big Thicket was designated a national preserve in 1974 by President Gerald Ford, establishing the first national preserve in the national park system. It is well worth the drive. The preserve contains eight hiking trails, with the longest being an 18-mile hike; but since most of the hikes are even farther from Houston than the Kirby Nature Trail, which is featured in this book, I left them out.

EAST (including Beaumont)

The hikes east of Houston visit coastal wetlands, with a few deep East Texas hikes, including the recently added Sheldon Lake State Park just east of downtown Houston. All of these hikes offer a variety of wildlife for observation, and most are a birder's paradise. Goose Creek Stream Greenbelt is an urban hike located in Baytown that gives you good views of the marina and parks just past the Baytown Bridge. Village Creek State Park and J. J. Mayes Wildlife Trace can flood after heavy rains, so watch the weather and call their respective offices to ask about trail conditions before heading out.

SOUTHEAST (including Galveston)

Hikes in Armand Bayou, although not very long, visit some of the most diverse ecosystems in the area. You will go through marshes, hike beside bayous, slog through forests, and step out into the prairie sun—all on the same hike. Challenger Seven Memorial is a park dedicated to the members of the Challenger Seven crew who perished in 1986 when the space shuttle exploded. This is a recreation park with a fine hike in the back of the park that takes you on boardwalks, through forests, and past open fields. One of my favorite hikes is the Galveston Island State Park hike. Although it is not in the woods or along a meandering creek, it is one of the most scenic hikes in the area. The hike is entirely on the coastal grasslands and sandy banks of the bay; and due to the low elevation, you can see for miles in all directions. Please try and save this hike for the cooler months, as there is no shade.

HIKING RECOMMENDATIONS

HIKES 1 TO 2.9 MILES

HIKES 3 TO 6 MILES

HIKES GREATER THAN 6 MILES

BEST FOR CHILDREN

BEST FOR SOLITUDE

BEST HIKES FOR BIRD-WATCHING

BUSY HIKES ON WEEKENDS

EASIEST HIKES

HIKES ALONG CREEKS, RIVERS, AND BAYOUS

GARDEN HIKES

LAKE HIKES

MOST DIFFICULT HIKES

MOST SCENIC HIKES

SUNNY HIKES

URBAN HIKES

WHEELCHAIR-ACCESSIBLE HIKES

WILDFLOWER HIKES

WILDLIFE HIKES

WOODED URBAN HIKES

60 HIKES
WITHIN 60 MILES

HOUSTON
INCLUDING
HUNTSVILLE, GALVESTON, AND BEAUMONT

INTRODUCTION

Welcome to *60 Hikes within 60 Miles: Houston*. If you're new to hiking or even if you're a seasoned hiker, take a few minutes to read the following introduction. We explain how this book is organized and how to use it.

HOW TO USE THIS GUIDEBOOK

THE OVERVIEW MAP AND OVERVIEW-MAP KEY

Use the overview map on the inside front cover to find the exact locations of each hike's primary trailhead. Each hike's number appears on the overview map, on the map key facing the overview map, and in the table of contents. Flipping through the book, a hike's full profile is easy to locate by watching for the hike number at the top of each page. The book is organized by region as indicated in the table of contents. A map legend that details the symbols found on trail maps appears on the inside back cover.

REGIONAL MAPS

The book is divided into regions and prefacing each regional section is an overview map of that region. The regional map provides more detail than the overview map, bringing you closer to the hike.

TRAIL MAPS

Each hike contains a detailed map that shows the trailhead, the route, significant features, facilities, and topographic landmarks such as creeks, overlooks, and peaks. The author gathered map data by carrying a Garmin eTrex Vista C GPS unit while hiking. This data was downloaded into the digital mapping program Topo USA and Garmin BaseCamp and processed by expert cartographers to produce the highly accurate maps found in this book. Each trailhead's GPS coordinates are included with each profile.

ELEVATION PROFILES

Corresponding directly to the trail map, each hike contains a detailed elevation profile. The elevation profile provides a quick look at the trail from the side, enabling you to visualize how the trail rises and falls. Key points along the way are labeled. Note the number of feet between each tick mark on the vertical axis (the height scale). To avoid making flat hikes look steep and steep hikes appear flat, height scales are used throughout the book to provide an accurate image of the hike's climbing difficulty.

GPS TRAILHEAD COORDINATES

To collect accurate map data, each trail was hiked with a Garmin eTrex Vista C GPS unit. Data collected was then downloaded and plotted onto a digital USGS topo map. In addition to highly specific trail outlines, this book also includes the GPS coordinates for each trailhead using latitude–longitude. Latitude–longitude coordinates tell you where you are by locating a point west (latitude) of the 0° meridian line that passes through Greenwich, England, and north or south of the 0° (longitude) line that belts the Earth, a.k.a. the Equator.

For readers who own a GPS unit, whether handheld or onboard a vehicle, the latitude–longitude coordinates provided on the first page of each hike may be entered into the GPS unit. Just make sure your GPS unit is set to navigate using WGS84 datum. Now you can navigate directly to the trailhead.

Most trailheads, which begin in parking areas, can be reached by car, but some hikes still require a short walk to reach the trailhead from a parking area. In those cases a handheld unit is necessary to continue the GPS navigation process. That said, however, readers can easily access all trailheads in this book by using the directions given, the overview map, and the trail map, which shows at least one major road leading into the area. But for those who enjoy using the latest GPS technology to navigate, the necessary data has been provided.

For more on GPS technology, the USGS offers a good deal of information on its website, **usgs.gov.**

HIKE DESCRIPTIONS

Each hike contains seven key items: an "In Brief" description of the trail, a Key At-a-Glance Information box, directions to the trail, trailhead coordinates, a trail map, an elevation profile, and a trail description. Many also include a note on nearby activities. Combined, the maps and information provide a clear method to assess each trail from the comfort of your favorite reading chair.

IN BRIEF

A "taste of the trail." Think of this section as a snapshot focused on the historical landmarks, beautiful vistas, and other sights you may encounter on the hike.

KEY AT-A-GLANCE INFORMATION

The information in these boxes gives you a quick idea of the statistics and specifics of each hike.

LENGTH The length of the trail from start to finish (total distance traveled). There may be options to shorten or extend the hikes, but the mileage corresponds to the described hike. Consult the hike description to help you decide how to customize the hike for your ability or time constraints.

CONFIGURATION A description of what the trail might look like from overhead. Trails can be loops, out-and-backs (trails on which one enters and leaves along the same path), figure eights, or a combination of shapes.

DIFFICULTY The degree of effort an "average" hiker should expect on a given hike. For simplicity, the trails are rated as "easy," "moderate," or "difficult."

SCENERY A short summary of the attractions offered by the hike and what to expect in terms of plant life, wildlife, natural wonders, and historic features.

EXPOSURE A quick check of how much sun you can expect on your shoulders during the hike.

TRAFFIC Indicates how busy the trail might be on an average day. Trail traffic, of course, varies from day to day and season to season. Weekend days typically see the most visitors. Other trail users, such as cyclists, who you may encounter on the trail are also noted here.

TRAIL SURFACE Indicates whether the trail surface is paved, rocky, gravel, dirt, boardwalk, or a mixture of surfaces.

HIKING TIME The length of time it takes to hike the trail. A slow but steady hiker will average 2 to 3 miles an hour, depending on the terrain.

DRIVING DISTANCE The length of time it takes to access the trail by car.

ACCESS A notation of any fees or permits that may be needed to access the trail or park at the trailhead.

Trails in the state parks require either a Texas State Parks Pass, which may be purchased yearly, or a day pass, which may be purchased at the entrance to each park. If you plan to hike frequently each year, it is worth buying the annual pass. You can purchase the Texas State Parks Pass at any state park or by calling the Customer Service Center in Austin, Texas ([512] 389-8900).

City and county parks typically do not require any permits or parking fees.

MAPS Here you'll find a list of maps that show the topography of the trail, including USGS topo maps.

WHEELCHAIR ACCESS Indicates whether or not the trail offers accommodations for persons with disabilities.

FACILITIES Indicates restrooms and water at the trailhead or nearby.

SPECIAL COMMENTS Lists any information that doesn't fit any other category.

DIRECTIONS

Used in conjunction with the overview map, the driving directions will help you locate each trailhead. Once at the trailhead, park only in designated areas.

GPS TRAILHEAD COORDINATES

These can be used in addition to the driving directions if you enter the coordinates into your GPS unit before you set out. See page 2 for more information.

DESCRIPTION

This is the heart of the hike profile: a summary of the trail's essence and highlights any special traits the hike has to offer. The route is clearly described, including landmarks, side trips, and possible alternate routes along the way.

NEARBY ACTIVITIES

Look here for information on nearby activities or points of interest. This includes parks, museums, restaurants, or even a brewpub where you can get a well-deserved beer after a long hike. Note that not every hike has a listing.

WEATHER

Although Houston has a reputation for hot, humid weather, hiking from October into early May is very pleasant and can, at times, be quite cold. Clear blue skies, crisp cool air, and low humidity in the winter allow you to hike when other parts of the country are knee deep in snow and slush. Because most southeast Texas forests contain evergreens along with some deciduous trees, there is not as much foliage change in the fall, creating a relatively green landscape all year.

While Houston has steady rainfall each month, at times the entire monthly average of 3–4 inches can occur during a single storm, causing flooding that may not drain for several days.

AVERAGE DAILY TEMPERATURES BY MONTH FOR HOUSTON, TEXAS					
	JAN	FEB	MAR	APR	MAY	JUN
HIGH	63	67	74	79	86	91
LOW	45	48	55	61	68	74
	JUL	AUG	SEP	OCT	NOV	DEC
HIGH	94	93	89	82	73	65
LOW	75	75	72	62	53	47

Hiking in the Houston area from late May to late September is best done in the early hours of the day, as temperatures can get quite high by noon. You will, however, have to contend with higher humidity in the morning hours. Late fall and winter offer the best weather and often the driest trail surfaces for hiking. Watch the weather for any late tropical storms that may drop several inches of precipitation in just a few hours. Winters in Houston are generally mild but temperatures can drop below freezing from November through April.

WATER

How much is enough? Well, one simple physiological fact should convince you to err on the side of excess when deciding how much water to pack: A hiker working hard in 90°F heat needs approximately ten quarts of fluid per day. That's 2.5 gallons—10 quart-sized water bottles or 16 20-ounce ones. In other words, pack along one or two bottles even for short hikes.

Some hikers and backpackers hit the trail prepared to purify water found along the route. This method, while less dangerous than drinking it untreated, comes with risks. Purifiers with ceramic filters are the safest. Many hikers pack along the slightly distasteful tetraglycine-hydroperiodide tablets to purify water (sold under the names Potable Aqua, Coughlan's, and others).

Probably the most common waterborne "bug" that hikers face is giardia, which may not hit until one to four weeks after ingestion. It will have you living in the bathroom, passing noxious rotten-egg gas, vomiting, and shivering with chills. Other parasites to worry about include E. coli and cryptosporidium, both of which are harder to kill than giardia.

For most people, the pleasures of hiking make carrying water a relatively minor price to pay to remain healthy. If you're tempted to drink "found water," do so only if you understand the risks involved. Better yet, hydrate prior to your hike, carry (and drink) six ounces of water for every mile you plan to hike, and hydrate after the hike.

CLOTHING

There is a wide variety of clothing from which to choose; and the type of hike you go on should determine what you wear. On all paved urban trails you can get away with wearing shorts and tennis shoes. However, you should wear long pants and hiking shoes or boots on all the trails in the state parks and in the Sam Houston National Forest. There are creeks to cross, low areas to slosh through, and poisonous plants and bugs to avoid. With shorts and sandals you may expose yourself to bites and rashes.

Always carry raingear and a jacket if the weather is predicted to change; however, most of the time, the weather in Houston is very predictable so you should be able to dress appropriately. During the winter, wear layers that you can take off as the temperature rises with the sun.

THE TEN ESSENTIALS

One of the first rules of hiking is to be prepared for anything. The simplest way to be prepared is to carry the "Ten Essentials." In addition to carrying the items listed below, you need to know how to use them, especially navigation items. Always consider worst-case scenarios like getting lost, hiking back in the dark, broken gear (for example, a broken hip strap on your pack or a water filter getting plugged), twisting an ankle, or a brutal thunderstorm. The items listed below don't cost a lot of money, don't take up much room in a pack, and don't weigh much, but they just might save your life.

1. **Water: durable bottles, and water treatment like iodine or a filter**

2. **Map: preferably a topo map and a trail map with a route description**

3. **Compass: a high-quality compass**

4. **First-aid kit: a high-quality kit including first-aid instructions**

5. **Knife: a multi-tool device with pliers is best**

6. **Light: flashlight or headlamp with extra bulbs and batteries**

7. **Fire: windproof matches or lighter and fire starter**

8. **Extra food: you should always have food in your pack when you've finished hiking**

9. **Extra clothes: rain protection, warm layers, gloves, warm hat**

10. **Sun protection: sunglasses, lip balm, sunblock, sun hat**

FIRST-AID KIT

A typical first-aid kit may contain more items than you might think necessary. These are just the basics. Prepackaged kits in waterproof bags (Atwater Carey and Adventure Medical make a variety of kits) are available. Even though there are quite a few items listed here, they pack down into a small space:

Ace bandages or Spenco joint wraps	**Gauze (one roll)**
Antibiotic ointment (Neosporin or the generic equivalent)	**Gauze compress pads (a half dozen 4 x 4-inch pads)**
Aspirin, ibuprofen, or acetaminophen	**Hydrogen peroxide, Betadine, or iodine**
Band-Aids	**Insect repellent**
Benadryl or the generic equivalent diphenhydramine (in case of allergic reactions)	**Matches or pocket lighter**
	Moleskin/Spenco "Second Skin"
Butterfly-closure bandages	**Sunscreen**
Epinephrine in a prefilled syringe (for people known to have severe allergic reactions to such things as bee stings)	**Whistle (it's more effective in signaling rescuers than your voice)**

HIKING WITH CHILDREN

No one is too young for a hike in the outdoors. Be mindful, though. Flat, short, and shaded trails are best with an infant. Toddlers who have not quite mastered walking can still tag along, riding on an adult's back in a child carrier. Use common sense to judge a child's capacity to hike a particular trail, and always count that the child will tire quickly and need to be carried.

When packing for the hike, remember the child's needs as well as your own. Make sure children are adequately clothed for the weather, have proper shoes, and are protected from the sun with sunscreen. Kids dehydrate quickly, so make sure you have plenty of fluid for everyone. To assist an adult with determining which trails are suitable for children, a list of hike recommendations for children is provided on page xvii.

GENERAL SAFETY

To some inexperienced hikers the deep woods can seem perilous and at times scary. But with proper planning and the following tips, your trip can be fun, easy, and, above all else, safe.

- **Always hike with a buddy. While most of these areas are safe, you should have someone else with you while hiking.**
- **Always carry food and water whether you are planning to go overnight or not. Food will give you energy, help keep you warm, and sustain you in an emergency situation until help arrives. You never know if you will have a stream nearby when you become thirsty. Bring potable water or treat water before drinking it from a stream. Boil or filter all found water before drinking it.**
- **Stay on designated trails. Most hikers who get lost do so because they leave the trail. Even on the most clearly marked trails, there is usually a point where you have to stop and consider which direction to head. If you become disoriented, don't panic. As soon as you think you may be lost, stop, assess your current direction, and then retrace your steps back to the point where you went awry. Using a map, compass, this book, and keeping in mind what you have passed thus far, reorient yourself, and trust your judgment on which way to continue. If you become absolutely unsure of how to continue, return to your vehicle the way you came in. Should you become completely lost and have no idea of how to return to the trailhead, remaining in place along the trail and waiting for help is most often the best option for adults and always the best option for children.**
- **Be especially careful when crossing streams. Whether you are fording the stream or crossing on a log, make every step count. If you have any doubt about maintaining your balance on a foot log, go ahead and ford the stream instead. When fording a stream, use a trekking pole or stout stick for balance**

and face upstream as you cross. If a stream seems too deep to ford, turn back. Whatever is on the other side is not worth risking your life.

- Standing dead trees and storm-damaged living trees pose a real hazard to hikers and tent campers. These trees may have loose or broken limbs that could fall at any time. When choosing a spot to rest or a backcountry campsite, look up.

- Know the symptoms of hypothermia. Shivering and forgetfulness are the two most common indicators of this insipid killer. Hypothermia can occur at any elevation, even in the summer, especially when the hiker is wearing lightweight cotton clothing. If symptoms arise, get the victim shelter, hot liquids, and dry clothes or a dry sleeping bag.

- Take along your brain. A cool, calculating mind is the single most important piece of equipment you'll ever need on the trail. Think before you act. Watch your step. Plan ahead. Avoiding accidents before they happen is the best recipe for a rewarding and relaxing hike.

- Ask questions. Park employees are there to help. It's a lot easier to gain advice beforehand and thereby avoid a mishap than to try to amend an error far away from civilization. Use your head out there.

ANIMAL AND PLANT HAZARDS

TICKS

Ticks like to hang out in the brush that grows along trails. Hot summer months seem to explode their numbers, but you should be tick-aware during all months of the year. Ticks, which are arthropods and not insects, need a host to feast on in order to reproduce. The ticks that light on you while hiking will be very small, sometimes so tiny that you won't be able to spot them. Primarily of two varieties, deer ticks and dog ticks, both need a few hours of actual attachment before they can transmit any disease they may harbor. Ticks may settle in shoes, socks, hats, and may take several hours to actually latch on. The best strategy is to visually check every half-hour or so while hiking, do a thorough check before you get in the car, and then, when you take a post-hike shower, do an even more thorough check of your entire body. Ticks that haven't attached are easily removed, but not easily killed. If you pick off a tick in the woods, just toss it aside. If you find one on your body at home, dispatch it and then send it down the toilet. For ticks that have embedded, removal with tweezers is best.

SNAKES

The venomous snakes found in the United States, which include the rattlesnake, cottonmouth, copperhead, and coral snake, all live in the Houston area and can be found on virtually every hike in this book. However, most of your snake encounters will be with the 100-plus nonvenomous species and subspecies. While hiking I only came across one snake on a trail surface and saw just a handful in the water along the Texas coast. Although you could spend some time studying the snakes in the area, the best rule is to leave all snakes alone and give them a wide berth as you hike past.

ALLIGATORS

Alligators are present on many of the Houston hikes along the bayous, in coastal wetlands, and in Brazos Bend State Park. While completing the hikes for this book I was within 15 feet of alligators on six different hikes, with the potential of seeing them on many others. They are beautiful animals to watch and are, in general, very docile. However, do not approach one, try to feed it, or go near a large mound of grass and mud that it may be protecting. This could be a nest and approaching one will cause an alligator to become aggressive. You are almost guaranteed seeing an alligator in the wild at Brazos Bend State Park due to the number of them in the park. Because of this, keep young children at your side at all times.

POISON IVY/POISON OAK/POISON SUMAC

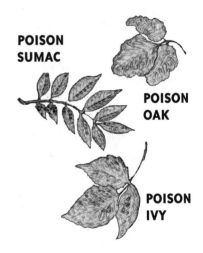

POISON SUMAC

POISON OAK

POISON IVY

Recognizing poison ivy, oak, and sumac and avoiding contact with them is the most effective way to prevent the painful, itchy rashes associated with these plants. In the South, poison ivy ranges from a thick, tree-hugging vine to a shaded groundcover, three leaflets to a leaf; poison oak occurs as either a vine or shrub, with three leaflets as well; and poison sumac flourishes in swampland, each leaf containing 7 to 13 leaflets. Urushiol, the oil in the sap of these plants, is responsible for the rash. Usually within 12 to 14 hours of exposure (but sometimes much later), raised lines and/or blisters will appear, accompanied by a terrible itch. Refrain from scratching because bacteria under fingernails can cause infection and you will spread the rash to other parts of your body. Wash and dry the rash thoroughly, applying a calamine lotion or other product to help dry the rash. If itching or blistering is severe, seek medical attention. Remember that oil-contaminated clothes, pets, or hiking gear can easily cause an irritating rash on you or someone else, so wash not only any exposed parts of your body but also clothes, gear, and pets.

MOSQUITOES

Although it's not a common occurrence, individuals can become infected with the West Nile virus by being bitten by an infected mosquito. Culex mosquitoes, the primary varieties that can transmit West Nile virus to humans, thrive in urban rather than in natural areas. They lay their eggs in stagnant water and can breed in any standing water that remains for more than five days. Most people infected with West Nile virus have no symptoms of illness, but some may become ill, usually 3 to 15 days after being bitten.

In the Houston area, late spring and summer are the times thought to be the highest risk periods for West Nile virus. At this time of year—and anytime you expect mosquitoes to be buzzing around—you may want to wear protective clothing, such as long sleeves, long pants, and socks. Loose-fitting, light-colored clothing is best. Spray clothing with insect repellent. Remember to follow the instructions on the repellent and to take extra care with children when using a repellent with DEET.

TIPS FOR ENJOYING HOUSTON

Before you go on any of the Sam Houston National Forest hikes, visit the Lone Star Hiking Trail Club (LSHTC) website at **lshtclub.com.** The LSHTC has mapped the entire 128-mile Lone Star Hiking Trail and provides information on the area and various sections of the hike. In addition, the following tips will make your hike enjoyable and more rewarding:

- **Get out of your car and onto a trail. Auto touring allows a cursory overview of the area, but only from a visual perspective. On the trail you can use your ears and nose as well. This guidebook recommends some trails over others, but any trail is better than no trail at all.**

- **Investigate different areas of each park. Many of these parks also include camping, fishing, biking, and picnic sites.**

- **Take your time along the trails. Pace yourself. The areas around Houston are diverse, offering many types of ecosystems, flora, and fauna. Take in the coastal wetlands; the deep East Texas forest; the prairies; the riparian landscapes along the bayous, rivers, and creeks; and the urban vistas of downtown Houston. Take your time on shorter hikes to identify the wildflowers, native plants, and birds you see; and on longer hikes, enjoy the solitude of several hours on the trail.**

- **Many of the hikes in Houston are not heavily traveled, so hike during the week or on weekends, whichever is more convenient. If at all possible hike from October to May, when the weather is cooler and bug-free.**

TOPO MAPS

The maps in this book have been produced with great care and, used with the hiking directions, will direct you to the trails and help you stay on course. However, you will find superior detail and valuable information in the United States Geological Survey's 7.5-minute series topographic maps. Topo maps are available online in many locations, including **topomaps.usgs.gov** and **msrmaps.com.** You can view and print topos of locations all over the United States from these websites, and you can view aerial photos of the same areas at TerraServer-USA. Online services such as **trails.com** charge annual fees for additional features such as shaded relief, which makes the topography stand out more. If you expect to print out many topo maps each year, it might be worth paying for such extras. The downside to USGS topos is that most are outdated, having been created 20 to 30 years ago. But they still provide excellent topographic detail.

Digital topographic-map programs such as Delorme's Topo USA enable you to review topo maps of the entire United States on your PC. Gathered while hiking with a GPS unit, GPS data can be downloaded into the software so you can plot your own hikes.

If you're new to hiking, you might be wondering, "What's a topographic map?" In short, a topo indicates not only linear distance but elevation as well, using contour lines. Contour lines spread across the map like dozens of intricate spider webs. Each line represents a particular elevation, and at the base of each topo, a contour's interval designation is given. If the contour interval is 20 feet, then the distance between each contour line is 20 feet. Follow five contour lines up on the same map, and the elevation has increased by 1,000 feet.

Let's assume that the 7.5-minute series topo reads "Contour Interval 40 feet," that the short trail we'll be hiking is two inches in length on the map, and that it crosses five contour lines from beginning to end. What do we know? Well, because the linear scale of this series is 2,000 feet to the inch (roughly 2.75 inches representing 1 mile), we know our trail is approximately four-fifths of a mile long (2 inches are 2,000 feet). But we also know we'll be climbing or descending 200 vertical feet (five contour lines are 40 feet each) over that distance. And the elevation designations written on contour lines will tell us if we're heading up or down.

TRAIL ETIQUETTE

Whether you're on a city, county, state, or national park trail, always remember that great care and resources (from nature as well as from your tax dollars) have gone into creating these trails. Treat the trail, wildlife, and fellow hikers with respect:

- **Hike on open trails only. Respect trail and road closures (ask if not sure), avoid possible trespassing on private land, and obtain all permits and authorization as required. Also, leave gates as you found them or as marked.**

- **Leave only footprints. Be sensitive to the ground beneath you. This also means staying on the existing trail and not blazing any new trails. Be sure to pack out what you pack in. No one likes to see the trash someone else has left behind.**

- **Never spook animals. An unannounced approach, a sudden movement, or a loud noise startles most animals. A surprised animal can be dangerous to you, to others, and to themselves. Give them plenty of space.**

- **Plan ahead. Know your equipment, your ability, and the area in which you are hiking—and prepare accordingly. Be self-sufficient at all times; carry necessary supplies for changes in weather or other conditions. A well-executed trip is a satisfaction to you and to others.**

- **Be courteous to other hikers, bikers, equestrians, and others you encounter on the trails.**

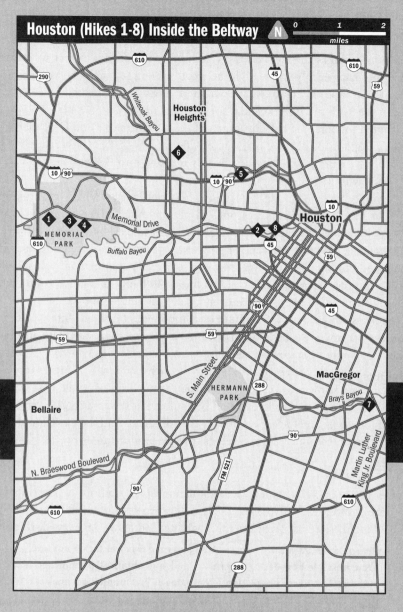

HOUSTON
(INSIDE BELTWAY 8)

1 HOUSTON ARBORETUM AND NATURE CENTER OUTER LOOP TRAIL

KEY AT-A-GLANCE INFORMATION

LENGTH: 2 miles

CONFIGURATION: Loop

DIFFICULTY: Very easy

SCENERY: Wide open trail with woods, meadows, and a pond

EXPOSURE: Very shady

TRAIL TRAFFIC: Light weekdays, moderate to heavy weekends

TRAIL SURFACE: Crushed granite

HIKING TIME: 1 hour

DRIVING DISTANCE: Inside the 610 Loop, approximately 0.25 miles from intersection of the 610 Loop and Woodway Drive

ACCESS: 7 a.m. to dusk (gates close at 7 p.m.; no fee but donations appreciated

MAPS: USGS Houston Heights; trail maps are available at the nature center.

WHEELCHAIR ACCESS: The trail is smooth enough for wheelchair and stroller access.

FACILITIES: Parking, benches, restrooms, nature center

SPECIAL COMMENTS: Mosquito spray is a must except during the winter months; they even offer it at the nature center free of charge; dogs on a leash are welcome.

GPS TRAILHEAD COORDINATES

LATITUDE: N 29° 45.915'
LONGITUDE: W 95° 27.143'

IN BRIEF

Located in an urban park, this is an easy trail that offers a glimpse of Houston before the days of concrete and skyscrapers. A new bridge just east of the Houston Arboretum connects the north side of Memorial Park to the south side.

DESCRIPTION

The Houston Arboretum and Nature Center's (HANC) 155 acres are part of the much larger 1,466-acre tract of land called Memorial Park. One of the largest urban parks in Texas, and formerly known as Camp Logan, the U.S. Army trained soldiers here during World War I. In 1924, the City of Houston set the land aside as a park in memory of those soldiers. The city acquired an additional 1,000 acres for the park from William C. Hobby and his brother Mike.

One of the first nature-education facilities built for children in the state of Texas, the HANC is a nonprofit urban nature sanctuary that includes 5 miles of trails through forest, pond, wetland, and meadow habitats. Originally, the arboretum spanned 265 acres of Memorial Park, but due to road building and other right-of-way issues, the park has been reduced to its current size.

To get to the Outer Loop Trail, take the sidewalk around the nature center to the right and locate the Alice Brown Trail. Follow the Alice Brown Trail to the right about 50 yards until you come to the intersection for the

----

Directions ⟶

From the 610 Loop south of I-10, exit onto Woodway Drive. Head east on Woodway Drive for 0.25 miles. The entrance is on the right, at 4501 Woodway Drive.

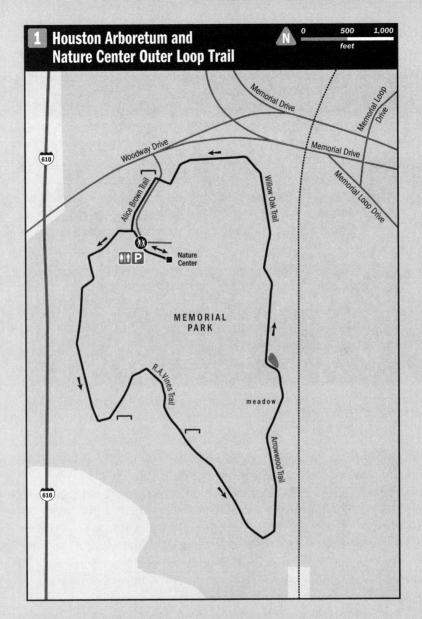

1 Houston Arboretum and Nature Center Outer Loop Trail

N

0   500   1,000
feet

Memorial Drive

Memorial Loop Drive

Memorial Drive

Memorial Loop Drive

610

Woodway Drive

Alice Brown Trail

Willow Oak Trail

Nature Center

MEMORIAL PARK

R.A. Vines Trail

meadow

Arrowwood Trail

610

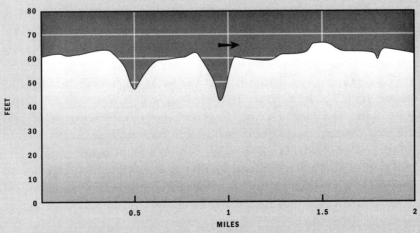

FEET

80
70
60
50
40
30
20
10
0

0.5   1   1.5   2

MILES

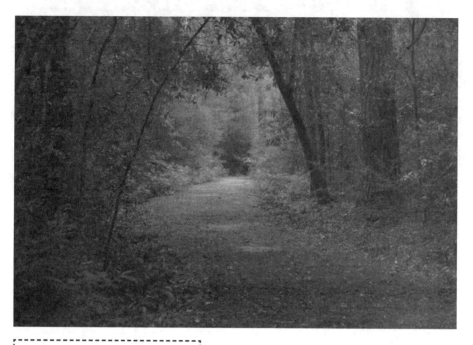

The deep forest of the Outer Loop Trail

Outer Loop Trail. At the intersection, turn left on the Outer Loop Trail (you will return to this junction near the end of the hike).

The trail is well marked every 0.25 miles along the 2-mile route. This is a nice shady trail to hike in the summer, but be prepared to fend off the mosquitoes by taking plenty of mosquito repellent and using it! In general the canopied trail feels cooler due to the shade, even though the humidity can be quite high.

Once on the Outer Loop Trail, continue past a bridge on your right. Several benches dot the trail, often placed near intersections with other trails. Stay on the Outer Loop Trail.

Pine, oak, and hickory trees border most of the trail. Other plants along the trail include parsley hawthorn, American beautyberry, snowdrop tree, sweet bay magnolia, eastern redbud, Texas mountain laurel, coral honeysuckle, coral bean, and southern wax myrtle. The most scenic time to hike here is in the spring when the flowers are in full bloom.

As you continue along the trail, cross the R. A. Vines Trail and then the Arrowwood Trail. The R. A. Vines Trail is named after ecologist and educator Robert A. Vines, who convinced the City Council to transform part of Memorial Park into a nature sanctuary. If you need to cut your hike short, both the R. A. Vines and Arrowwood trails are shortcuts back to the nature center.

Stay on the Outer Loop Trail, eventually reaching a three-acre meadow on your left. Inside this meadow is a small artificial pond where you may encounter copperheads, coral snakes, toads, and other wildlife.

Approach the meadow quietly and you may see the family of coyotes that lives here. While these coyotes are welcome in the HANC, they are breeding in numbers that cannot be supported by the limited habitat and are moving into some of the urban neighborhoods. Because they are native to Houston and moved into the arboretum from the outlying areas, the HANC has chosen to keep them in the park.

Other wildlife common to the area include Virginia opossum, gray squirrel, eastern mole, fox squirrel, evening bat, nine-banded armadillo, raccoon, and swamp rabbit. Like most areas around Houston, the bird population is quite large. A few of the birds you might see include the yellow-crowned night heron, the pileated woodpecker (the model for Woody Woodpecker), and, during winter months, the great horned owl.

After leaving the pond, continue down the Outer Loop Trail. The Willow Oak Trail, which is a shortcut to the parking lot, intersects the Outer Loop Trail at 1.5 miles into the hike. Continue down the Outer Loop Trail and at the 1.75-mile mark, cross the entrance road to the HANC (*Note:* trail markings can be a bit confusing here).

Cross over the road and turn left onto the Alice Brown Trail, which will soon join the Outer Loop Trail at the original T-junction. At the sign indicating the Outer Loop Trail, bear left, staying on the Alice Brown Trail back to the nature center.

The nature center offers restrooms and benches along with a Discovery Room for kids and a small gift shop. The Discovery Room has an interactive environment where kids can work puzzles, solve mysteries, touch animal skins and pelts, and peek through a microscope. Just behind the nature center is the Wildlife Garden where you can sit and watch the birds, bees, and butterflies.

There are numerous educational opportunities available at the HANC, including school programs, Scouting programs, and teacher workshops. A unique feature of the HANC is the Marie Vann Memorial Library. This 3,000-volume library, open seven days a week from 10 a.m. to 4 p.m., contains books on natural history, nature education, and natural history for children.

The nature center is open 9 a.m.–5 p.m., seven days a week. Check the website at **houstonarboretum.org** for building-closure days.

NEARBY ACTIVITIES

The HANC is on the western edge of Memorial Park, one of the most heavily used parks in Houston. Besides picnic facilities, the park offers an 18-hole golf course (one of the top municipal courses in Texas), tennis, softball, swimming, track, croquet, volleyball, in-line skating, a 3-mile running course, and cycling. The almost 6 miles of bike trails are also open to hikers and runners.

2 BUFFALO BAYOU PARK HIKE AND BIKE TRAIL

KEY AT-A-GLANCE INFORMATION

LENGTH: 5.1 miles

CONFIGURATION: Loop

DIFFICULTY: Moderate

SCENERY: Woodlands, downtown Houston, bayou, cemetery, art sculptures, parkland, skate park

EXPOSURE: Sunny

TRAIL TRAFFIC: Light to moderate

TRAIL SURFACE: Asphalt and concrete

HIKING TIME: 2 hours

DRIVING DISTANCE: Inside the 610 Loop, approximately 4.8 miles from the intersection of Memorial Drive and the 610 Loop

ACCESS: Free

MAPS: USGS Houston Heights and Settegast

WHEELCHAIR ACCESS: Yes

FACILITIES: Parking, benches, water fountains, playground, canoe and kayak launches, skate park

SPECIAL COMMENTS: Close to downtown Houston, this hike is in an area that has been revitalized in the past few years. After heavy rains, be cautious of water levels in Buffalo Bayou, as it is one of the main flood-control channels in Houston and water levels will stay high for days after a heavy rain.

GPS TRAILHEAD COORDINATES

LATITUDE: N 29° 45.706'
LONGITUDE: W 95° 22.770'

IN BRIEF

This urban hike offers some of the best views of downtown Houston. As you hike west, away from the parking lot, you can see the Federal Reserve Bank building to the south and town homes on both sides of the bayou. Buffalo Bayou Park was originally created in 1929 to link downtown Houston with the suburban development of River Oaks, one of the more exclusive neighborhoods in Houston today. The 124-acre park includes Eleanor Tinsley Park, Police Officers Memorial, Glenwood Cemetery, Beth Yeshurun Cemetery, the Lee and Joe Jamail Skate Park, and the Sandy Reed Memorial Trail.

DESCRIPTION

Once in the parking lot, head west toward Allen Parkway to get to the trail. There are benches, a playground, and picnic tables at Eleanor Tinsley Park, east of the parking lot. Head along the trail with Allen Parkway directly on your left and the park on your right. Most of the park is adorned with art sculptures, making this one of the more eclectic urban parks in Houston. Cross the exit road from the parking lot and get back on the trail by going straight. Although the trail surface is concrete at the start, it changes to asphalt and stays this way

----

Directions ————————————————————→

From the intersection of the 610 Loop and Memorial Drive, go east on Memorial Drive 3 miles to Shepherd Drive and turn right. At the first stoplight, turn left onto Allen Parkway. Go 2.4 miles to Bagby Street (passing the parking lot on the opposite side of Allen Parkway) and turn left. Turn left again at the first light to get back onto Allen Parkway heading west. The parking lot is 0.5 miles on the right.

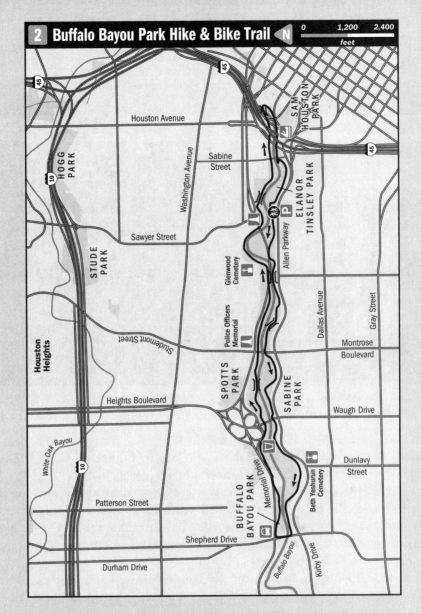

0   1,200   2,400
feet

Houston Avenue

Sabine
Street

Washington Avenue

HOGG
PARK

SAM
HOUSTON
PARK

ELANOR
TINSLEY PARK

Sawyer Street

Allen Parkway

STUDE
PARK

Glenwood
Cemetery

Dallas Avenue

Gray Street

Police Officers
Memorial

Sudemont Street

Montrose
Boulevard

Houston
Heights

SPOTTS
PARK

SABINE
PARK

Waugh Drive

Heights Boulevard

White Oak Bayou

Dunlavy
Street

Beth Yeshurun
Cemetery

BUFFALO
BAYOU PARK

Memorial Drive

Patterson Street

Shepherd Drive

Buffalo Bayou

Kirby Drive

Durham Drive

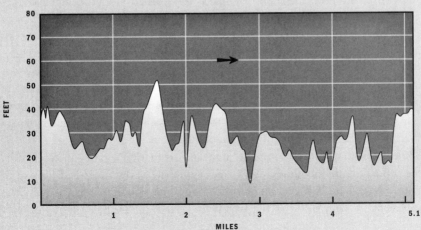

FEET

80
70
60
50
40
30
20
10
0

1   2   3   4   5.1

MILES

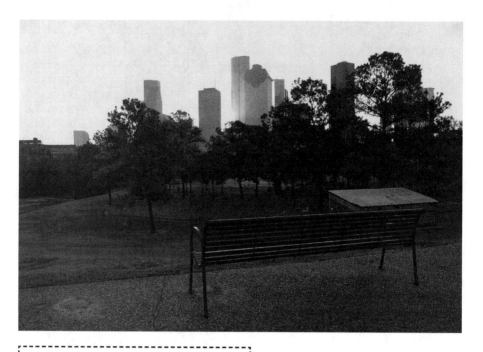

for most of the hike. This is a hiking and biking trail, so be cautious of bikers. Stay to the right when hiking and listen for bikers behind you.

Buffalo Bayou is on your right, between you and Memorial Drive to the north. Stay to the right on the trail with Allen Parkway directly on your left. The trail heads right, away from the road, and down into the park. As it does, look to your left across Memorial Drive for the Police Officers Memorial, a monument dedicated to officers killed in the line of duty. Dedicated in 1992, the memorial is shaped like a cross and consists of five levels of stepped pyramids. To the west of the memorial is a granite stone etched with the names of the slain officers. Once down into the park, the trail curves left beside benches and a planted garden. Past the garden the trail swings right and takes you back to Allen Parkway. Hike along the road until it turns right and takes you closer to the bayou. Cross a bridge and head uphill. Although the bayou is on your right, visibility of it is hampered greatly by overgrown kudzu vines, a plant that was brought from Japan in 1876 and heavily propagated throughout the South in the 1930s for foliage and to control soil erosion. It is one of the most invasive non-native plants in the southeastern United States, growing up to a foot a day in the summer months and killing many native plants.

Buffalo Bayou Park is a popular dog and recreational park on weekends, but the trails remain only moderately used. Continue as the trail heads downhill and curves right among trees below the road. The elevation change with the embankment on your left and the bayou on your right creates a much quieter part of the hike. Cross another bridge and head uphill and left to a clearing on your left. Much of the park is mowed regularly, creating open green spaces, hills, and shade trees. As the trail winds back and forth it heads uphill and then under Studemont Road. Past Studemont Road the trail swings left and uphill toward Allen Parkway. There are large open spaces (and a few garbage cans) on the right. The trail continues steeply uphill and then goes right, with a bench on the right and a railing on the left between the trail and the road. Go past a water fountain on the left and a sign for the WAUGH DRIVE BAT COLONY. About 250,000 Mexican free-tailed bats make the crevices of the Waugh Drive bridge their permanent home—this is the largest year-round bat colony in Texas. The bats can be seen leaving the bridge to eat each evening just after dusk. After the sign head right and back into the park around a large geodesic water fountain. The trail passes the fountain and then heads back uphill to Allen Parkway.

To the right is a metal fence separating the trail from the bayou; before you reach Waugh Drive there is a bat viewing stand. Take the right fork and follow the smell to go under Waugh Drive. The presence of 250,000 bats makes for a very strong odor. Go left after Waugh Drive and head back uphill toward the road. After winding back and forth, the trail goes downhill and curves right. After heading back uphill, continue past the Beth Yeshurun Cemetery, on your right. Follow the trail right and back down into the park to a large green space, where you cannot hear the road traffic. Continue past a bench on the left and head back uphill by two benches on your right. At the intersection of Allen Parkway and Shepherd Drive, continue on the trail, hiking along the Shepherd Drive bridge over Buffalo Bayou. Once over the bridge, head right and past a Metro bus stop to continue the hike. Memorial Drive is now on your left, with the bayou on your right. Go past a water fountain on the right and head downhill following the asphalt trail. The trail surface, although narrower and older here, and perhaps covered in places with sand, is still easy to see.

Continue uphill and toward Memorial Drive. There is a planted garden to your right followed by a sign for the Sandy Reed Memorial Trail. Stop at the sign and look southwest to see the Beth Yeshurun Cemetery across the bayou. Continue uphill, hiking by a bench on the right, and past another bat-colony sign. Go straight on the trail past a set of stairs to the right. The trail swings right, taking you beside the exit ramp for Waugh Drive. Take the right fork to head back into the park, toward the bayou and under Waugh Drive. There is another bat viewing stand, and the undeniable smell of bats, before you reach the underpass. Hike under Waugh Drive and listen for high-pitched bat sounds. The trail curves right, past a water fountain on the left. High embankments on the left keep the traffic sounds away as you continue downhill.

Cross a bridge and hike past an exercise station on the right and a bench on the left. The trail starts back uphill past another bench and then under Studemont Road. The bayou is much more visible on your right as you go by a bench and head back downhill. As the trail bends left, go under Memorial Drive and hike for about 150 yards before exiting and going left. The trail angles right; from here you can see the Police Officers Memorial over the trees to your right. Cross another bridge before going back under Memorial Drive to get back to the park between Allen Parkway and Memorial Drive. The trail goes left and takes you under one of the sculptures that was created specifically for the park. Continue on the trail over two small bridges and then go left past a disc-golf marker on the right. Stay on the trail past all exits to streets, parking lots, canoe and kayak launches, and other landmarks. At the exit for Sabine Street, the trail surface changes to concrete and the landscape is more maintained. The Lee and Joe Jamail Skate Park is located close to Sabine Street and the Fonde Recreation Center. The section from Sabine Street to Bagby Street underwent a revitalization that was completed in late 2006 and included new lights, trail surface, plantings, and artwork. Go under many of the downtown underpasses, past all intersections, until you reach a bridge on the right that takes you back to the other side of the trail. Take a right once off the bridge and head west toward the parking lot. Go past a canoe and kayak launch on your right and take the left fork up a set of stairs. Continue right after the stairs and then go straight toward the parking lot, which is only a few hundred yards ahead.

Note: Allen Parkway and Memorial Drive are high-traffic roads, so do not park on either of them. Park in one of the lots along Allen Parkway or on a side street.

NEARBY ACTIVITIES

The downtown Houston entertainment district is within walking distance of the Sabine Street to Bagby Street section of the hike, along with the Aquarium, an amusement park, and restaurant. Minute Maid Park, home of the Houston Astros, and Toyota Center, home of the Houston Rockets and the Houston Aeros, are just east of the hike. Sam Houston Park and Tranquility Park are also east of Buffalo Bayou Park.

MEMORIAL PARK: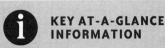
Ho Chi Minh Trail West

IN BRIEF

Memorial Park, the largest urban park in Texas, is often called the Central Park of Houston. It includes an 18-hole golf course, tennis courts, baseball and softball fields, football/soccer fields, picnic sites, a 3-mile jogging trail, swimming pool, croquet, volleyball, in-line skating, cycling, and hiking. The 1,600-acre park was acquired by William C. Hogg from the U.S. government in 1918; he subsequently turned it over to the City of Houston. While the park already contains many hiking and biking trails, there are plans to add additional trails. All the wooded areas on the south side of the park are crisscrossed by trails, many of which run along Buffalo Bayou and other smaller creeks.

DESCRIPTION

Start on the west side of the Ho Chi Minh Trail behind the parking lot and to the right of the map signboard. Go over the bridge and then turn left to get on the trail. There is a large football/soccer field to the right of the trail, and woodlands on the left. The trail surface is dirt with some old asphalt at the beginning, but once you get into the trees, it remains predominantly dirt with exposed tree roots. These trails are used heavily on weekends by cyclists, so stay to the right of the trail and listen for their approach. Once past the football/soccer field, the vegetation gets dense on both sides of the trail and stays that way, creating a very shady environment that is often cooler than the surrounding area.

- -

Directions ———————————————→

From the 610 Loop and Woodway Drive, drive 0.5 miles west to the first stoplight. Turn right and park in the first parking lot on the right.

KEY AT-A-GLANCE INFORMATION

LENGTH: 2 miles
CONFIGURATION: Loops
DIFFICULTY: Easy
SCENERY: Creek beds, woodlands, fields
EXPOSURE: Shady
TRAIL TRAFFIC: Moderate to heavy
TRAIL SURFACE: Dirt
HIKING TIME: 1 hour
DRIVING DISTANCE: Inside the 610 Loop, 0.5 miles from intersection of the 610 Loop and Woodway Drive
ACCESS: Free
MAPS: USGS Houston Heights; trail map available at trailhead
WHEELCHAIR ACCESS: None
FACILITIES: Restrooms, picnic tables, baseball fields, trail signs
SPECIAL COMMENTS: The Ho Chi Minh Trail, which is heavily used on the weekends by cyclists, is much less used during the week. Although there seemed to be a large number of people in the park, I did not feel crowded on the trails during the hike.

GPS TRAILHEAD COORDINATES

LATITUDE: N 29° 45.901'
LONGITUDE: W 95° 26.705'

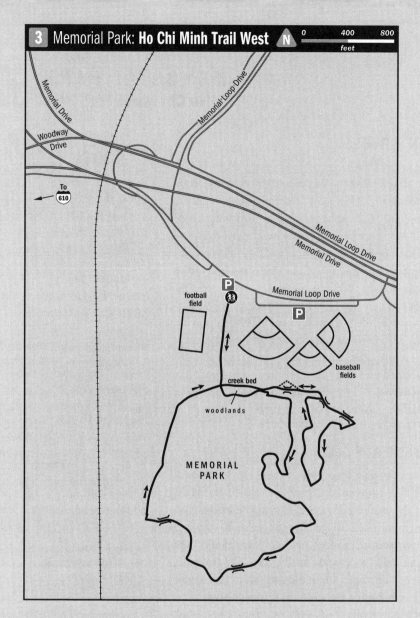

N

0   400   800
feet

To
610

Memorial Drive

Woodway
Drive

Memorial Loop Drive

Memorial Loop Drive

Memorial Drive

Memorial Loop Drive

football
field

P

P

baseball
fields

creek bed

woodlands

MEMORIAL
PARK

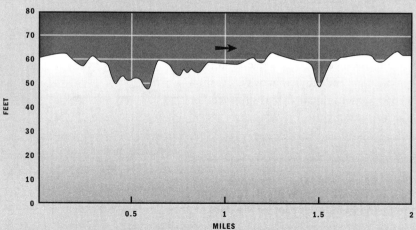

80
70
60
50
40
30
20
10
0

FEET

0.5   1   1.5   2

MILES

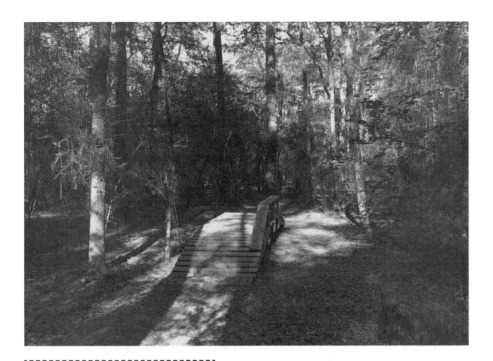

A small bridge on the Ho Chi Minh Trail

At the first intersection, there are color-coded markers: a red marker pointing right, a purple marker pointing left, and a yellow marker pointing straight. Follow the yellow marker and go straight. These mixed pine-and-oak woodlands, which are hemmed in by urban sprawl from all directions, contain a diverse population of birds, including the yellow-crowned night heron, the pileated woodpecker, and during winter months, the great horned owl. With pine, oak, and hickory trees bordering most of the trail, you can also find parsley hawthorn, American beautyberry, snowdrop tree, sweet bay magnolia, eastern redbud, Texas mountain laurel, coral honeysuckle, coral bean, and southern wax myrtle. Animals to watch for include Virginia opossum, gray squirrel, eastern mole, fox squirrel, evening bat, nine-banded armadillo, raccoon, swamp rabbit, coyote; venomous snakes here are coral snakes and copperheads.

The yellow trail narrows and winds back and forth through dense woodlands. Continue past another yellow marker on your right and look left to see the red trail as it briefly runs parallel to the yellow trail. There is a deep ditch to your left, so stay on the trail to prevent stepping off the loose embankment. The trail continues to go back and forth with a creek bed now on your left. The trail is not wide enough for hikers and cyclists at the same time, so look ahead and listen from behind at all times. Stay on the trail past another marker on the left. The vegetation on the right is dense, with a steep drop-off on the left. As the trail curves considerably to the right, you go away from the creek before the trail bends left again. Continue toward the creek and downhill over tree roots.

Watch your footing as some of the roots are quite large. Go past another yellow marker on your right and downhill steeply to a small bridge. Cross the bridge and then head uphill and left. The trail swings right and heads downhill slightly before winding back and forth toward the creek. Continue past a yellow marker on your right.

Go past another marker on the right and cross a small channel that feeds into the creek on your left. The trail heads right and uphill before coming to a washed-out part of the trail. The center is deeper than the sides and has considerable water damage for about 15 yards. Past the damaged area, the trail heads downhill and left over a small bridge. Continue to the right to get back on the trail and go past a marker on the right before going downhill. Hike past a tree in the middle of the trail before heading downhill steeply to the right and then back uphill. Go through an intersection past a yellow marker and head downhill very steeply. Again, watch your footing and take this section slowly if you do not have on proper hiking shoes. Cross a bridge and head uphill to another yellow marker. Go right to get on a wider, more roadlike part of the trail. This section is much straighter and you can see for some distance ahead.

Pass a yellow marker on your right and head to the right onto a narrower trail. The trail curves left and downhill before winding back and forth. Go across a small concrete bridge and then uphill. Continue past the next yellow marker and then head left. The trail is now only about 3 feet wide here but still easy to follow. You are no longer hiking along a creek and the trail surface is much flatter, with very little elevation change. Cross another bridge and then head right to stay on the trail. At an intersection go right and follow the yellow marker. The trail is much wider now and heavily used by bikers. Follow the markers for the purple trail. You can hear the hum of traffic on the 610 Loop, which is just west of Memorial Park. This is one of the most traveled roads in the United States.

Follow the purple marker and head right to a flatter part of the trail void of tree roots. Once you reach the initial intersection from the beginning of the hike, head right and follow the red trail marker. The trail is now winding back and forth and has narrowed considerably. You are again hiking along creeks and ditches. Hike past a red marker on the right and look farther to your right to see the yellow trail. At the intersection, head straight and downhill. Cross a small bridge and then head uphill on a very steep incline. You can see the baseball field's lights over the tops of the trees to the left of the trail. The trail goes right and downhill before going back uphill and over another long bridge followed directly by a shorter bridge. Follow a blue trail marker and head straight. The trail turns sharply right and then goes back and forth. Cross another small bridge that seems to be built for cyclist fun only, since it does not actually bridge anything. Continue past a blue marker on the right and then a red marker on the left. Follow the next red marker to the right and downhill over additional tree roots. The creek is now on your left and the trail bends right. Go past another red marker on the right and continue straight. Once the trail takes a big bend to the right, look left for a stone wall that was erected to help with erosion. Go left at an intersection and head down into a creek bed before ascending the other side. You can now see the baseball field on your right. Turn right at the next intersection and then head left at a red marker. Now head left at a fork in the trail. Go right at the next intersection and then straight until you see a red marker ahead. At this red marker, go slightly right. At the last red marker, head left and then take a quick right to go back toward the parking lot and past the football/soccer field on your left. At the trail signboard cross the bridge and end the hike at the parking lot.

Note: There are additional trails throughout the park that are longer and more challenging; however, this hike is a fine beginner hike through a park that gives no evidence of being just miles from downtown Houston and the very urban Galleria Uptown area. All the trails have color-coded trail markers to help you navigate through the park. There is heavy car traffic on weekends, so any hiker with a respiratory condition should exercise caution.

NEARBY ACTIVITIES

Houston Arboretum and Nature Center, (713) 681-8433, is only 0.25 miles west of the trailhead, off Woodway Drive. Additional Memorial Park activities include the Memorial Park Golf Course, (713) 862-4033, Memorial Park Tennis Center, (713) 867-0440, and the Memorial Park Swimming and Fitness Center, (713) 802-1662. The Galleria, one of the top shopping areas in the United States, is just west of the park with downtown Houston located to the east. Buffalo Bayou Park, White Oak Bayou Hike and Bike Trail, and Tranquility Park are also close by.

4 MEMORIAL PARK: Cambodia Trail

KEY AT-A-GLANCE INFORMATION

LENGTH: 3.4 miles

CONFIGURATION: Out-and-back

DIFFICULTY: Moderate

SCENERY: Creek beds, woodlands, kudzu field

EXPOSURE: Shady

TRAIL TRAFFIC: Moderate

TRAIL SURFACE: Dirt

HIKING TIME: 2 hours

DRIVING DISTANCE: Inside the 610 Loop, 0.6 miles from the intersection of the 610 Loop and Woodway Drive.

ACCESS: Free

MAPS: USGS Houston Heights; trail map available at trailhead

WHEELCHAIR ACCESS: None

FACILITIES: Restrooms, picnicking, baseball fields, trail signs

SPECIAL COMMENTS: The Cambodia Trail is heavily used on the weekends by cyclists but is used only sparingly during the week. This up-and-down trail can be challenging for those with limited abilities but is still easily hiked by most people. The trail has numerous color-coded trail markers to help you navigate the park. There is heavy car traffic on weekends, so those with a respiratory condition should be cautious.

GPS TRAILHEAD COORDINATES

LATITUDE: N 29° 45.822'
LONGITUDE: W 95° 26.380'

IN BRIEF

Memorial Park, the largest urban park in Texas, is often called the Central Park of Houston. It includes an 18-hole golf course, tennis courts, baseball and softball fields, football and soccer fields, picnic sites, a 3-mile jogging trail, swimming pool, croquet, volleyball, in-line skating, cycling, and hiking. The 1,600-acre park was acquired by William C. Hogg from the U.S. government in 1918; he subsequently turned it over to the City of Houston. The park already contains many hiking and biking trails, but there are plans to add additional trails. All the wooded areas on the south side of the park are crisscrossed by trails, many of which run along Buffalo Bayou and other smaller creeks.

DESCRIPTION

The Cambodia Trail starts from the next entrance off Memorial Drive, but because this entrance is often closed, park at the entrance directly past the second stoplight. There are restrooms and water fountains near the parking lots. Once parked, go east toward the park road that runs parallel to Memorial Drive. Hike along the road past a small parking lot on the right until you come to an entrance gate farther along Memorial Drive. Go around the front of the gate to the green trailhead marker across the entrance road. Head straight into the woods and then go left, following the trail. The dirt trail surface is only about 3 feet wide and is not wide enough for hikers and cyclists at

Directions ———————————→

From the 610 Loop and Woodway Drive, drive 0.6 miles west to the second stoplight. Turn right and then left. Parking is available on both sides of the Memorial Park Picnic Loop.

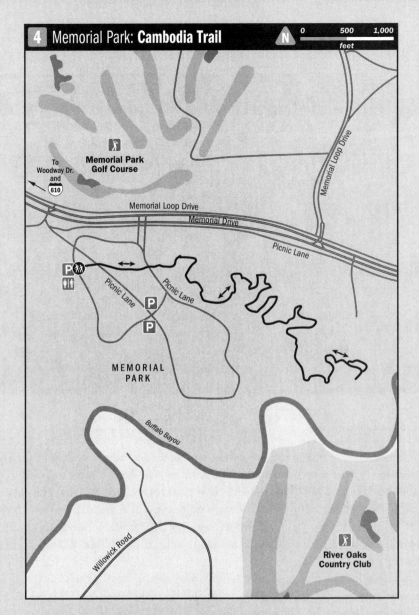

N

0   500   1,000
feet

Memorial Loop Drive

To
Woodway Dr.
and
610

Memorial Park
Golf Course

Memorial Loop Drive

Memorial Drive

Picnic Lane

Picnic Lane

Picnic Lane

MEMORIAL
PARK

Buffalo Bayou

Willowick Road

River Oaks
Country Club

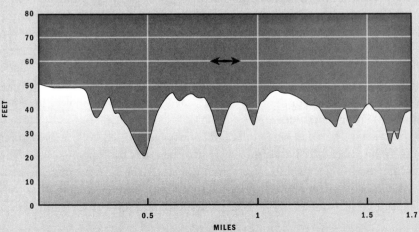

80
70
60
50
40
30
20
10
0

FEET

0.5   1   1.5   1.7

MILES

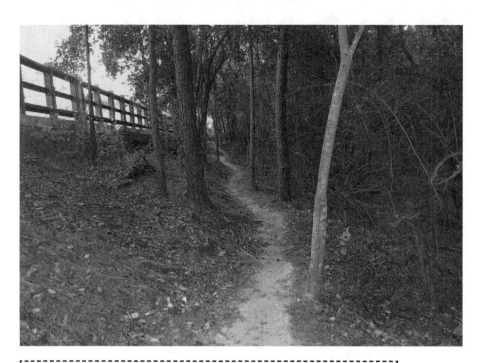

The Cambodia Trail heads toward Memorial Drive before going back into the trees

the same time, so look ahead and listen from behind at all times. Step to the right if you see or hear a cyclist coming. The winding trail has a deep creek bed to the right and Memorial Drive to the left. As it goes toward Memorial Drive, the trail heads downhill and right. This descent is quite steep in some areas, so watch your footing and take it slowly if you are not wearing proper hiking shoes. Continue on the trail uphill and to the right as it takes you away from Memorial Drive and back into the trees.

These mixed pine and oak woodlands, which are hemmed in by urban sprawl from all directions, contain a diverse population of birds, including the yellow-crowned night heron, the pileated woodpecker, and during winter months, the great horned owl. Pine, oak, and hickory trees border most of the trail, and you can also find parsley hawthorn, American beautyberry, snowdrop tree, sweet bay magnolia, eastern redbud, Texas mountain laurel, coral honey-suckle, coral bean, and southern wax myrtle. Animals to watch for include Virginia opossum, gray squirrel, eastern mole, fox squirrel, evening bat, nine-banded armadillo, raccoon, swamp rabbit, coyote; venomous snakes here are coral snakes and copperheads.

Go past a trail marker on your left and one on your right. Follow the marker on your right to head back into the trees with the creek bed on your right. The ground on the left goes uphill, away from the trail. The trail narrows slightly, so be even more vigilant about watching for cyclists. Continue past another trail marker and go left and downhill over numerous tree roots. As the trail takes a big bend to the right, go through the next intersection heading straight ahead. At the next trail marker on the left, continue straight. The trail winds right and then sharply left, with a lot of accumulated sand on the trail surface. Head downhill and then back up the other side of the hill, hiking over tree roots and packed dirt. At the next intersection, go left. The cyclists like to take the steeper right fork, but it's best for hikers to take the high embankment on the left. Continue straight at the next intersection where the two trails meet.

The trail bends sharply left and uphill over an eroded stretch. The center of the trail is at least two feet below the sides. The trail then curves right with the creek bed still on your right. You can still clearly hear the traffic on Memorial Drive, to your left. Continue past a trail marker on your right and go straight to stay on the trail. There are numerous vines hanging from the trees, and the vegetation is thick; however, visibility into the trees is good. Go past another trail marker on the left and head downhill over another eroded part of the trail. Once downhill, go to the right and head back uphill. The trail continues to wind back and forth going up and downhill many times before coming to another trail marker on the right. Head downhill and to the right, past the marker. Go uphill and follow the trail as it winds uphill over big tree roots. Pass another trail marker on the right. The trail, which levels some, is not quite so up and down here. Go between two trees—hard for a bike but on foot quite easy. As the trail takes a big turn to the left, it heads downhill before leveling again.

Continue past another marker as you step up and over a small embankment. The trail takes a quick left and then goes right, heading downhill. A big bend left takes the trail uphill. Head slightly left to stay on the trail and then climb steeply uphill. Go around a fallen tree and then head right. Cross a small bridge and then follow the trail as it winds back and forth. After a big bend to the left, the trail heads uphill gradually to another trail marker on the right. Go straight to the next trail marker and a sign on the right that states no bikes beyond this point. After the sign the trail winds left and then right passing more no-bikes signs on the left. The trail is much flatter here with little elevation change. Continue straight past another trail marker on the right. As the trail curves left, it narrows some. Hike past a nursery on your left and follow the marker on the right. The trail takes a big right turn before going past two benches and another trail marker. Go right onto a narrower part of the trail and then past another trail marker on the right before a big bend to the left.

Go over a fallen tree in the middle of the trail and past a marker on the right and another no-bikes sign. Continue past another marker and no-bikes sign as the trail winds back and forth, downhill and then back uphill the other side. As the trail bends right and then takes a quick left, head downhill steeply. Look to your right and you can see the trail that you will be on shortly. Hike past more no-bikes signs on the left and some houses that you can see just over the trees on the left. As the trail swings back to the right, head away from the creek bed and into an opening with a trail marker pointing straight ahead. Go straight into a large field of overgrown kudzu vines, a plant that was brought over from Japan for erosion in 1876 and heavily propagated throughout the South in the 1930s. It is one of the most invasive nonnative plants in the southeastern United States, growing up to a foot a day in summer and killing many native plants. Head through the kudzu on both sides of the trail to the next intersection and take the left fork. Head downhill steeply and to the right before going back to the left. Go straight up the trail over rocks and dirt as you leave the kudzu field. At the next intersection, go left until you come to the opening you were in at the start of the kudzu field. Head to the right at the intersection and head back up the trail the same way you came.

NEARBY ACTIVITIES

Houston Arboretum and Nature Center, (713) 681-8433, is only 0.25 miles west of the trailhead, off Woodway Drive. Additional Memorial Park activities include the Memorial Park Golf Course, (713) 862-4033, Memorial Park Tennis Center, (713) 867-0440, and the Memorial Park Swimming and Fitness Center, (713) 802-1662. The Galleria, one of the top shopping areas in the United States, is just west of the park with downtown Houston located to the east. Buffalo Bayou Park, White Oak Bayou Hike and Bike Trail, and Tranquility Park are also close by.

WHITE OAK BAYOU HIKE AND BIKE TRAIL

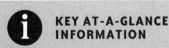

IN BRIEF

The White Oak Bayou watershed covers about 111 square miles and includes three primary streams: White Oak Bayou, Little White Oak Bayou, and Cole Creek. Located in Houston Heights, the White Oak Bayou Hike and Bike Trail is located in one of the oldest neighborhoods in Houston. Chosen for its higher elevation (23 feet higher than downtown Houston), Houston Heights was started in 1890 by Oscar Martin Carter, a self-made millionaire. He created a utopian neighborhood at a time when Houston was plagued with yellow fever and annual floods. Houston Heights was the location of residences, businesses, schools, open spaces for parks, libraries, civic clubs, and churches—all necessary elements for a close-knit community. Starting in the 1940s, the exodus to the suburbs began a deterioration of the Heights, and by 1970 the neighborhood was known for poverty and crime. In 1973 the Houston Heights Association was established to revitalize the community and preserve its historic buildings.

DESCRIPTION

Start the hike from the parking lot across from the Stude Community Center. Once on the asphalt trail, go left toward the baseball fields and swimming pool. At the fork, go right, past a bench on the left. You are now hiking between the baseball fields on your left and the

KEY AT-A-GLANCE INFORMATION

LENGTH: 2 miles

CONFIGURATION: Loop

DIFFICULTY: Easy

SCENERY: Bayou, woodlands, downtown skyline

EXPOSURE: Sunny

TRAIL TRAFFIC: Light

TRAIL SURFACE: Asphalt and dirt

HIKING TIME: 1 hour

DRIVING DISTANCE: Inside the 610 Loop, 4.2 miles from the intersection of the 610 Loop West and I-10

ACCESS: Free; open 6 a.m.–11 p.m.

MAPS: USGS Houston Heights and Settegast

WHEELCHAIR ACCESS: Yes

FACILITIES: Restrooms, baseball fields, picnic tables

SPECIAL COMMENTS: This hike and bike trail starts in Stude Park next to the Stude Community Center and is located between I-10 and Houston Heights. Stude Park, which includes ball fields, a swimming pool, playground, and picnic tables, can be crowded during warm-weather months, but this trail is often less crowded than other parts of the park. Pets must be on a leash at all times.

Directions

From the 610 Loop West and I-10, drive 4 miles east to the Studemont exit. Turn left, go 0.25 miles to Stude Street, and turn right. The parking lot is straight ahead.

GPS TRAILHEAD COORDINATES

LATITUDE: N 29° 46.734'
LONGITUDE: W 95° 23.126'

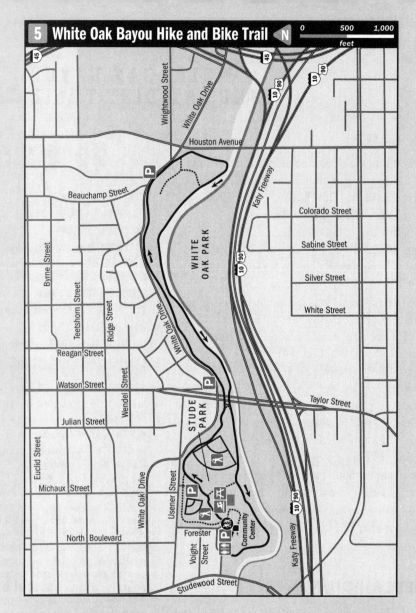

0   500   1,000
feet

N

45

45

90

10 90

10 90

Wrightwood Street

White Oak Drive

Houston Avenue

P

Beauchamp Street

Katy Freeway

Colorado Street

Sabine Street

90

10 90

Silver Street

WHITE OAK PARK

White Street

Byrne Street

Teetshorn Street

Ridge Street

White Oak Drive

Reagan Street

Watson Street

Wendel Street

P

Taylor Street

Julian Street

STUDE PARK

Euclid Street

Michaux Street

White Oak Drive

Usener Street

P

10 90

North Boulevard

Forester

P

Community Center

Voight Street

Katy Freeway

Studewood Street

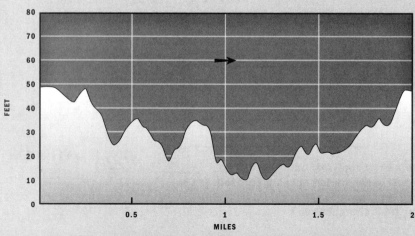

80
70
60
50
40
30
20
10
0

FEET

0.5   1   1.5   2

MILES

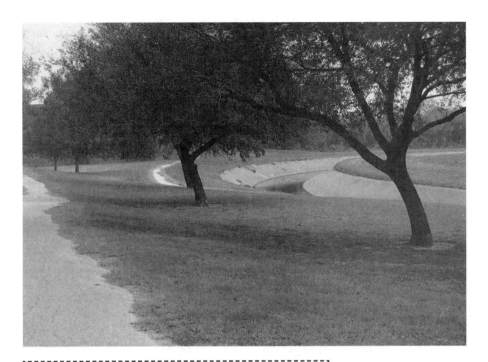

The concrete sides of White Oak Bayou on the right side of the trail

swimming pool on the right. In the distance to your right is the Houston downtown skyline, just past I-10. Continue down the trail as it takes a right turn and then curves left. Go through the next intersection and then past another parking lot and bench on the left. There are more baseball fields on the right as you hike gently downhill, past another bench on the left and toward some houses ahead.

As you get closer to White Oak Drive, the trail swings right. Continue past a bench and then the baseball fields, both right. Go past a bench on the left and then a third parking lot on the left, just across from the last baseball fields. As the trail heads away from the baseball fields, it goes downhill. At a fork, bear left keeping White Oak Bayou on your right. The sides of White Oak Bayou were hardened with concrete in the 1970s to control flooding—a common practice in Houston until the value of natural bayous was realized. As the trail heads uphill slightly, you pass under the Taylor Street underpass. Once past Taylor Street, the trail winds left and uphill, with houses on your left and the bayou still on your right. Although the right side of the trail has thick vegetation, this is a very sunny trail and you should wear sunscreen at all times.

Continue downhill and straight for some distance. As you pass an old park sign, look right to see a footbridge below in the flood overflow area of the bayou. You can also see a trail to your right—you use this to finish the hike. The area between the trail and bayou here are mowed, creating a large open area. Look far to your right for the freeway system that runs into Houston from the north. The trail continues to follow White Oak Drive and curves right. The area on the right contains thick vegetation, obscuring the view of the bayou. Head uphill steeply and continue through the next intersection. Look right for the overflow flood area of the bayou, which is overgrown with vegetation and often contains debris from recent floods. As you pass the King Biscuit Patio Café on the left (a great local spot), head down the trail past a fence on the left. Take the right fork at the next intersection to head downhill and into the trees. The trail surface changes to dirt as you enter the bayou's overflow flood area. Go straight through the next intersection and then head right, following the trail. Downtown Houston is now on your left, and you are headed back in the direction you came from. Once you start back, the trail surface changes back to asphalt. At the intersection, take the right fork and go over a small spillway with a culvert for drainage.

White Oak Bayou is now left, and a wooded area is on your right, just past a large swath of mowed grass. As the trail heads uphill, you can see the trail you came down earlier on the right. Go straight through the next intersection. The trail surface gets a little rough with eroded asphalt before changing back to smooth asphalt. As the trail narrows to no more than three feet wide, a high embankment on the left obscures views of downtown Houston. Continue as the trail bends right and downhill, allowing you to hike atop the concrete side of the bayou. Once off the concrete wall, the trail curves left and uphill. Cross a bridge over a small drainage channel and then follow a winding course. Continue as the trail heads downhill and onto another part of the bayou's concrete wall before heading back under Taylor Street. Continue through the next intersection, past a bench on the right. The baseball fields are now on your right, with the bayou still on your left. The route heads uphill and through an intersection, with the community pool on your right. Go by two benches and then head steeply uphill toward a large sculpture. Stude Community Center and picnic tables are now on your right. The trail bends right, passing the sculpture and a playground, both right. Go past another bench on the right and continue toward the parking lot to finish the hike.

NEARBY ACTIVITIES

Houston Arboretum and Nature Center, (713) 681-8433, Memorial Park Golf Course, (713) 862-4033, Memorial Park Tennis Center, (713) 867-0440, and the Memorial Park Swimming and Fitness Center, (713) 802-1662, are just 3.5 miles west. The Galleria, one of the top shopping areas in the United States, is just southwest of the park and downtown Houston is directly southeast of the park, only minutes away. Buffalo Bayou Park and Tranquility Park are also close by. The Heights Hike and Bike Trail (described in detail on pages 37–40), which connects Houston Heights to downtown Houston, is just west of the trail.

HEIGHTS HIKE AND BIKE TRAIL

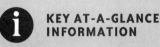

IN BRIEF

Located in one of the oldest neighborhoods in Houston, the Heights Hike and Bike Trail offers glimpses of some of the most beautiful examples of Victorian and turn-of-the-century architecture Houston has to offer. Chosen for its higher elevation (23 feet higher than downtown Houston), Houston Heights was started in 1890 by Oscar Martin Carter, a self-made millionaire. He created a utopian neighborhood at a time when Houston was plagued with yellow fever and annual floods. After years of blight, the Houston Heights Association was established in 1973 to revitalize the community and preserve its historic buildings.

DESCRIPTION

Start the hike by parking at Lawrence Park near North Shephard and 7th Street in The Heights. There is a basketball court, baseball field, and a portable restroom. Head east toward the concrete trail and then south toward downtown Houston and the heart of the Heights Historic District. The cottages, early-19th-century homes, and newer town homes present a glimpse into the architecture of Houston both past and present.

The Heights Hike and Bike Trail is part of the national Rails-Trails program created in 1986 to turn former railroad tracks into public trails. The Heights trail is relatively

KEY AT-A-GLANCE INFORMATION

LENGTH: 6.8 miles

CONFIGURATION: Out-and-back

DIFFICULTY: Moderate

SCENERY: Cottages, bayou, downtown, beautiful architecture

EXPOSURE: Sunny with some shade

TRAIL TRAFFIC: Heavy on weekends

HIKING TIME: 3 hours

DRIVING DISTANCE: 3.9 miles

ACCESS: Free

MAPS: USGA Houston Heights and Settegast

WHEELCHAIR ACCESS: Yes

FACILITIES: None, but local restaurants and shops

SPECIAL COMMENTS: This trail is one of the recent additions to the local Rails-Trails projects. It runs along the top of an old railroad connecting one of the original suburbs of Houston to the downtown district. There are numerous local restaurants and shops in the area that make for great diversions from the trial.

Directions

From Beltway 8 and I-10, drive 2.67 miles east to the Shephard Drive exit. Turn left, go .96 miles to 10th Street, and turn right. Drive 1.7 miles to Lawrence and turn right. Lawrence Park and the parking lot are .3 miles straight ahead.

GPS TRAILHEAD COORDINATES

LATITUDE: N 29° 47.046'
LONGITUDE: W 95° 24.431'

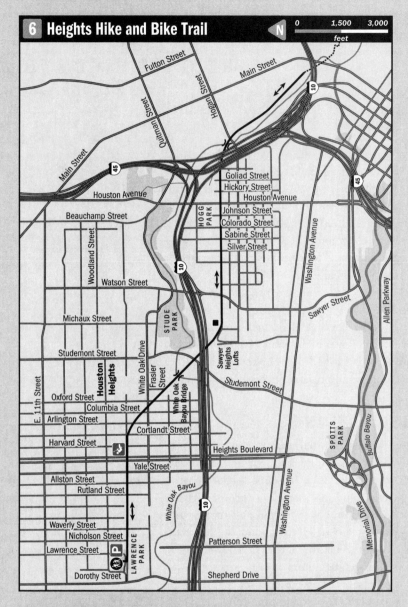

0   1,500   3,000
feet

Fulton Street
Main Street
Quitman Street
Hogan Street
Main Street
Houston Avenue
Beauchamp Street
Woodland Street
Watson Street
Michaux Street
Studemont Street
Houston Heights
E. 11th Street
Oxford Street
Columbia Street
Arlington Street
Harvard Street
Yale Street
Allston Street
Rutland Street
Waverly Street
Nicholson Street
Lawrence Street
Dorothy Street

Goliad Street
Hickory Street
Houston Avenue
Johnson Street
Colorado Street
Sabine Street
Silver Street
HOGG PARK
STUDE PARK
White Oak Drive
Frasier Street
White Oak Bayou Bridge
Cortlandt Street
Heights Boulevard
White Oak Bayou
Sawyer Heights Lofts
Studemont Street
Washington Avenue
Sawyer Street
Allen Parkway
SPOTTS PARK
Buffalo Bayou
Memorial Drive
LAWRENCE PARK
Patterson Street
Shepherd Drive

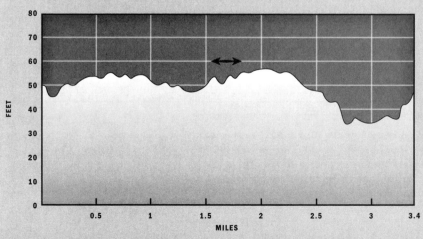

FEET
80
70
60
50
40
30
20
10
0

0.5   1   1.5   2   2.5   3   3.4
MILES

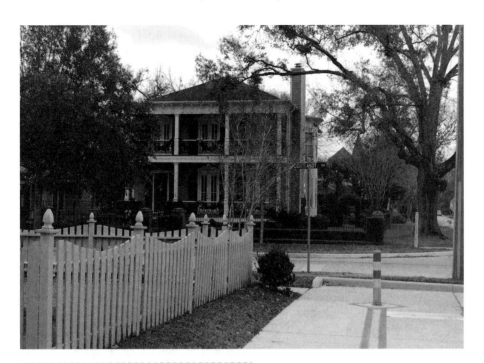

Historic turn-of-the-century houses in The Heights

new, having been completed in 2010. Part of the Missouri, Kansas, Texas Southern Pacific railroad, this trail connects The Heights to downtown Houston on a well-maintained 8-foot-wide trail accessible to hikers, runners, cyclists, and skaters.

As you hike, be aware of cyclists and make sure you stay on the right side of the trail. You will cross numerous roads, so be cautious and look both ways before crossing. Continue down the trail past industrial buildings on the right and beautiful, quaint cottages on the left. The trail is quite straight and very smooth to allow for wheelchair and stroller access. Cross several small streets, passing by a large complex on the left with white silos and a shallow ditch on your right.

As you hike, take time to look at the Victorian homes on both sides of the trail. This very exclusive area of Houston was home to urban blight less than 40 years ago but has had a renewal of spirit, and the homes and businesses definitely reflect the change. Continue past some new town homes on the left and an open field on the right before you approach Koelsch Gallery on the left. Cross Yale Street, making sure to look both ways as this is a very busy four-lane road. The next major road is Heights Boulevard, one of the more stunning streets in Houston with houses that are on an annual home tour in the Heights. While this is also a very congested road, it is split with a tree-lined boulevard in the middle.

Once you cross Heights Boulevard, pass a playground on the left. The next major street is Cortlandt Street, where you must cross the street diagonally to the right to get back on the trail. Pause to look at some of the French-inspired architecture and Victorian homes on Cortlandt. Continue crossing more minor roads and follow the trail as it winds slightly, giving you a good view of downtown Houston.

Cross White Oak Drive, watching for traffic. This four-lane drive is home to some of the best restaurants, clubs, and shops in The Heights, including Onion Creek Cafe only a few hundred yards to the left of the trail. Once you cross, you can see the trail extend in a straight line toward downtown. Past White Oak Drive, the trail enters a small industrial area with old Quonset huts and small businesses as you leave the heart of The Heights.

Leaving The Heights, cross a large bridge over White Oak Bayou, where you can easily see the White Oak Bayou Trail (featured in this book on pages 33–36) to the left and downtown Houston straight ahead. This massive bayou is often the source of Houston flooding during hurricanes and storms. Continue straight as the trail goes under I-10 and into a newly developed area with chain stores and restaurants. There is an oil derrick sign to the right reminding you that you are in Texas.

Continue on the trail past restaurants, shops, and new businesses. Pay attention to traffic entering and leaving the parking lots of these shops because the trail does pass in front of several of these entrances. Cross Sawyer Street, watching for traffic from all directions. Once past Sawyer, many of the newer developments give way to warehouses and old structures. Cross Henderson, Spring, Ring, Colorado, and Johnson streets before arriving at a bridge over Houston Avenue (one of the main streets into The Heights from I-10).

Hike past an old church on the right and cross over both Hickory and Goliad before going under I-45 and the many overpasses above. Cross another bridge over White Oak Bayou as you now enter an open part of the hike with the freeway far to your right. This is the newest part of the trail and will eventually connect to other trails in Houston, including the Sabine to Bagby Trail (also featured in this book on pages 46–49). Head slightly uphill toward the University of Houston downtown and the end of the hike. Turn around and head back in the direction you came.

NEARBY ACTIVITIES

White Oak Bayou Hike and Bike Trail, Houston Arboretum and Nature Center ([713] 681-8433), Memorial Park Golf Course ([713] 862-4033), Memorial Park Tennis Center ([713] 867-0440), and the Memorial Park Swimming and Fitness Center ([713] 802-1662) are just 3 miles west. The Galleria, one of the top shopping areas in the United States, is just southwest, and downtown Houston is at the end of the hike. Buffalo Bayou Park and Tranquility Park are just a short walk from the end of the Heights Hike and Bike Trail.

BRAYS BAYOU UPPER BANK HIKE AND BIKE TRAIL

7

IN BRIEF

The Brays Bayou Hike and Bike Trail was initially developed in the early 1970s when the bayou channel was paved. Although this hike is just over 9.7 miles, you can continue to Stella Link, making the out-and-back route more than 20 miles long. This is a moderate to difficult hike because of the length. The trail is often used by both hikers and cyclists, so watch out for bikes at all times.

DESCRIPTION

To begin the Brays Bayou Upper Bank Trail, park at MacGregor Park and head west across Calhoun Street to the trailhead. There is a sign for the Levi Vincent Perry Jr. Jogging Trail, which is part of the Upper Bank Trail. Brays Bayou has upper bank and lower bank trails that run along the bayou from MacGregor Way to Brompton. That 15-mile trek can be done in a day, but this hike only takes you on an out-and-back, 9.8-mile hike. Once on the trail, you pass an exercise station on your left. Brays Bayou is on your right and South MacGregor Way is on your left. The trail has an elevated asphalt surface, with a steep embankment down into the bayou on your right and a green space on your left. The University of Houston is in the distance on your right, less than 0.25 miles away. Continue past another exercise station on your left and follow the trail as it heads uphill slightly and curves left. From here, you can see the bayou

----

Directions ———————————→

From the 610 Loop and Beechnut Street, drive 8 miles east to Calhoun Street. Go past Calhoun Street and park at MacGregor Park, which is straight ahead.

KEY AT-A-GLANCE INFORMATION

LENGTH: 9.8 miles
CONFIGURATION: Out-and-back
DIFFICULTY: Moderate to difficult
SCENERY: Bayou, urban landscape, Texas Medical Center skyline; meadow, urban forest, downtown skyline
EXPOSURE: Very sunny with no shade; be sure you wear sunscreen and bring plenty of water.
TRAIL TRAFFIC: Moderate weekdays, heavy weekends
TRAIL SURFACE: Asphalt
HIKING TIME: 4.5 hours
DRIVING DISTANCE: Inside the 610 Loop, 8 miles from intersection of the 610 Loop and Beechnut Street
ACCESS: Free; open 6 a.m.–10 p.m.
MAPS: USGS Bellaire and Park Place
WHEELCHAIR ACCESS: Yes, but there are some steep inclines, so make sure you can maneuver up and down steep hills before venturing out.
FACILITIES: None
SPECIAL COMMENTS: Pets on leash no longer than 6 feet at all times. Although there are no restrooms on the trail, there are businesses that you can stop at and have coffee or a soft drink and use their restrooms.

GPS TRAILHEAD COORDINATES

LATITUDE: N 29° 42.662'
LONGITUDE: W 95° 20.453'

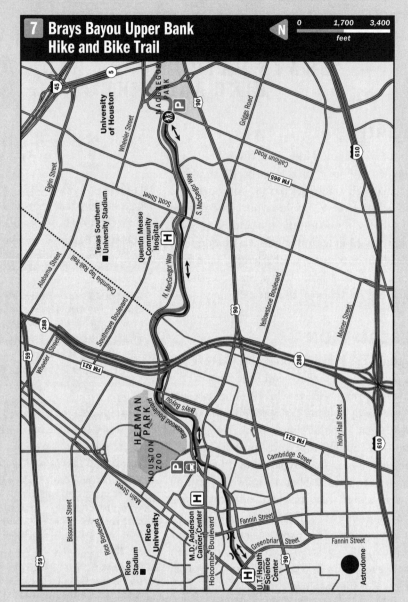

N

| 0 | 1,700 | 3,400 |

feet

University of Houston

MACGREGOR PARK

P

5

45

90

Griggs Road

Calhoun Road

FM 865

610

Wheeler Street

Elgin Street

Scott Street

S. MacGregor Way

Texas Southern University Stadium

Columbia Tap Rail-Trail

Alabama Street

Quentin Mease Community Hospital

H

N. MacGregor Way

Southmore Boulevard

90

Yellowstone Boulevard

Mainer Street

288

59

Wheeler Street

FM 521

HERMAN PARK

HOUSTON ZOO

Braeswood Boulevard

Brays Bayou

288

Holly Hall Street

FM 521

610

Cambridge Street

Main Street

Bissonnet Street

Rice Boulevard

Rice University

P

H

M.D. Anderson Cancer Center

Holcombe Boulevard

Fannin Street

Greenbriar Street

Fannin Street

59

Rice Stadium

H

U.T. Health Science Center

90

Astrodome

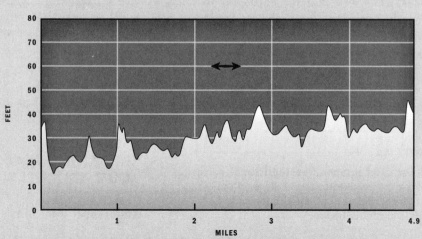

FEET

80
70
60
50
40
30
20
10
0

1   2   3   4   4.9

MILES

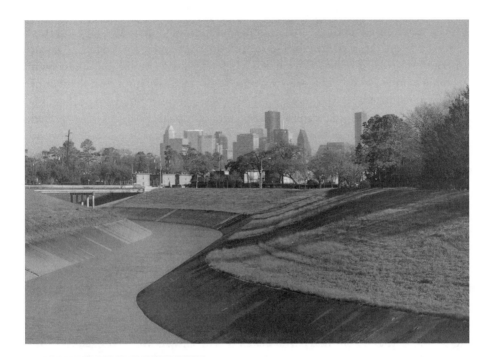

Dowtown Houston looking to the west

up ahead for quite some distance. This is a hiking and biking trail, so be cautious of cyclists at all times. Traffic on weekends can be heavy, so be very watchful of cyclists where the trail takes big bends. There are some blind spots, and cyclists can come up on you quickly.

Brays Bayou was channeled or paved in 1972, creating a concrete-lined bayou with paved walls that extend 30 to 40 feet above the bottom of the bayou. Due to the paving of the bayou, the only wildlife visible on the trail are birds. You can expect to see herons, egrets, and songbirds. The bayou runs through an older neighborhood with large mansion-style houses. Make sure to look at the architectural styles, as there are many beautiful homes on this hike. Continue as the trail heads uphill and bends right. Go by two more exercise stations on the left as the trail levels. After a long straight stretch the trail swings left and goes by two more exercise stations on the left. Again the trail straightens and levels out before heading uphill and under a large oak. In addition to oaks, there are oleanders, palms, and pines along the trail. There is also a considerable amount of moss growing on the oak trees, indicating much healthier air quality now than in the 1970s, when most of the moss started to die.

Continue until you reach the top of a hill with a large green space on the left. Now the trail heads back downhill and right. Look to your right across the bayou to see many of the palm trees that have been planted by homeowners. As the trail heads back uphill it swings left and toward Scott Street. Cross Scott

Street, watching for traffic—this is a busy intersection and there is no stoplight. Once back on the trail, the bayou is still on your right but there are houses instead of a road directly on your left. The trail heads uphill and under some telephone poles, whose lines are very close to the trail. Do not touch them under any circumstances.

As the trail continues uphill it veers left, affording you great views of the Texas Medical Center in the distance. Continue as the trail heads back downhill and then bends right. There are concrete steps on the sides of the bayou that allow you to walk down to the lower level, but watch for high water as the lower level is often under water. Go past another exercise station on the left as the trail heads downhill and left. Pass by another exercise bench on the left. There are large culverts on the left side of the trail that drain water into the bayou. Stay away from these, since the openings are large enough for you to fall into. Continue as the trail heads uphill and zigzags left, then right. You can look across the bayou and see another trail on its north side that runs parallel to the one you are on. Your trail takes a big rightward bend, following the curve of the bayou, and then passes a bench on the left. As the trail goes right, you get a good view of the Houston skyline to your right. Go through an intersection with a trail departing left, and continue past a bench on the left. As you approach Ardmore Street, the trail swings left and goes by a bench on the left. Cross Ardmore at the stoplight and get back on the trail headed west.

The trail now zigzags uphill. You pass by some old bridge columns in the bayou on your right, and then draw near a road on your left. As the trail continues to curve left, you head back toward the Texas Medical Center, which you can see in the distance. Pass a guardrail on your left as you head downhill and onto the top of the concrete wall of Brays Bayou. Cross under I-288, hiking atop the paved wall. This part of the hike is much quieter due to the embankment on your left that muffles the sound of traffic. Watch your step around the edge of the bayou because the embankment down to the water is very steep. Once past the interstate, the trail heads uphill and out of the bayou. The incline out of the bayou is very steep, so watch your footing.

Continue along the trail as it heads toward Almeda Road. Cross the road at a stoplight, take an immediate left, and then cross South MacGregor Way. Once across the street, turn right and walk to the first intersection. Here turn left to get back on the asphalt trail. The Houston Zoo and Hermann Park Golf Course are on your right. The trail heads downhill and bends left before going back uphill. At the next intersection, where a trail departs left, continue straight. The trail curves left past a sign about the Hermann Park Urban Forest. Here there are picnic tables and a small forest for a nature walk. Continue past another sign about a meadow and more picnic tables. There is a water fountain on the left, just before another intersection, where a trail goes left into the park. Here continue straight, passing a sign about Brays Bayou and a bayou restoration project on the left. As you hike past the restoration project, the trail swings right. At the next intersection, go straight toward a large bridge over the bayou. Go across the bridge to get on the north side of the bayou. Now go left, toward the Texas Medical Center. Look to your right, through the trees and across the street, for the Hermann Park Golf Course. Continue to follow the trail to Holcombe Boulevard. At Holcombe Boulevard, go left past the Metro bus stop, cross a bridge, and go left again to get back on the trail. The trail winds downhill toward the paved bayou. At a fork, bear left to reach the top of the bayou. Go under Holcombe Boulevard and then make a big bend to the right. Brays Bayou is left; a high grass embankment is on your right. Go under a road and bear left at the next fork. Go under another road as you approach Fannin Street and the rail line. The trail winds toward Greenbriar Street. When you reach the fork heading up to Greenbriar Street turn around and retrace your route to complete the hike.

NEARBY ACTIVITIES

The University of Houston, Rice University, Hermann Park, the Houston Zoo, Houston Museum of Natural Science, Holocaust Museum, Medical Museum, Museum of Fine Art, Children's Museum, Miller Outdoor Theater, Reliant Stadium, and the Houston Astrodome are all within five minutes of Brays Bayou.

8 SABINE TO BAGBY TRAIL

KEY AT-A-GLANCE INFORMATION

LENGTH: 2.4 miles

CONFIGURATION: Out-and-back

DIFFICULTY: Easy

SCENERY: Downtown Houston, bayou, Theater District, Downtown Aquarium, parkland, University of Houston Downtown, historic buildings

EXPOSURE: Sunny

TRAIL TRAFFIC: Light to moderate

TRAIL SURFACE: Concrete

HIKING TIME: 1 hour

DRIVING DISTANCE: Inside the 610 Loop, approximately 4.5 miles from the intersection of Memorial Drive and the 610 Loop

ACCESS: Free; open 6 a.m.–11 p.m.

MAPS: USGS Settegast

WHEELCHAIR ACCESS: Yes

FACILITIES: Parking, benches, water fountains, lights, canoe/kayak launches

SPECIAL COMMENTS: After heavy rains, be aware of water levels in Buffalo Bayou; it is one of the main flood-control channels in Houston, and water levels may stay high for days. There are no restrooms on this hike, but numerous restaurants and businesses in the area would appreciate your patronage.

GPS TRAILHEAD COORDINATES

LATITUDE: N 29° 45.733'
LONGITUDE: W 95° 22.429'

IN BRIEF

This urban hike offers some of the best views of downtown Houston and the Theater District. It includes hiking and biking trails on both sides of Buffalo Bayou, which link the Buffalo Bayou Park Trails to Sesquicentennial Park in downtown. There are 23 new street-to-bayou access points, new canoe/kayak launches, and a new lighting system that allows hiking until 11 p.m. Much of the lighting was created with a blue-to-white color scheme, giving this section of the bayou its new nickname, "Blue Bayou." The lights change in tandem with the phases of the moon.

DESCRIPTION

To start the hike, from City of Houston Lot H head east toward the Buffalo Bayou Walk sign. Hike down the paved path past a park sign. At a fork, bear left to get on the trail. There are benches to the right that overlook Buffalo Bayou. This trail is part of the 23-acre, $15 million Sabine to Bagby Waterfront Park that links Buffalo Bayou Park in the west with Sesquicentennial Park in downtown Houston. This trail is beautiful in the daytime because of native landscaping, and even more beautiful at night with blue-to-white lights that change with the phases of the moon.

In 2002, the Buffalo Bayou Partnership and the City of Houston devised a 20-year master plan to bring Buffalo Bayou back to life and create a waterfront of parks, canals,

- -

Directions ───────────────►

From the intersection of the 610 Loop and Memorial Drive, go east on Memorial Drive 4.5 miles to the Houston Avenue exit. After exiting, turn into the first parking lot on the right.

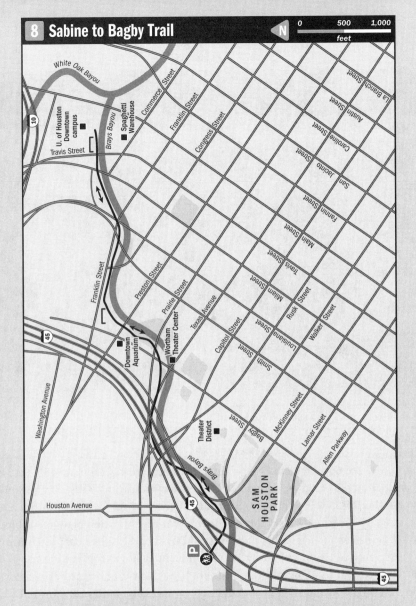

8 Sabine to Bagby Trail

0   500   1,000
feet
N

White Oak Bayou

U. of Houston Downtown campus

Spaghetti Warehouse

Brays Bayou

Commerce Street

Franklin Street

Congress Street

La Branch Street

Austin Street

Caroline Street

San Jacinto Street

Fannin Street

Main Street

Travis Street

Milam Street

Rusk Street

Walker Street

10

Travis Street

Franklin Street

Preston Street

Prairie Street

Texas Avenue

Capitol Street

Louisiana Street

Smith Street

McKinney Street

Lamar Street

Allen Parkway

45

Downtown Aquarium

Wortham Theater Center

Washington Avenue

Theater District

Bagby Street

Brays Bayou

SAM HOUSTON PARK

Houston Avenue

45

P

45

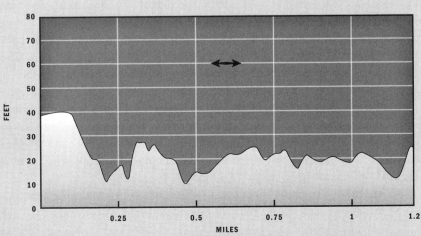

FEET

80
70
60
50
40
30
20
10
0

0.25   0.5   0.75   1   1.2

MILES

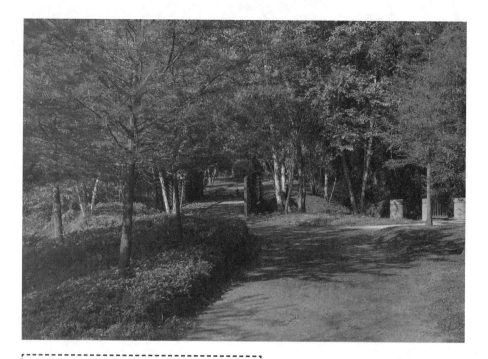

One of the bridges on the Sabine to Bagby Trail

and mixed-use development. The plan focuses on a 10-square-mile area that will create 850 acres of new parkland in downtown Houston. Trails now reconnect neighborhoods to the waterway, expanding access to the bayou from numerous locations. Part of the City of Houston downtown-revitalization plan, the Sabine to Bagby Trail now connects the parks west of downtown to the heart of Houston.

As you hike, you will go by Wortham Center, home of the Houston Ballet and Houston Grand Opera. Built entirely through private donations at a cost of $66 million, Wortham Center was the first opera house built in the United States in more than 25 years. It was built during the height of the oil bust, and was completed four months ahead of schedule and $5 million under budget. Other attractions along the "Blue Bayou" include The Downtown Aquarium, Spaghetti Warehouse Restaurant, and the University of Houston Downtown. The Downtown Aquarium redeveloped two Houston landmarks, Fire Station No. 1 and The Central Waterworks Building. It is a 6-acre entertainment and dining complex with full-service restaurants, rides, shopping, and a 500,000-gallon aquarium which is home to more than 200 species of aquatic life. Founded in 1974 and part of the University of Houston System, the Downtown campus was instrumental in revitalizing the north end of downtown Houston with its new and innovative architecture.

Once on the paved path, hike under numerous overpasses and roads that lead into downtown Houston. Buffalo Bayou and the Theater District are directly on your right. Go by some benches on the left and follow the trail as it goes downhill and then swings left. Although the bayou is often used by canoeists and kayakers, use caution—alligators and poisonous snakes do exist in this part of the bayou. Go by a railing on your right before the trail heads steeply uphill. There is a road now on your left and many roads above your head. At a fork, bear right on the lower trail to get away from the road on your left. This trail takes you farther down into the bayou. It curves slightly left and then heads uphill. Continue straight where the upper trail rejoins from the left, then swing right, hiking under more roads.

When you reach another set of steps on your left, continue straight. At the next intersection, go right and downhill. Look to your right and across the bayou for the Wortham Center. Cyclists also use this trail, so stay to the right at all times. While they are supposed to yield to pedestrians, you should still give them plenty of room to get by. Follow the trail as it winds uphill. The Downtown Aquarium is now on your left, just past the road columns that are painted like waves. At the steps to the aquarium, continue straight. Hike beneath more overpasses and then go past a sign for the start of Sesquicentennial Park. Go past benches on the right and bike racks on the left.

Continue past steps and another park sign, both left. At an upcoming fork, bear right and head under another road. Pass some steps and concrete benches on your left. Cross a small bridge, go under another road, and pass a large concrete wall on the left. Go under another major road and past two benches on the right. This trail is patrolled by Houston Police on horses, so you should watch where you step. Look right, across the bayou, for the Old Spaghetti Warehouse. To the left is the University of Houston Downtown campus. Turn around at the U-turn sign and retrace your route.

Note: All of the roads near this hike are high-traffic roads, so do not park on any of them. Park your car in City of Houston Lot H, at the start of the trail.

NEARBY ACTIVITIES

The downtown Houston entertainment district is located along the walk at ground level and includes the aquarium, an amusement park, and restaurant. Minute Maid Park, home of the Houston Astros, and Toyota Center, home of the Houston Rockets and Houston Aeros, are just east of the trail. Sam Houston Park and Tranquility Park are also east of the trail. The Houston Theater District runs along the south side of the bayou, as do restaurants, clubs, and downtown parks.

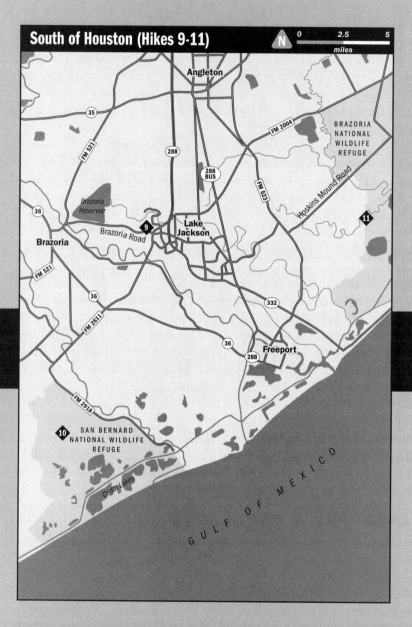

South of Houston (Hikes 9-11)

N

0   2.5   5

miles

Angleton

35

FM 521

288

288 BUS

FM 2004

BRAZORIA
NATIONAL
WILDLIFE
REFUGE

FM 523

Hoskins Mound Road

36

Brazoria
Reservoir

Lake
Jackson

Brazoria Road

9

11

Brazoria

FM 521

36

FM 2611

332

36

Freeport

288

FM 2918

10

SAN BERNARD
NATIONAL WILDLIFE
REFUGE

Cedar Lakes

G U L F   O F   M E X I C O

SOUTH of HOUSTON

9 LAKE JACKSON WILDERNESS PARK

KEY AT-A-GLANCE INFORMATION

LENGTH: 2.8 miles

CONFIGURATION: Out-and-back

DIFFICULTY: Easy

SCENERY: Bayou, woodlands, bottomland forest

EXPOSURE: Shady with some sun

TRAIL TRAFFIC: Light

TRAIL SURFACE: Grass and dirt

HIKING TIME: 1.5 hours

DRIVING DISTANCE: 39.5 miles from the intersection of Beltway 8 and I-288

ACCESS: Free; open every day 6 a.m.–10 p.m.

MAPS: USGS Lake Jackson

WHEELCHAIR ACCESS: None

FACILITIES: Parking, picnic areas, fishing, boat ramp

SPECIAL COMMENTS: This very small park is used mainly for hiking and for launching small boats, kayaks, or canoes. Biking is permitted on the trails, so stay to the right at all times. While there is a round-trip hike of 8 miles along the bayou, the bridge at the 1.43-mile marker has been damaged, so this hike has been shortened until the bridge is fixed.

GPS TRAILHEAD COORDINATES

LATITUDE: N 29° 2.902'
LONGITUDE: W 95° 28.667'

IN BRIEF

Lake Jackson Wilderness Park is bordered by Buffalo Camp Bayou and the Brazos River bottomland forest. It also parallels The Wilderness Golf Course, but you can only vaguely see the course during the hike. Primitive camping is allowed with approval, and there is one interpretive nature loop in the park. Other activities here include boating, fishing, picnicking, and bird-watching. The Gulf Coast Bird Observatory is just across the bayou from the entrance to Wilderness Park. Do not veer off onto any small paths that take you into the forest. These are not part of the park's trail system and it is best to stay on the marked trails.

DESCRIPTION

Start the hike in the parking lot just to the right of the boat ramp. There are picnic tables and good views of Buffalo Camp Bayou. Continue into the trees past the trail sign and through the gate. The trailhead sign is to the right of the trail and lists the various hikes in the park. As you hike into the trees, the bayou is on your left and the forest is on your right. This is a wide dirt trail that winds through the trees following the path of the bayou. Go past a trail marker on the right and continue as the trail takes a big bend to the left. Stay out of the water and away from the banks of the bayou, as alligators and poisonous snakes exist

----

Directions ⟶

From Beltway 8 and I-288, head south 38 miles to FM 2004 and take a right. Go 1.3 miles to FM 332 and turn right. The entrance to the park is on the left, just after you cross Buffalo Camp Bayou.

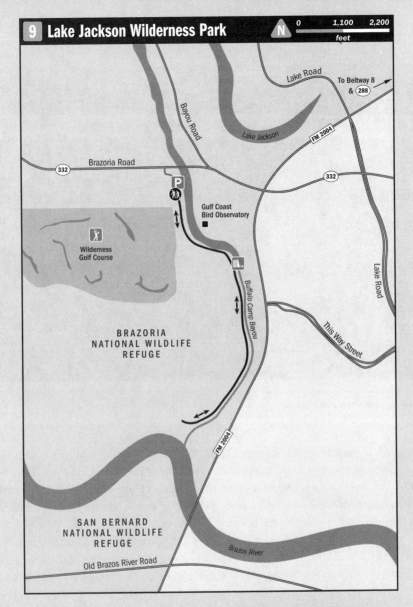

N

0   1,100   2,200

feet

Lake Road

To Beltway 8
& 288

Bayou Road

Lake Jackson

FM 2004

Brazoria Road

332

332

P

Gulf Coast
Bird Observatory

Wilderness
Golf Course

Lake Road

BRAZORIA
NATIONAL WILDLIFE
REFUGE

Buffalo Camp Bayou

This Way Street

FM 2004

SAN BERNARD
NATIONAL WILDLIFE
REFUGE

Brazos River

Old Brazos River Road

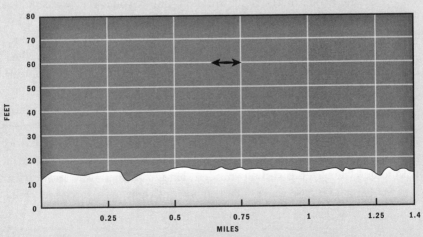

FEET						
80						
70						
60						
50						
40						
30						
20						
10						
0	0.25	0.5	0.75	1	1.25	1.4

MILES

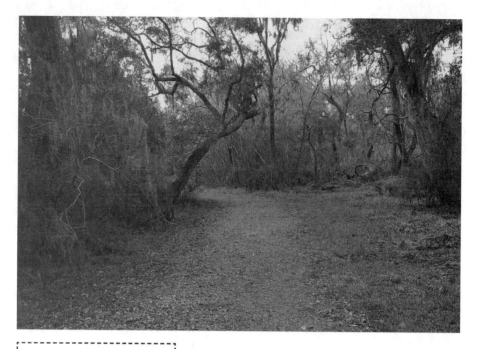

Coastal vegetation along the trail

along all the bayous in this part of Texas. As the trail bends right, the trail surface changes to grass; however, it is still easy to follow because it was cut out of the forest. Look to your left across the bayou for the Gulf Coast Bird Observatory headquarters on the opposite bank. It has a large picnic pavilion and a small fishing pier, along with nature trails and picnic sites.

Following the trail over a drainage pipe, look to your right to get a brief glimpse of The Wilderness Golf Course. The vegetation on the right is very thick and impenetrable. The foliage on the left can be thick enough in some areas to obscure views of the bayou. Continue as the trail narrows and gets even grassier. Go by a 0.25-mile marker on the right. Buffalo Camp Bayou is very wide and the water can run swiftly after heavy rains, so stay on the trail at all times. While hiking, you may see kayakers and canoeists on the bayou. Also look for birds such as neotropical migrants, such as warblers and wood ducks. Besides alligators, wild pigs are also found in the area, as evidenced by the tracks on the trail. Common plants are sawtooth palmettos, moss-draped oaks, and fan palms.

Continue on the trail as it heads uphill and bends right, past some large oak trees covered in moss. The trail then heads left, taking you briefly away from the bayou. At a fork, bear left to view the concrete spillway for the bayou. Turn around, head back to the fork, and then head sharply left to get back on the main route. The bayou is still on your left, but it is farther away and you can only see the banks, not the water. The trail swings right, past some low spots.

Hike around them if they are too wet or muddy to get through. This is a bike trail also, so watch for cyclists at all times and stay to the right.

The trail winds through the trees and then past a large stand of fan palms on the right. Although the trail surface is grass, it looks like an old road with parallel ruts on each side. Continue as the trail bends right and downhill, over a drainage pipe, and then to the left and uphill. You can hear the traffic on the highway to your left. Once up the hill the trail swings right. The bayou is still on your left but is not visible. The trail heads uphill out of the trees and into a sunny opening between the vegetation on the right and the bayou on the left. Pass a large oak tree on your left. The bayou is directly on your left now with the road just to the left of the bayou. You are hiking on the bank of the bayou in an opening that is not a well-defined part of the trail. The route is still easy to follow—just stay between the vegetation on the right and the bayou on the left. Continue as the trail heads downhill off the embankment and then back uphill on the other side.

Look to your right to see how the trees grow in twisted, knotty fashion. They are works of art created by the prevailing winds of the Gulf Coast. Follow the trail as it veers right into the trees, away from the bayou, and then left through a wide opening in the forest. This part of the trail is more defined, because it has been cut through the middle of the trees. There is thick foliage on both sides with the bayou farther on your left. At a fork, bear left toward the bayou. Now veer right as you pass a trail marker on the right. At a large oak tree on your left, the trail bends to the right, back into the trees. Up ahead you can see the remnants of an old bridge. Turn around and retrace your route to complete the hike.

NEARBY ACTIVITIES

San Bernard National Wildlife Refuge, the Gulf Coast Bird Observatory, and Brazoria National Wildlife Refuge are less than 15 miles from Lake Jackson Wilderness Park. Brazos Bend State Park and the George Ranch are also close by. The Brazos River Trail, a 125-mile trail through Fort Bend and Brazoria counties, is part of the Sam Houston Trail & Wilderness Preserve. Hiking, biking, paddling, and horseback riding trails abound along this trail that heads through 18 different parks and refuges, including Lake Jackson Wilderness Park. The northernmost point is Brazos Park, while the southernmost is San Bernard National Wildlife Refuge.

10 SAN BERNARD NATIONAL WILDLIFE REFUGE: Cowtrap Marsh Trail

KEY AT-A-GLANCE INFORMATION

LENGTH: 1.74 miles

CONFIGURATION: Out-and-back

DIFFICULTY: Easy

SCENERY: Shallow lakes, marshes, prairies, freshwater ponds

EXPOSURE: Sunny

TRAIL TRAFFIC: Light

TRAIL SURFACE: Grass

HIKING TIME: 1 hour

DRIVING DISTANCE: 51 miles from the intersection of Beltway 8 and I-288

ACCESS: Free; open every day, sunrise–sunset

MAPS: USGS Cedar Lane NE and Cedar Lakes West; trail signs and trail map

WHEELCHAIR ACCESS: None

FACILITIES: Picnic tables, restrooms, hiking information, and parking at refuge headquarters on CR 306; fishing piers

SPECIAL COMMENTS: While on a levee, the trail is not very high above the bordering marshes and lakes (i.e., alligators and snakes are very close). Leave pets and small children at home. Separate hunting areas total 9,000 acres of the refuge; check with headquarters about hunting locations and seasons.

GPS TRAILHEAD COORDINATES

LATITUDE: N 28° 52.852'
LONGITUDE: W 95° 33.470'

IN BRIEF

San Bernard National Wildlife Refuge is open year-round for wildlife observation, hiking, photography, and fishing. Fishing is allowed in many of the open lakes within the tidelands and Cedar Lake Creek. Hunting for waterfowl is also permitted within a public hunting area and a permit-hunt area. A boat ramp at Cedar Lake Creek provides boat access to the Cedar Lake area. Canoes, kayaks, and small motorboats are welcome to launch from the ramp.

DESCRIPTION

To get to the trails, head out the gate and turn left on CR 306. Drive another mile on the dirt road to the next San Bernard Refuge sign and turn left. Drive a mile to the auto-tour trail on the left. To reach the Cowtrap Marsh Trail trailhead, park at the viewing platform on the Moccasin Pond auto-tour loop. Although there is handicap parking at the viewing platform, the Cowtrap Marsh Trail is not accessible to wheelchairs or strollers. Head toward the trailhead sign and a nature sign describing some of the birds you might see during your hike. During the winter months you can see more than 1,000 Canada and greater white-fronted geese in the salt marshes and numerous saltwater lakes. The duck species include pintail, teal, gadwall, widgeon, and mottled

Directions

From Beltway 8 and I-288, head south 38 miles to FM 2004 and take a right. Go 7 miles until FM 2004 becomes FM 2611 and then go another 4 miles. Turn left onto FM 2918 and go 1 mile to County Road 306 and turn right. The entrance to San Bernard National Wildlife Refuge is approximately 1 mile on the left.

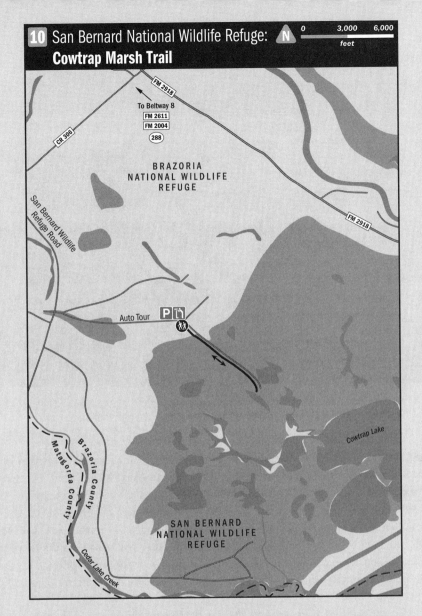

N

0   3,000   6,000
feet

FM 2918

To Beltway 8
FM 2611
FM 2004
288

CR 306

BRAZORIA
NATIONAL WILDLIFE
REFUGE

FM 2918

San Bernard Wildlife
Refuge Road

Auto Tour   P

Cowtrap Lake

Brazoria County

Matagorda County

Cedar Lake Creek

SAN BERNARD
NATIONAL WILDLIFE
REFUGE

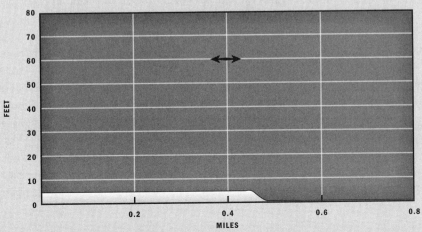

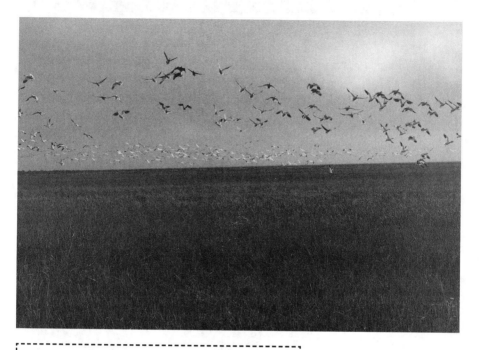

Thousands of migrating geese taking flight over the marshes

ducks. Other birds that are prevalent in the refuge include herons, ibis, sandpipers, stilts, yellow rails, roseate spoonbills, reddish egrets, white-faced ibis, wood storks, gulls, royal terns, black skimmers, barred owls, clapper and king rails, and brown pelicans. The marine life includes spotted sea trout, redfish, black drum, flounder, oysters, shrimp, and crabs. In the upland part of the park are bobcats, coyotes, wild pigs, and white-tailed deer. Other frequent inhabitants of the marshes and lakes are alligators and snakes (many of them poisonous). Cyclists are welcome on all refuge roads open to public vehicles. They are not allowed on any of the trails.

At the trailhead, go around the car barrier to get on the wide grassy trail atop the levee. While the barrier prevents visitors' cars from getting on the trail, the refuge does use the trail as a road to access remote parts of the refuge. As a result, there are deep ruts and tracks, making for uneven footing. Watch your step and stay in the middle of the levee at all times, keeping a safe distance from the water. This is a very sunny trail with no shade, so take sunscreen, a hat, and plenty of water. Also, due to the marshes and lakes, there is a profusion of mosquitoes even during the winter months. The levee, which is 30–35 feet wide, is only about a foot or so above the surrounding marshes.

Look to either side to see for miles across rippling marshes and ponds toward stands of trees that are more than a mile away. This is what much of coastal Texas looked like before settlement. Less than half of the refuge is open to the public, so much of what you see is a vast landscape of wild undeveloped land. As you continue along the straight and flat trail, you may see thousands of geese and ducks. When they take flight, the sound is almost deafening as they screech and squawk. Continue on the trail past a fence on your right that is about 40 yards away. Between the trail and the fence are a series of small ponds that house snakes, alligators, mosquitoes, and ducks. Be cautious at all times.

Continue toward a lone tree on the trail, past several more ponds on both sides of the trail. While I was hiking, I saw several alligators on the left side of the trail. These ponds are home to many of the local ducks, whereas the marshes are home to most of the migrating waterfowl, such as the snow geese. The mowed trail atop the levee becomes less traveled and less distinct 0.7 of a mile into the hike. The trail narrows some but there are no longer any deep ruts on the surface, making for an easier hike. There is more sand on this part of the trail, which may contain many animal tracks. This part of the levee is even lower than before, making for very little elevation change between the marsh and the trail surface. Continue as the trail narrows to only a footpath. The grass is more overgrown and the trail surface less distinct. Look straight ahead and you can see a tall structure but not much of anything else. At a yellow metal stake on the right side of the trail, turn around and retrace your route. This turnaround is 0.87 miles from the start of the hike. While hiking, you can see Olney's bulrush, salt-marsh plants, and some prickly pear cactus. The tree line for much of the bottomland forests of the refuge is straight ahead and to the left, but several miles away.

When you get back to your car, continue on the auto tour, heading past a viewing platform on the right. This is a one-way road. While heading back on the auto tour, notice the willow trees, which attract high numbers of warblers migrating north. If the weather is warm, the moist air from the Gulf collides with cold, dry air heading south creating heavy rain and wind. During spring's northward migration, this results in a warbler "fallout," causing hundreds of these tiny birds to drop into the shelter of the willow trees, too tired to fly any farther.

NEARBY ACTIVITIES

Lake Jackson Wilderness Park, the Gulf Coast Bird Observatory, and Brazoria National Wildlife Refuge are less than 15 miles from San Bernard. Brazos Bend State Park and the George Ranch are also close by. Brazos River Trail, a 125-mile trail through Fort Bend and Brazoria counties, is part of the Sam Houston Trail & Wilderness Preserve. Hiking, biking, paddling, and horseback riding trails abound along this trail that heads through 18 different parks and refuges. The northernmost point is Brazos Park, while the southernmost is San Bernard National Wildlife Refuge.

11 BRAZORIA NATIONAL WILDLIFE REFUGE: Big Slough Trail

KEY AT-A-GLANCE INFORMATION

LENGTH: 1.2 miles

CONFIGURATION: Loop

DIFFICULTY: Easy

SCENERY: Slough, marshes, prairies, woodlands

EXPOSURE: Sunny

TRAIL TRAFFIC: Light

TRAIL SURFACE: Grass

HIKING TIME: 1 hour

DRIVING DISTANCE: 52 miles from the intersection of Beltway 8 and I-288

ACCESS: Free; open every day, sunrise–sunset

MAPS: USGS Oyster Creek; trail signs and trail map

WHEELCHAIR ACCESS: None

FACILITIES: Restrooms, Discovery Center, parking, picnic areas, fishing piers

SPECIAL COMMENTS: A picnic area and restrooms are available at the Discovery Center, but there is no water, so bring drinking water along with sunscreen, mosquito repellent, and a hat. There are poisonous snakes and alligators in the refuge so exercise caution at all times. Do not let young children run ahead of you during the hike.

GPS TRAILHEAD COORDINATES

LATITUDE: N 29° 3.588'
LONGITUDE: W 95° 16.077'

IN BRIEF

Brazoria National Wildlife Refuge, which opened in the late 1980s, is home to more than 400 species of wildlife. Its marshes and prairies create some of the richest environments on Earth. Two hunting areas exist—the Christmas Point Public Waterfowl Hunting Area and the Middle Bayou Public Waterfowl Hunting area. Check with headquarters for restrictions and seasons. Fishing is also available, and the Bastrop Bayou Public Fishing Area has a wheelchair-accessible fishing pier. Bank fishing is available at the Clay Banks and Salt Lake public fishing areas.

DESCRIPTION

The Big Slough Trail is named after a freshwater lifeline that runs through the prairie, marsh, and woodland habitats. Start the hike in the Discovery Center parking lot. Hike toward the marsh and boardwalk behind the building, passing under the picnic pavilion. Once on the boardwalk, go to the right past some newly constructed pylons on the left. There is a sign on the right describing the butterfly garden habitat that exists just off the slough. The boardwalk is several feet above the water and a safe distance from any alligators. Follow the boardwalk as it wanders over the slough. Stop to see how many ducks, snakes, and alligators you can spot. Continue

Directions

From Beltway 8 and I-288, head south 38 miles to FM 2004 and take a left. Go 6.3 miles to FM 523 and turn right. Drive 5.6 miles to County Road 227 and turn left, driving 2 miles to the entrance of the refuge, on the right. The Discovery Center is 3 miles ahead.

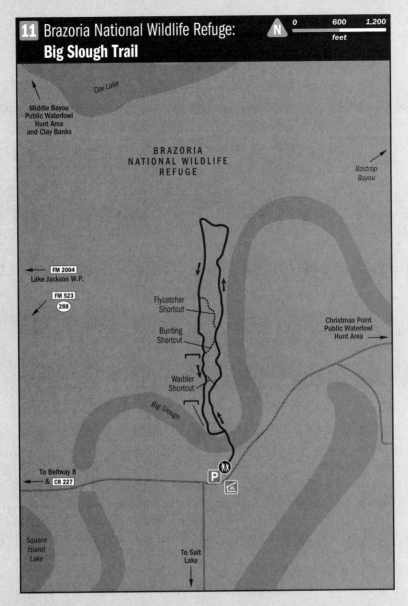

N

0   600   1,200
feet

Cox Lake

Middle Bayou
Public Waterfowl
Hunt Area
and Clay Banks

BRAZORIA
NATIONAL WILDLIFE
REFUGE

*Bastrop
Bayou*

FM 2004
Lake Jackson W.P.

FM 523
288

Flycatcher
Shortcut

Bunting
Shortcut

Christmas Point
Public Waterfowl
Hunt Area

Warbler
Shortcut

Big Slough

P

To Beltway 8
& CR 227

*Square
Island
Lake*

To Salt
Lake

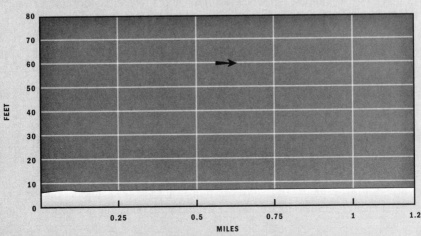

80
70
60
50
40
30
20
10
0

FEET

0.25   0.5   0.75   1   1.2

MILES

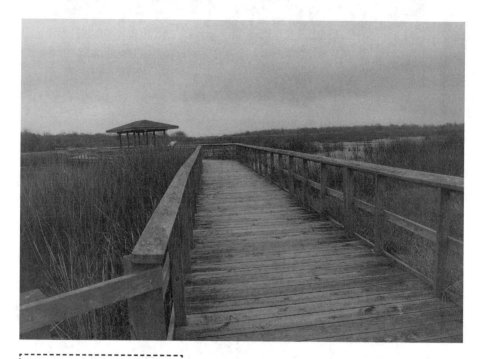

A long boardwalk over Big Slough

under another pavilion with benches and past a nature sign about the coastal wetlands on the right. Go by a platform on the right that takes you closer to the water and the wildlife.

Continue along the boardwalk past a sign about the American alligator, and then get off the boardwalk heading to the right. Go by a bench on the left as the trail surface changes to grass. Follow a trail sign for the Big Slough Trail and go by trail marker 1. These markers coincide with the information in the Big Slough Trail Guide, which you can pick up at the information center. Some of the plants on this trail include grasses, sedges, rushes, cattails, water lilies, palmetto, prickly pear cactus, ash trees, Chinese tallow trees, yaupon bushes, and willows. Continue past trail maker 2, where the vegetation on both sides of the trail is thick and impenetrable. Go by a nature sign on the right about songbirds, neotropical migrants that include kingbirds, yellow warblers, gray catbirds, and common yellowthroats. As the trail heads right and into the trees, watch where you step, as there are cows that frequently use this trail. The slightly elevated trail curves right and then passes the Warbler Shortcut, which joins from the left. Continue straight, passing a sign about the wildlife signs, which include tracks, feathers, and scat.

Wildlife you may see include coyotes, bobcats, raccoons, opossums, swamp rabbits, skunks, armadillos, feral hogs, alligators, and snakes. The eastern cottonmouth and rattlesnake are two of the poisonous snakes found in the refuge, but there are also nonpoisonous snakes, including the rat snake and water snake.

Continue past trail marker 3 and then curve right. Now swinging left, go by trail marker 4 and then through the next intersection, with the Bunting Shortcut. The route then veers left past a bench on the left and goes through the intersection with the Flycatcher Shortcut. Go straight to find trail marker 5. Swing left to trail marker 6.

The wide trail passes trail marker 7, then winds to trail marker 8. Now head uphill, past trail marker 9 and a viewing platform on the right. There is a bench on the platform that overlooks a small marsh. Continue as the trail bends to the left; to the right is a closed section of the refuge. Follow the sign for the Big Slough Trail and go left and uphill. Look to your right for a large stand of trees in the distance, past the coastal prairie. Throughout the hike, look for refuge birds such as great blue herons, moorhens, northern cardinals, mockingbirds, quail, snow geese, roseate spoonbills, and black-necked stilts.

Continue past trail markers 10, 11, and 12, and through an intersection with a trail on the left. The refuge boundary fence is now on your right, just beyond the vegetation. After trail marker 13, the trail bends left and then takes a quick turn right. Continue past a bench on the left and an intersection with a trail on the left. Go past trail marker 14. The stand of trees on the right includes the Osage orange and the sugar hackberry. Wander back and forth to the next intersection, with a trail on the left, and then follow the trail exit sign. The boundary fence is still on your right as you go by a bench on the left.

After trail marker 15, the trail goes slightly uphill and left. You can see the Discovery Center straight ahead, past a small lily pond. Curve left, keeping the pond on your right. You are headed back to the boardwalk and the Big Slough. At the boardwalk, head to the right and retrace your route to the trailhead.

NEARBY ACTIVITIES

Lake Jackson Wilderness Park, the Gulf Coast Bird Observatory, and San Bernard National Wildlife Refuge are less than 15 miles from Brazoria National Wildlife Refuge. Brazos Bend State Park and the George Ranch are also close by.

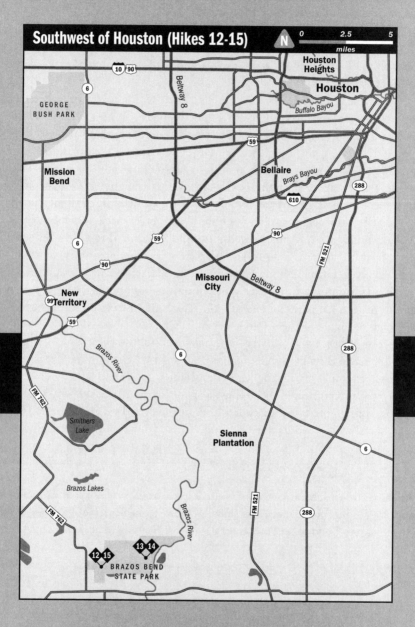

Southwest of Houston (Hikes 12-15)

N

0   2.5   5
miles

Houston
Heights

Houston

Buffalo Bayou

GEORGE
BUSH PARK

Beltway 8

Mission
Bend

Bellaire

Brays Bayou

Missouri
City

Beltway 8

New
Territory

Brazos River

Smithers
Lake

Brazos Lakes

Sienna
Plantation

Brazos River

BRAZOS BEND
STATE PARK

SOUTHWEST OF HOUSTON

12

BRAZOS BEND STATE PARK:
40-Acre Lake Loop Trail/Elm Lake Loop Trail

KEY AT-A-GLANCE INFORMATION

LENGTH: 5.2 miles

CONFIGURATION: Loops

DIFFICULTY: Easy

SCENERY: Prairie, marshes, lakes, woodlands, alligators

EXPOSURE: Sunny with some shady stretches

TRAIL TRAFFIC: Light weekdays, moderate weekends

TRAIL SURFACE: Crushed granite and dirt

HIKING TIME: 2.5 hours

DRIVING DISTANCE: 25.14 miles from the intersection of Beltway 8 and I-59

ACCESS: $4 per person, age 13 and older; open 8 a.m.–10 p.m. in summer and 8 a.m.–5 p.m. in winter

MAPS: USGS Thompsons, Damon, and Otey; trail signs and trail map

WHEELCHAIR ACCESS: No

FACILITIES: Restrooms, parking, water fountains, dog fountains, benches, camping, picnic areas, playgrounds

SPECIAL COMMENTS: The trail, which is wide enough to accommodate both hikers and bikers comfortably, is one of the better trails for viewing water birds.

GPS TRAILHEAD COORDINATES

LATITUDE: N 29° 22.239'
LONGITUDE: W 95° 37.633'

IN BRIEF

Brazos Bend State Park has more than 22 miles of hiking trails within its roughly 5,000 acres. It is one of the best camping and day-use parks in the area and is less than an hour from Houston. The 40-Acre Lake Loop Trail and the Elm Lake Loop Trail are located in the southwest section of the park, with the majority of the park stretching to the east and north. The trails are on elevated crushed-granite walkways, which get you as close to the wildlife as possible while still being at a safe distance. If you are interested in birds, more than 290 species have been sighted here. A nature center near the center of the park houses exhibits that pertain to the major ecosystems (marshes and woodlands) in the park. The center is free and open on weekends and most holidays 9 a.m.–5 p.m.

Safety note: The most prominent feature of Brazos Bend State Park is the alligators, which can be as close as five feet with no fence or barrier separating you from them. Be very aware of your surroundings and do not let small children run ahead. Most of these alligators are acclimated to people, but it is best to err on the side of caution. Pets on leash are allowed, but do not let them drink from the lake or enter the water under any circumstances. There are water stations located on the trails for both people and dogs.

Directions ⟶

From Beltway 8 and I-59, headwest 10.75 miles on I-59 and exit at Crabb River Road. Turn left and drive 8.69 miles to Tadpole Road and turn left. Drive 5.7 miles to the park entrance, which is left. The parking lot is just inside the park entrance, on the left, at 40-Acre Lake.

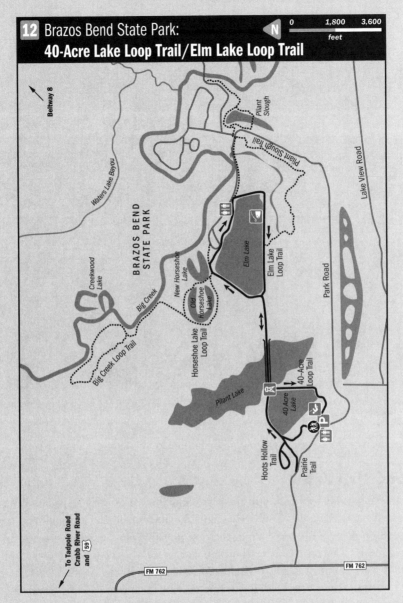

Beltway 8

Pilant Slough

Pilant Slough Trail

Lake View Road

Waters Lake Bayou

BRAZOS BEND STATE PARK

Elm Lake

Elm Lake Loop Trail

Park Road

Creekwood Lake

New Horseshoe Lake

Old Horseshoe Lake

Big Creek

Horseshoe Lake Loop Trail

Big Creek Loop Trail

Pilant Lake

40-Acre Loop Trail

40 Acre Lake

Hoots Hollow Trail

Prairie Trail

To Tadpole Road
Crabb River Road
and 59

FM 762   FM 762

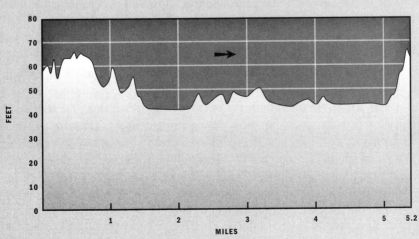

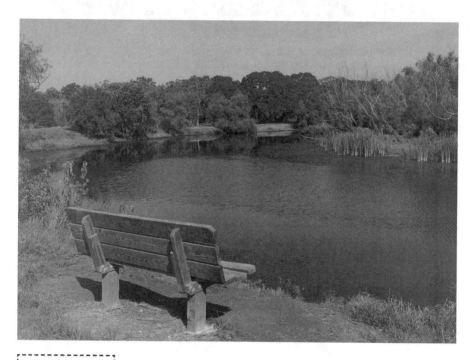

A view of Elm Lake

DESCRIPTION

From the parking lot, walk past the restrooms toward 40-Acre Lake and the trail-head. At the Observation Tower sign, go left. The trail surface is dirt and sand with towering oak trees on each side of the trail. Spanish moss hangs from most of the trees, creating an eerie look to the trail. At the fork beside a bench, bear right. A prairie with tall grass is left, with deep woods on the right. At the next fork, bear left to get on the Prairie Trail, a 0.3-mile out-and-back trail. (This is one of the few prairies left in the area—a worthwhile side trip.) The trail surface is grassy, with truck tracks indicating this is an access road to other parts of the park.

Continue along the trail until you reach the park road. From the road, the park headquarters are straight ahead. Turn around and head back up the Prairie Trail to get on the Hoots Hollow Trail. At the trailhead, take the left fork to get on the Hoots Hollow Trail, a 0.9-mile loop. A bench is located at the trailhead with thick undergrowth on both sides of the trail. Continue along the trail until you reach a tree with a small arrow pointing straight ahead. Take the left fork to get on the loop and start heading uphill on a dirt-and-grass trail surface. The trail is a bit rough on this loop but is easy to follow. Continue past a bench and around a tree on the left. Cross a wood bridge and then go slightly uphill. Be aware of banana spiders, a large nonpoisonous black and yellow spider, from spring to late fall on some parts of the trail.

Head past a very large oak tree and continue down the grass-covered trail. Where the trail surface changes to dirt, there is a bench on the left and then the end of the Hoots Hollow Loop. Continue past the arrow you saw earlier and go right to head back up the trail toward the 40-Acre Lake Loop Trail. Take the left fork at the trailhead for the 40-Acre Lake Loop Trail. A sign about the alligators is on the left warning you not to feed or approach them. You *will* see alligators from this trail: you do not need to go off the trail to look for them.

Continue past a bench on your left and 40-Acre Lake on your right. The trail surface is now an elevated crushed-granite walkway accessible to both walkers and cyclists. Walk in the center of the trail if possible, staying away from the edges, where alligators are known to sun themselves. A lake is on the right and a marsh is on the left. Continue along the trail until you get to an observation tower. 40-Acre Lake and Elm Lake are the best places in the park to view alligators—the observation tower is an excellent place to view them from a safe distance. At the tower, head straight ahead to get to the Elm Lake Loop Trail. Continue along the trail and over the Pilant Lake spillway. Pilant Lake is a freshwater marsh shared by both the park and private landowners. On the other side of the spillway, the trail is more open, with benches scattered along the trail to view the alligators and birds. As part of the Great Texas Coastal Birding Trail, Brazos Bend State Park is home to migratory waterfowl, a variety of shorebirds, wading birds, songbirds, and raptors.

The trail turns into a tree-canopied walkway, with oaks lining both sides and reaching out to completely shade the trail. Continue on the trail to a bench and an alligator-information sign warning you not to approach a pile of rotting grass, which may be an alligator nest. While hiking, I encountered a nine-to-ten foot alligator just off the trail, impeding my progress briefly. Continue past the sign and go left to get on the Elm Lake Loop Trail. There is a water station for people and dogs, as well as benches and informational signs. As you head left, Elm Lake is on your right and a marsh is on your left. The trail is very sunny and has the same surface as the 40-Acre Lake Loop Trail. Continue past the Horseshoe Lake Loop Trail trailhead. New Horseshoe Lake is on your left. Fork right into a big grassy field and head through one of the park's picnic and camping areas. Elm Lake is now 40–50 feet away on your right. Cross over a bridge and continue to a concrete walkway heading left to restrooms.

Wheelchair-accessible camping sites, a recent addition to Brazos Bend State Park, are connected to the parking lot by concrete paths. Continue until you come to an Elm Lake Loop Trail trailhead sign and a bench, then go right. Where the trail bends right, you'll see a series of fishing piers jutting out from the trail. Although the fishing here is good, be aware that the alligators are also in these waters and like to come after your line. Do not under any circumstances enter the water and do not use a stringer. Perch, crappie, sunfish, black bass, bowfin, gar, and catfish are all found in both 40-Acre Lake and Elm Lake.

Continue past several more fishing piers, the trailhead for the Pilant Slough Trail, two outhouses, and various benches until you get back to the intersection to the 40-Acre Lake Loop Trail. While hiking, look up into the trees on the right side of the trail and you may see dozens of banana spiders seemingly suspended in the air above your head. Once at the trailhead, go left along the 0.6-mile trail to the 40-Acre Lake Loop Trail. Back at the observation tower, take the left fork. 40-Acre Lake is now on your right, with a marsh on your left. Cross a small bridge and continue past several benches until you get to a 40-Acre Lake Loop Trail sign. Take the right fork and get on a dirt trail, leaving the lake behind. Cross a bridge, go past a large fallen tree, and wander along a shady and more typically woodland trail. When you come to the parking lot, head right past a playground and around the back of the restrooms. Continue past a large fishing pier to your right, and the restrooms and parking lot on your left, to your car.

NEARBY ACTIVITIES

The George Observatory, operated by the Houston Museum of Natural Science, is located in the park and is open on Saturdays 3–10 p.m. George Ranch, a working ranch since 1824, is only 12 miles from Brazos Bend State Park. Open 9 a.m.–5 p.m. every day, it is located at 10215 FM 762. For more information, go to **georgeranch.org**. Brazos River Trail, a 125-mile trail through Fort Bend and Brazoria counties, is part of the Sam Houston Trail & Wilderness Preserve. Hiking, biking, paddling, and horseback riding trails abound along this trail that heads through 18 different parks and refuges, including Brazos Bend State Park.

BRAZOS BEND STATE PARK:
Hale Lake Loop Trail

13

IN BRIEF

Brazos Bend State Park has more than 22 miles of hiking trails within its roughly 5,000 acres. It is one of the best camping and day-use parks in the area and is less than an hour from Houston. Hale Lake Loop Trail is one of the more popular hikes in the park. It borders a large picnic area and is relatively short, making it a good hike for smaller children. A nature center, located near the center of the park, houses exhibits that pertain to the major ecosystems (marshes and woodlands) in the park. The center is free and open on weekends and most holidays 9 a.m.–5 p.m.

Safety note: The most prominent feature of Brazos Bend State Park is the alligators, which can be as close as five feet with no fence or barrier separating you from them. Because of this, be very aware of your surroundings and do not let small children run ahead. Most of these alligators are acclimated to people, but it is best to err on the side of caution. Pets on leash are allowed, but do not let them drink from the lake or enter the water under any circumstances. There are water stations located on the trails for both people and dogs.

KEY AT-A-GLANCE INFORMATION

LENGTH: 2.2 miles

CONFIGURATION: Loop

DIFFICULTY: Easy

SCENERY: Wetlands, marshes, Big Creek, picnic area

EXPOSURE: Sunny

TRAIL TRAFFIC: Light weekdays, moderate weekends

TRAIL SURFACE: Dirt

HIKING TIME: 1.5 hours

DRIVING DISTANCE: 25.14 miles from the intersection of Beltway 8 and I-59

ACCESS: $4 per person, age 13 and older; open 8 a.m.–10 p.m. in summer and 8 a.m.–5 p.m. in winter

MAPS: USGS Thompsons and Otey; trail signs and trail map

WHEELCHAIR ACCESS: None

FACILITIES: Restrooms, parking, water fountains, benches, camping, picnic areas, playgrounds, fishing piers

SPECIAL COMMENTS: The trail is wide enough to accommodate both hikers and bikers comfortably.

Directions

From Beltway 8 and I-59, head west 10.75 miles on I-59 and exit at Crabb River Road. Turn left, go 8.69 miles to Tadpole Road, and turn left. Go 5.7 miles to the entrance of the park on the left. The parking lot is at the back of the park. Get a map from headquarters and head to the parking lot at the Group Camp Area and Fishing Pier for Hale Lake.

GPS TRAILHEAD COORDINATES

LATITUDE: N 29° 22.706'
LONGITUDE: W 95° 35.044'

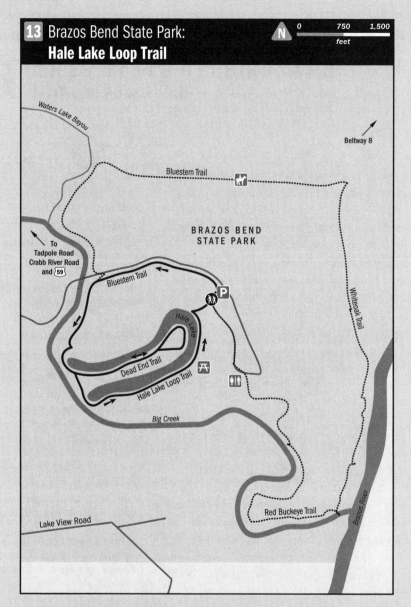

N

0   750   1,500
feet

Waters Lake Bayou

Beltway 8

Bluestem Trail

BRAZOS BEND
STATE PARK

To
Tadpole Road
Crabb River Road
and 59

Bluestem Trail

Whiteoak Trail

P

Hale Lake

Dead End Trail

Hale Lake Loop Trail

Big Creek

Red Buckeye Trail

Brazos River

Lake View Road

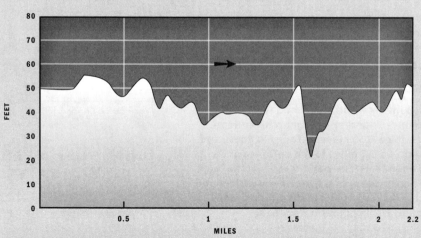

FEET	
80	
70	
60	→
50	
40	
30	
20	
10	
0	

0.5   1   1.5   2   2.2

MILES

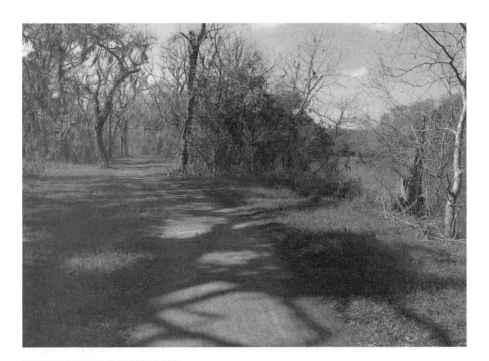

View of Big Creek from the trail

DESCRIPTION

From the Hale Lake parking lot, head to your right toward a trail opening in the trees. This trail is part of the Bluestem Trail that runs parallel to the park road. The vegetation on both sides of the trail is thick, but you can easily see the road on your right. The dirt trail, which winds through the woods for 0.5 miles, ends at the park road and a bridge over Big Creek. At the bridge, go left at the trailhead sign to get on the Hale Lake Loop Trail. The trail heads downhill and past a bench on the right. Big Creek is flowing on your right, just past the bench and down a steep incline. Pass by a sign alerting you to the presence of alligators and warning you to keep a safe distance. The vegetation on the right is thick and very close to the trail; however, there is a 15-to-20 yard open area between the trail and the thick vegetation on the left.

You can easily see Big Creek on your right past the trees. As the trail curves right, the vegetation on the left becomes closer but the right side opens up. Go straight at the Hale Lake Loop Trail sign, past a bench on the right. The trail now curves slightly left. At a fork, head right and downhill. Hale Lake is on your left, with Big Creek still on your right. Continue past a steep drop-off on the right. The trail heads uphill and left, toward a sign for the Hale Lake Point Dead End. Take the left fork toward the dead end. The lake is still on your left and there is thick vegetation on your right. Big Creek is behind you. The trail winds through the trees with considerable Spanish moss growing in many of the oaks.

Be aware of banana spiders from spring to late fall on some parts of the trail. You may also see bobcats, coyotes, raccoons, gray and red foxes, river otters, feral hogs, white-tailed deer, and rodents. There are about 21 species of reptiles and amphibians here, including American alligators, snakes (some poisonous), turtles, lizards, and frogs. Brazos Bend State Park is home to 290 species of birds such as migratory waterfowl, shorebirds, wading birds, songbirds, and raptors.

Continue past a bench on the right, with better views of the lake on the left. The trail bends left following the contour of the lake. Go straight through the next intersection, with a trail on the right. You can see the dead end ahead, where a gazebo, picnic table, and several benches await. The dead-end peninsula juts into Hale Lake, providing fine views of various parts of the lake. Look across the lake for a fishing pier and part of the Hale Lake Loop Trail. Turn around and retrace your route on the Dead End Trail. At the intersection of the Dead End Trail and the Hale Lake Loop, bear left. The trail heads uphill and then curves right.

The vegetation is very thick where the trail goes back downhill and then left. Go by a bench on the left that overlooks Hale Lake, then head left and downhill. Big Creek is still on your right and Hale Lake is on your left. As you go downhill, you head away from the creek, which is now behind you. Although the lake is still on your left, the vegetation is thick enough to obscure good views of it. The trail veers right and uphill, taking you by a small prairie on your right. Go past an inlet into the lake on the left and follow the trail as it winds through the trees. Continue uphill; a clearing on the right slopes downhill, away from the trail. The trail curves right before leveling atop a hill. Go left, toward the lake, passing an alligator-caution sign on the left and a bench on the right.

A large picnic area and restrooms are to the right. The trail bends left around the lake and past a mowed picnic area. Look for the fishing pier, which you saw from the Dead End Trail, ahead. Go by another alligator-caution sign on the left and then look right for a large covered pavilion. Across the lake to your left is the gazebo at the end of the Dead End Trail. Continue to a trail sign for the Hale Lake Loop Trail and take the right fork to get on the concrete path that links the fishing pier to the parking lot. Once in the parking lot and at the end of the concrete path, head left toward your car and the end of the hike.

NEARBY ACTIVITIES

George Observatory, operated by the Houston Museum of Natural Science, is located in the park and open on Saturdays, 3–10 p.m. George Ranch is only 12 miles from Brazos Bend State Park on Crabb River Road. In use since 1824, the ranch is now open to the public as a living-history museum. It's open daily, 9 a.m.–5 p.m. and located at 10215 FM 762. For more information, go to **george ranch.org**. Brazos River Trail, a 125-mile trail through Fort Bend and Brazoria counties, is part of the Sam Houston Trail & Wilderness Preserve. Hiking, biking, paddling, and horseback riding trails abound along this trail that heads through 18 different parks and refuges, including Brazos Bend State Park.

BRAZOS BEND STATE PARK: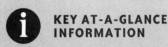
Red, White, and Blue Trail

IN BRIEF

Brazos Bend State Park has more than 22 miles of hiking trails within its roughly 5,000 acres. It is one of the best camping and day-use parks in the area and is less than an hour from Houston. The Red, White, and Blue Trail is a combined hike along the Red Buckeye Trail, the Whiteoak Trail, and the Bluestem Trail. This hike runs along the banks of the Brazos River and then beside the wetlands in the east end of the park. If you are interested in birds, more than 290 species have been sighted here. A nature center, located near the center of the park, houses exhibits that pertain to the major ecosystems (marshes and woodlands) in the park. The center is free and open on weekends and most holidays 9 a.m.–5 p.m.

Safety note: The most prominent feature of Brazos Bend State Park is the alligators, which can be as close as five feet with no fence or barrier separating you from them. Because of this, be very aware of your surroundings and do not let small children run ahead. Most of these alligators are acclimated to people, but it is best to err on the side of caution. Pets on leash are allowed, but do not let them drink from the lake or enter the water under any circumstances. There are water stations located on the trails for both people and dogs.

Directions ➔

From Beltway 8 and I-59, head west 10.75 miles on I-59 and exit at Crabb River Road. Turn left, go 8.69 miles to Tadpole Road, and turn left. Go 5.7 miles to the entrance of the park on the left. The parking lot is at the back of the park. Get a map from headquarters and head to the parking lot at the Whiteoak trailhead.

KEY AT-A-GLANCE INFORMATION

LENGTH: 4.3 miles

CONFIGURATION: Loop

DIFFICULTY: Easy

SCENERY: Wetlands, marshes, Big Creek, Brazos River, woodlands

EXPOSURE: Red Buckeye Trail is shady, Whiteoak and Bluestem trails are sunny

TRAIL TRAFFIC: Light weekdays, moderate weekends

TRAIL SURFACE: Dirt

HIKING TIME: 2.5 hours

DRIVING DISTANCE: 25.14 miles from the intersection of Beltway 8 and I-59

ACCESS: $4 per person, age 13 and older; open 8 a.m.–10 p.m. summer and 8 a.m.–5 p.m. winter

MAPS: USGS Thompsons and Otey; trail signs and trail map

WHEELCHAIR ACCESS: No

FACILITIES: Restrooms, parking, water fountains, dog fountains, benches, camping, picnic areas, playgrounds

SPECIAL COMMENTS: The trail is wide enough to accommodate both hikers and bikers comfortably. After recent rain, parts of this hike may be muddy, so watch your footing and wear appropriate hiking boots.

GPS TRAILHEAD COORDINATES

LATITUDE: N 29° 22.706'
LONGITUDE: W 95° 35.044'

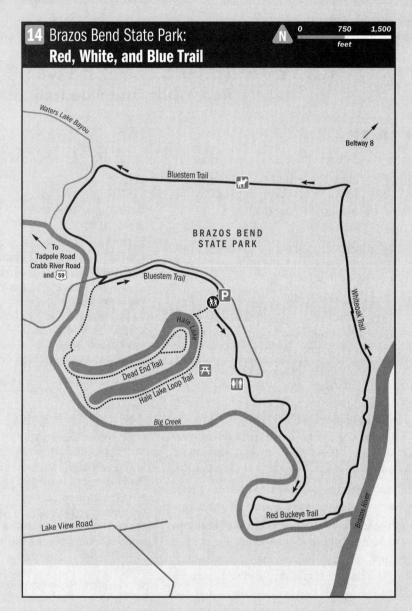

N

0   750   1,500
feet

Beltway 8

Waters Lake Bayou

Bluestem Trail

BRAZOS BEND
STATE PARK

To
Tadpole Road
Crabb River Road
and 59

Bluestem Trail

P

Whiteoak Trail

Hale Lake

Dead End Trail

Hale Lake Loop Trail

Big Creek

Red Buckeye Trail

Brazos River

Lake View Road

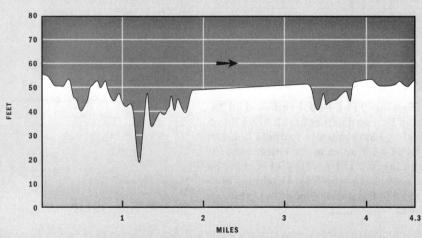

FEET

80
70
60
50
40
30
20
10
0

1   2   3   4   4.3

MILES

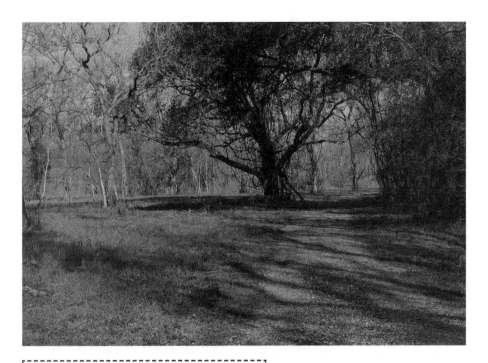

A view of the riparian landscape of the Brazos River

DESCRIPTION

From the parking lot, head left, away from the restrooms and toward the White-oak Trail trailhead sign on the right side of the park road. At the sign, go right to get on a dirt-and-gravel trail. The trail curves left, away from picnic tables on your right. As the trail continues curving left, you pass a pipeline easement on the left and woodlands on your right. Go by a bench on the right and a sign for the Red Buckeye Trail and Big Creek. At a fork, bear right to get on the Red Buckeye Trail. The trail narrows to only about 4–5 feet wide and becomes more primitive than the Whiteoak Trail. Be aware of banana spiders from spring to late fall on some parts of the trail. Most of them are high in the trees, allowing you to duck under their webs. Some are not as high, so be on the lookout. Other wildlife you may see includes bobcats, coyotes, raccoons, gray and red foxes, river otters, feral hogs, white-tailed deer, and rodents. There are about 21 species of reptiles and amphibians, including American alligators, snakes (some poisonous), turtles, lizards, and frogs. Brazos Bend State Park is home to 290 species of birds such as migratory waterfowl, shorebirds, wading birds, songbirds, and raptors.

The trail winds through trees and thick vegetation. There are exposed roots here, so watch your footing. Cross a small bridge and soon look right for the banks of Big Creek through the trees. This hike follows Big Creek to where it meets up with the Brazos River. Go through an intersection where a trail joins from the right. Past the intersection the trail winds uphill, then downhill, toward the creek. At a fork, bear right to stay on the Red Buckeye Trail, headed toward Big Creek. You can still see Big Creek on your right and now a wetlands on your left. Go through the next intersection, following the sign to Big Creek.

Soon the trail takes a big rightward bend and widens. A sign on the right warns you to keep your distance from the creek, because its loose, sandy banks could cause you to fall in. Where the trail widens even more, Big Creek is directly on your right. Notice the hanging vines, Spanish moss, and lichen growing in the trees along the creek. Go past a bench on the right and follow the trail as it bends to the right and past a trail marker on the right.

At a fork, bear right, toward Big Creek. The trail heads uphill through the trees as you travel on the left bank of the creek. The trail roller-coasters along, passing through a stand of tall grasses. After the trail heads downhill again, there is a high embankment on the left side of the trail. You are in a low reedy area beside the creek. Head uphill and across a small culvert. At the next fork, again bear right, soon enjoying views of the Brazos River, ahead and right. Head toward a bench on the right that overlooks the Brazos River. This is where Big Creek meets up with the Brazos River. To your right is a sign about the Bottomlands of the Brazos, indicating that this is the lowest point in the park—only a few inches lower than the picnic area at Hale Lake. Turn around and retrace your route to the previous intersection; here turn right to get back on the trail.

The trail winds uphill and out of the lower area. The Brazos River is now on your right with a high embankment on your left. Follow the trail as it takes another big bend left and uphill, away from the river. As it heads back downhill and toward the river, the trail widens. Pass a trail marker on the left and then curve right. At the next fork, bear right, heeding a DO NOT ENTER WATER sign. To visit a bench overlooking the river, turn right at the next intersection. Otherwise go straight, passing another trail marker on the right. After a long straight stretch, the trail winds into the trees. Go by a bench on the right and a number of trail markers. At a fork, bear right on the Whiteoak Trail. There is a bench at right and a large open field at left. The river is now farther away on your right.

After another long straight stretch, look left, beyond the open field, for a swamp, or wetland, in the trees. Go by another bench on the right and a sign for the Whiteoak Trail. Past the open field on the left, the trees are closer to the trail. Cross a small bridge and hike past a trail marker on the right, just before the trail bends right. At a T-intersection, turn left on the Bluestem Trail. This part of the trail has the appearance of a road that runs straight for 0.6 miles. After that, the trail bends left at a sign for the Bayou Trail on the right. There is a gate and sign indicating that the Bayou Trail is closed. Go past a bench on the right, then look right and through the trees to see the banks of Cottonwood Bayou. The vegetation is thick on both sides of the trail here until you exit the woods at the park road. Just before you get to a bridge, head right, toward the trailhead signs across the street. At the trailhead signs, go left to get back on the Bluestem Trail, which now runs parallel to the park road. This narrow dirt trail, less than 40 feet from the park road, runs past some picnic areas on the right. Although the trail ends at a parking lot, you must continue through this and several other small parking lots to return to your car. Go past a sign on the right for a youth group camp and a sign for a fishing pier. Continue along the park road toward the restrooms, your car, and the end of the hike.

NEARBY ACTIVITIES

George Observatory, operated by the Houston Museum of Natural Science, is located in the park and is open on Saturdays, 3–10 p.m. George Ranch is only 12 miles from Brazos Bend State Park. In use since 1824, the ranch is now open to the public as a living-history museum. It's open daily, 9 a.m.–5 p.m. and located at 10215 FM 762. For more information, go to **georgeranch.org**. Brazos River Trail, a 125-mile trail through Fort Bend and Brazoria counties, is part of the Sam Houston Trail & Wilderness Preserve. Hiking, biking, paddling, and horseback riding trails abound along this trail that heads through 18 different parks and refuges, including Brazos Bend State Park.

15 BRAZOS BEND STATE PARK:
Big Creek Loop Trail

KEY AT-A-GLANCE INFORMATION

LENGTH: 3.8 miles

CONFIGURATION: Two loops

DIFFICULTY: Easy

SCENERY: Wetlands, lakes, Big Creek, woodlands, prairie

EXPOSURE: Sunny

TRAIL TRAFFIC: Light weekdays, moderate weekends

TRAIL SURFACE: Dirt and grass

HIKING TIME: 2 hours

DRIVING DISTANCE: 25.14 miles from the intersection of Beltway 8 and I-59

ACCESS: $4 per person, age 13 and older; open 8 a.m.–10 p.m. in summer and 8 a.m.–5 p.m. in winter.

MAPS: USGS Thompsons and Otey; trail signs and trail map

WHEELCHAIR ACCESS: None

FACILITIES: Restrooms, parking, water fountains, dog fountains, benches, camping, picnic areas, playgrounds, fishing piers

SPECIAL COMMENTS: The trail is wide enough to accommodate both hikers and bikers comfortably.

GPS TRAILHEAD COORDINATES

LATITUDE: N 29° 22.239'
LONGITUDE: W 95° 37.633'

IN BRIEF

Brazos Bend State Park has more than 22 miles of hiking trails within its roughly 5,000 acres. It is one of the best camping and day-use parks in the area and is less than an hour from Houston. Big Creek Loop Trail departs from the Horseshoe Lake Loop Trail and extends to the park boundary. Big Creek Loop Trail is not on the regular park map but is on a trail map available by request at park headquarters. Watch closely for alligators along the edge of New Horseshoe Lake and always be cautious of snakes, as many of them here are of the poisonous variety. If you are interested in birds, more than 290 species have been sighted here. A nature center, located near the center of the park, houses exhibits that pertain to the major ecosystems (marshes and woodlands) in the park. The center is free and open on weekends and most holidays 9 a.m.–5 p.m.

Safety note: The most prominent feature of Brazos Bend State Park is the alligators, which can be as close as five feet with no fence or barrier separating you from them. Because of this, be very aware of your surroundings and do not let small children run ahead. Most of these alligators are acclimated to people, but it is best to err on the side of caution. Pets on leash are allowed, but do not

----

Directions ⟶

From Beltway 8 and I-59, head west 10.75 miles on I-59 and exit at Crabb River Road. Turn left, go 8.69 miles to Tadpole Road, and turn left. Go 5.7 miles to the entrance of the park on the left. The parking lot is at the north end of the park, past the nature center and Elm Lake.

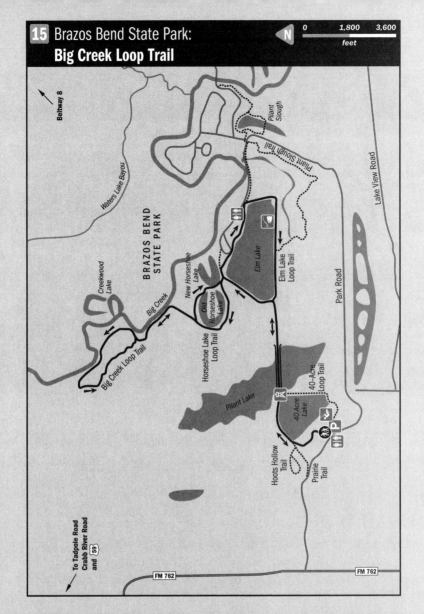

N

0   1,800   3,600
feet

Beltway 8

Pilant Slough

Pilant Slough Trail

Lake View Road

Waters Lake Bayou

BRAZOS BEND STATE PARK

Elm Lake

Elm Lake Loop Trail

Park Road

Creekwood Lake

Big Creek

New Horseshoe Lake

Old Horseshoe Lake

Horseshoe Lake Loop Trail

Big Creek Loop Trail

Pilant Lake

40-Acre Loop Trail

40-Acre Lake

P

Hoots Hollow Trail

Prairie Trail

To Tadpole Road
Crabb River Road
and 59

FM 762   FM 762

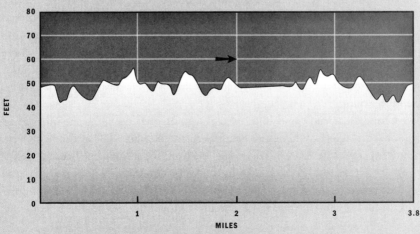

FEET

80
70
60
50
40
30
20
10
0

1   2   3   3.8

MILES

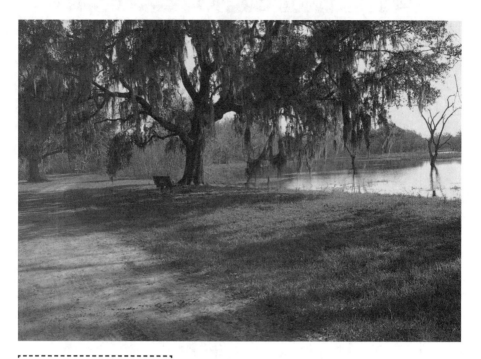

Elm Lake to the right of the trail

let them drink from the lake or enter the water under any circumstances. There are water stations located on the trails for both people and dogs.

DESCRIPTION

To find the Big Creek Loop Trail, park in the last parking lot heading toward New Horseshoe Lake. Once you've parked, head toward the Horseshoe Lake Loop Trail trailhead. Go left out of the parking lot toward a FISHING UP AHEAD sign and then go right to get on a concrete walkway. Continue past a trailhead sign on the right and get on a gravel trail, hiking past a bench on the left and a sign on the right describing the canebrake. The trail is wide, well defined, and heavily used in the spring and summer. New Horseshoe Lake is on your right and Old Horseshoe Lake is on your left. Continue past a bench on the left and curve left. Go by another bench, on the right, which overlooks New Horseshoe Lake. Go straight through an intersection, where a trail joins from the left, and pass a bench on the right.

At a fork, bear right and hike past a sign, on the right, for the Horseshoe Lake Loop Trail. Go by a bench on the right and then bear left at the next fork. While hiking past the water, be on the lookout for alligators sunning themselves on the banks at all times. Also be aware of banana spiders from spring to late fall on some parts of the trail. Most of them are high in the trees, allowing you to duck under their webs. Some are not as high, so be on the lookout.

Other wildlife you may see includes bobcats, coyotes, raccoons, gray and red foxes, river otters, feral hogs, white-tailed deer, and rodents. There are about 21 species of reptiles and amphibians here, including American alligators, snakes (some poisonous), turtles, lizards, and frogs. Brazos Bend State Park is home to 290 species of birds such as migratory waterfowl, shorebirds, wading birds, songbirds, and raptors.

The vegetation on the left side of the trail is thick; there is riparian vegetation on the right, along the shore of the lake. Follow the trail as it bends right and then passes a bench on the right. The area on the left opens up considerably, with the trail curving right again, past a bench on the right. As you move farther from the lake, the trailside vegetation closes in. The dirt trail follows the contour of the lake. The trail surface changes to a grass-and-dirt surface as you head away from the lake. Soon you pass a sign for the Big Creek Loop Trail on the left. At a fork, bear left to get on the Big Creek Loop Trail and head into the woods. The trail, hemmed in by foliage, is nevertheless easy to follow. The trail surface looks more like an old road that has grass growing on it. There is a clearing on the left and a very old oak tree whose limbs overarch the trail.

The trail takes a big leftward bend, giving you a fine view of Big Creek, which is now on your right. There is a steep slope beside Big Creek that can be slippery and conceal poisonous snakes, so stay on the trail at all times. The trail curves right, now atop the bank of Big Creek. Follow the trail as it winds toward a spillway for the creek. Cross the spillway and go past a bench on the right that overlooks Big Creek and then continue past a small pond on the left. At the next Big Creek Loop Trail sign, go straight, keeping the creek on your right. There is a large open field on your left. The trail heads uphill, bending left. Here the vegetation is denser and the trail surface is predominantly grass, but still easy to follow.

Continue as the trail bends left under a canopy of trees. The creek is on your right and there is a large clearing on the left. As the trail bends right, you go by trail markers hanging in the trees on the left. Near a state-park boundary sign on a fence ahead, the trail bends left and passes under some trees. At an upcoming fork, bear left; a barrier prevents your going straight. This part of the trail is very grassy and can be muddy or overgrown due to lack of use. The area on the right is low and can be under water, so stay on the trail.

Once out of the trees the trail wanders through a large clearing. From where it bends left, you can see the elevated trail you hiked on earlier before getting on this loop. Go left toward the Big Creek Loop Trail sign and then go right to get on the elevated trail. This is the same trail you took to get to the Big Creek Loop Trail. Now Big Creek is on your left, as you clamber up the creek bank. At the end of the Big Creek Loop Trail, take the left fork to get on the Horseshoe Lake Loop Trail. The trail heads downhill and left, with New Horseshoe Lake on your right. There is a low marsh on your left and then a short viewing platform on the right. Go past a bench and a wetlands, both left.

Hike on the now grassy trail past a bench on the left and then one on the right. Look left for a small lake through the trees. The trail heads uphill and left, with water on both sides. At the next intersection, go straight and slightly left toward Elm Lake, which is ahead. At the intersection beyond, go left and continue to the parking lot.

NEARBY ACTIVITIES

Brazos River Trail, a 125-mile trail through Fort Bend and Brazoria counties, is part of the Sam Houston Trail & Wilderness Preserve. Hiking, biking, paddling, and horseback riding trails abound along this trail that heads through 18 different parks and refuges, including Brazos Bend State Park.

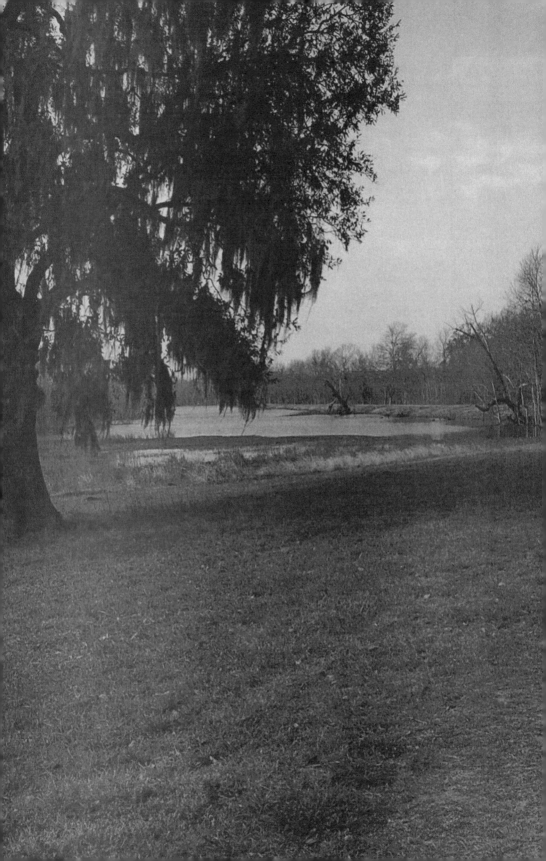

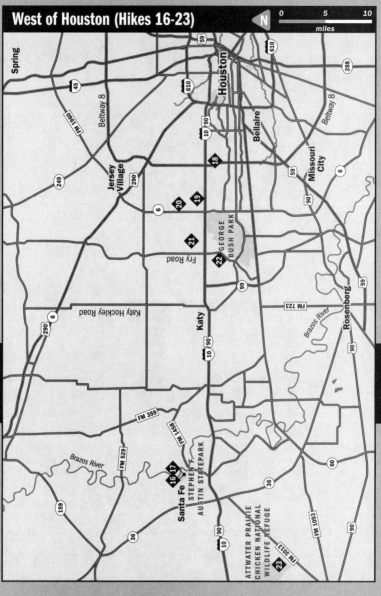

West of Houston (Hikes 16-23)

N

0   5   10

miles

Spring

Houston

Bellaire

Missouri City

Jersey Village

GEORGE BUSH PARK

Fry Road

Katy Hockley Road

Katy

Rosenberg

Brazos River

FM 723

FM 359

FM 1458

Brazos River

FM 529

Santa Fe

STEPHEN F. AUSTIN STATE PARK

ATTWATER PRAIRIE CHICKEN NATIONAL WILDLIFE REFUGE

FM 1093

FM 3013

WEST of HOUSTON

16 STEPHEN F. AUSTIN STATE PARK:
Main Loop

KEY AT-A-GLANCE INFORMATION

LENGTH: 3 miles

CONFIGURATION: Loop

DIFFICULTY: Moderate

SCENERY: Forest, campgrounds, creek beds, golf course

EXPOSURE: Partly shaded to very shaded

TRAIL TRAFFIC: Light weekdays, moderate weekends

TRAIL SURFACE: Dirt and some over-grown grassy areas

HIKING TIME: 1.5 hours

DRIVING DISTANCE: 36 miles from the intersection of Beltway 8 and I-10

ACCESS: Day use, $3 per person age 13 and older, or buy a yearly Texas State Parks Pass; open 8 a.m.– 10 p.m.

MAPS: USGS San Felipe; trail maps available at park headquarters

WHEELCHAIR ACCESS: None

FACILITIES: Restrooms, picnic tables, campsites, showers, state-park store, trail signs

SPECIAL COMMENTS: Dogs must be leashed at all times. Please be aware of poisonous snakes and a large population of deer.

GPS TRAILHEAD COORDINATES

LATITUDE: N 29° 48.850'
LONGITUDE: W 96° 6.503'

IN BRIEF

Stephen F. Austin State Park is bordered on the north and east by the Brazos River, which provides a natural habitat for many native plants and animals. While most of the park has been developed for camping, the undeveloped areas are great for hiking and fishing. During the week there is very little activity in the park, allowing for quiet, undisturbed hiking.

DESCRIPTION

Turn right out of the parking lot and walk back up the road for about 100 feet and locate the trailhead to your left. Cross the road to find the trailhead. At the trailhead, you can see the Stephen F. Austin Golf Course on your right and the park road on your left. About 20 feet along the trail is a fork. Bear right at the fork, down into a creek ravine.

At the bottom of the ravine is a metal bridge. Cross the bridge and start back up the other side of the creek. Be aware that if it is raining, even a small creek can turn into a flash flood fairly quickly. Once out of the ravine the trail becomes quite primitive and not as well defined as at its start. The trail continues in and out of several creek beds and through grassy, overgrown areas. The trail is very narrow and winding but still easy to follow. Watch out for large spider webs from

- -

Directions ─────────────────────→

From Beltway 8 and I-10, head west on I-10 for 33 miles. Exit and turn right onto FM 1458. Drive 2 miles to Park Road 38 and turn left. The park entrance is 1 mile ahead, at the end of the road. From the parkheadquarters, take Park Road 38 straight and park in the first lot on the left.

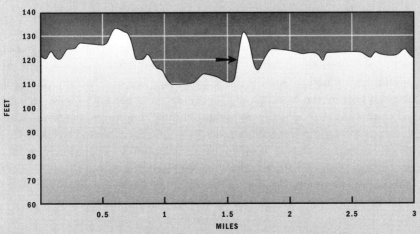
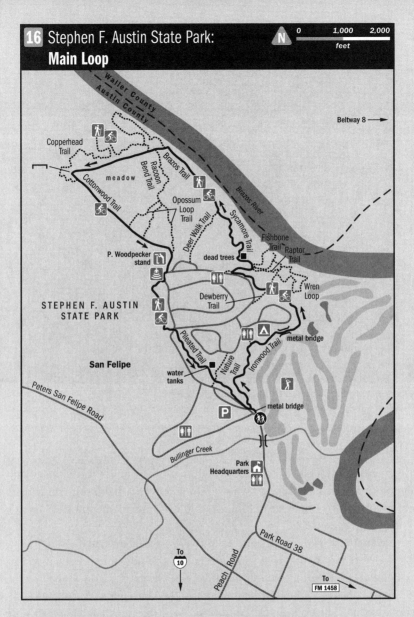

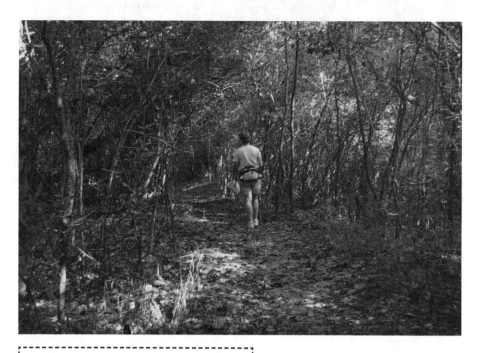

My hiking buddy, Pam Johnson, on the Main Loop

spring through early fall. Some of the spiders are banana spiders (also called yellow golden spiders), which can grow up to four inches in diameter and can seem quite menacing. However, they are not poisonous and pose no threat. The webs are generally about head high, so you can duck below most of them without disturbing the web.

Although the trail is still quite primitive, you can navigate by watching for the large concrete blocks that have been placed on it to help hikers maneuver through low-lying areas. Beyond the first set of blocks, the trail is grassy and weedy, and the canopy opens to allow sunlight. The trail becomes more defined as you cross a small bridge. The golf course is still visible on the right, and campsites are visible on the left. The main loop trail continues to alternate between primitive and more defined. Be careful of the poison ivy, oak, and sumac that grow prodigiously in this part of Texas. As you continue along the trail, the golf course fades out of sight while the campsites continue to be visible on your left. Cross another small creek, walking on concrete "stones" in the creek bed, and hike back up the other side. Once away from the creek, a water treatment plant becomes visible on your right. After crossing another creek and hiking through long grass, the trail opens. When you reach a fork in the trail, bear left to access the trailhead for the Sycamore Trail. You are now about a mile into the hike, on a dirt trail surface that becomes wider and more maintained the farther along you go.

Once on the Sycamore Trail, head downhill for about 40 yards to a ravine, then climb the other side. This part of the trail is shady and well maintained. At the next fork, bear left. The trail now is reminiscent of a path through an antebellum estate: straight, wide, shaded, and very pleasant. Even in August, this area is considerably cooler than other parts of the park. Soon the trail becomes more winding and the flora becomes more lush.

Now deep into the woods and in the undeveloped part of the park, go left at the next fork, where the trail surface changes to leaf-flecked dirt. Cross over several dead trees that have fallen over the trail. Regarding poison ivy vines, which may be present here, remember the Scout motto, "If it's hairy, it's scary." Although dead poison ivy vines might seem safe, they can still cause a rash if touched, so step under or over trees without touching the vines.

At the intersection, turn right on the Brazos Bend Trail, which is even wider and more pleasing than the Sycamore Trail. This trail is often used by Scout groups, so it could get a bit crowded on weekends during autumn and spring. Once on this trail, you leave the creek beds for good and head uphill to a flat part of the trail. At an intersection, continue straight to stay on the Brazos Trail. Look high for scissor-tailed flycatchers and pileated woodpeckers, and low for deer, raccoons, foxes, opossums, and squirrels.

Where the Brazos Trail ends, take a left onto the Cottonwood Trail. Surrounded by large oaks and pecan trees, listen for the very loud, quick, staccato drumming of the pileated woodpecker high above. This straight trail heads uphill to a bench, where you turn left at the next intersection. This is the only steep hill in the park and, if the trail is muddy and slippery, use the wooden steps provided on the left side of the trail. Past the bench, the trail becomes roadlike. There is even a trace of asphalt on some sections. Continue past the Possum Loop and Raccoon Bend trails, both left. At a fork, bear right. A pileated woodpecker stand is set up for viewing, with benches and a viewing wall containing cutouts at varying levels. Just past the stand is a small amphitheater on the right. The trail goes left of the amphitheater and joins the park road. Turn right on the road and go past campsites, left, to where a road joins on the left. Cross the park road on your left and regain the trail.

This part of the trail is well maintained, taking you over several newly constructed wooden bridges. Go through the Nature Trail intersection and continue down the trail. Cross one last bridge and bear right at the next fork to the parking lot and the end of the hike.

Note: The first mile of the trail is very primitive, so wear long pants. Be aware of numerous spider webs on the first mile of the trail: anywhere there are two trees flanking the path, look for webs and active spiders. If you wish for a more groomed trail, start this hike at the Sycamore trailhead.

NEARBY ACTIVITIES

Included in the Stephen F. Austin State Park system is the San Felipe State Historic Site. San Felipe is where Stephen F. Austin brought the first 297 families to colonize Texas in 1824. It was the capital of the American colonies in Texas and is called the "Cradle of Texas Liberty," as the conventions of 1832 and 1833 and the Consultation of 1835 were held here. These meetings led to the Texas Declaration of Independence. San Felipe is home to the first settler newspaper (the *Texas Gazette*), the home of the Texas postal system, and the original home of the Texas Rangers. Historical tours are given every Saturday and Sunday at 1 p.m. Also nearby is the Stephen F. Austin Golf Course, an 18-hole golf course, at the entrance to the park. The San Felipe Trail, a 21-mile trail running through post oak savannah and coastal prairie ecosystems is part of the Sam Houston Trail & Wilderness Preserve. Starting at the San Felipe de Austin State Historic Site, the trail heads north through Stephen F. Austin State Park, Katy Prairie Conservancy Preserve System, and the Cypress Creek Trail.

STEPHEN F. AUSTIN STATE PARK:
Sycamore to Cottonwood Trail

IN BRIEF

Stephen F. Austin State Park is bordered on the north and east by the Brazos River, which provides a natural habitat for many native plants and animals. While most of the park has been developed for camping, the undeveloped areas are great for hiking and fishing. During the week there is very little activity in the park, allowing for quiet, undisturbed hiking.

DESCRIPTION

From park headquarters, drive to the head of the Sycamore Trail using Park Road 38. There are restrooms and another small parking lot about 30 feet east of the trailhead. Turn right out of the parking lot and walk to the Sycamore Trail sign. Once on the trail, take a left at the first fork. Watch out for large spider webs on the trail from spring to early fall. Some of the spiders are banana spiders (also called yellow golden spiders), which can grow up to 4 inches in diameter and can seem quite menacing. However, they are not poisonous and pose no threat. The webs are generally about head high, so you can duck below most of them without disturbing the web.

The trail is easy to follow, with a thick bed of leaves guiding the way. Head downhill into a creek bed bordered by dense undergrowth and overhung by eastern cottonwoods,

KEY AT-A-GLANCE INFORMATION

LENGTH: 3 miles

CONFIGURATION: Loop

DIFFICULTY: Easy to moderate

SCENERY: Dense thickets, wetlands, the Brazos River, towering trees, bottomland forest, creek beds

EXPOSURE: Partly shaded to very shaded

TRAIL TRAFFIC: Light weekdays, moderate weekends

TRAIL SURFACE: Dirt and heavy leaf cover; overgrown grassy areas

HIKING TIME: 1.5 hours

DRIVING DISTANCE: 36 miles from the intersection of Beltway 8 and I-10

ACCESS: Day use, $3 per person age 13 and older, or buy a yearly Texas State Parks Pass; open 8 a.m.– 10 p.m.

MAPS: USGS San Felipe; trail maps available at park headquarters

WHEELCHAIR ACCESS: None

FACILITIES: Restrooms, picnic tables, campsites, showers, state-park store, trail signs

SPECIAL COMMENTS: Dogs must be leashed at all times. Please be aware of poisonous snakes and a large population of deer.

Directions ⟶

From Beltway 8 and I-10, head west on I-10 for 33 miles. Exit and turn right onto FM 1458. Drive 2 miles to Park Road 38 and turn left. The park entrance is 1 mile ahead, at the end of the road. From the park headquarters, take Park Road 38 straight and park in the first lot on the left.

GPS TRAILHEAD COORDINATES

LATITUDE: N 29° 48.850'
LONGITUDE: W 96° 6.503'

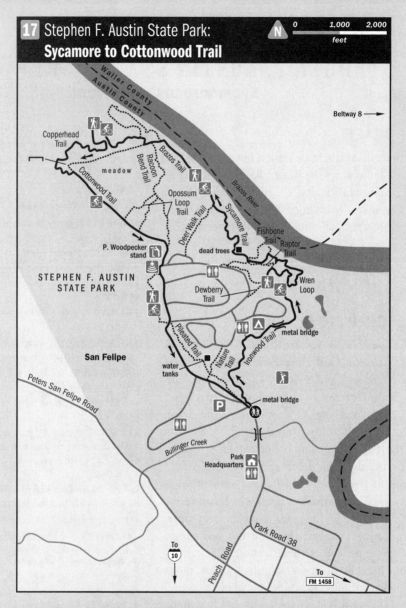

N

0   1,000   2,000
feet

Beltway 8 →

Waller County
Austin County

Brazos River

Copperhead
Trail

Brazos Trail

Racoon Bend Trail

meadow

Cottonwood Trail

Opossum
Loop
Trail

Deer Walk Trail

Sycamore Trail

Fishbone
Trail

Raptor
Trail

P. Woodpecker
stand

dead trees

Wren
Loop

STEPHEN F. AUSTIN
STATE PARK

Dewberry
Trail

metal bridge

San Felipe

Pileated Trail

Nature Trail

Ironwood Trail

water
tanks

P

metal bridge

Peters San Felipe Road

Bullinger Creek

Park
Headquarters

Park Road 38

To
10

Peach Road

To
FM 1458

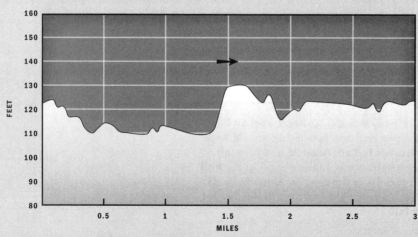

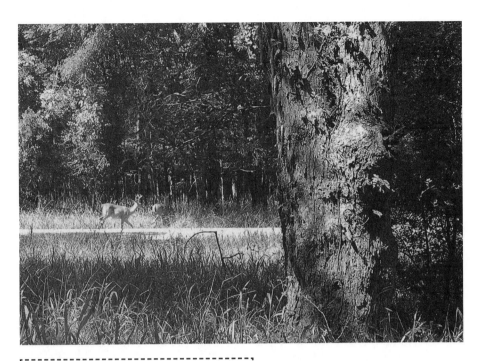

Deer along the trail in Stephen F. Austin State Park

sycamores, and box elder maples. Take the right fork into the creek bed and cross a small metal bridge. Be aware of the weather, as these small creeks can flood quickly during downbursts.

The trail is well defined, with considerable leaf clutter on its surface. Take the next fork right and then a quick left. A brief detour, right, provides a view of the Brazos River. Soon the undergrowth becomes denser and the trail becomes more primitive. The river is on your right but not visible.

At an intersection, turn left, away from the river. (Going right here leads to river-access points for anglers.) Where the trail becomes slightly overgrown, go left and keep a deep creek on your right. Stay away from the creek, because its sandy sides may collapse beneath your weight. Continue straight through an intersection where a trail joins on the left. The trail narrows and becomes less defined but is still easy to follow. Cross another small metal bridge, head downhill into a creek bed, and then hike up the other side. The terrain here changes to tall grasses and towering trees, with fewer vines and other underbrush. Grasses in this area include pinehill bluestem, purpletop, wild rye, and brownseed paspalum.

Beyond the grassy area, the trail winds through dense foliage. Go left at the next fork and cross a fallen tree trunk. In reference to poison ivy vines, which may be present here, remember the Scout motto, "If it's hairy, it's scary." Although dead poison ivy vines might seem safe, they can still cause a rash if touched, so step under or over trees without touching the vines. Continue down the trail as it opens more and becomes less primitive.

When you come to another Sycamore Trail sign, head right, toward a Brazos Bend Trail sign. At the Brazos Bend Trail, turn left. This trail is often used by Scout groups, so it could get a bit crowded on weekends during autumn and spring. Once on this trail, you leave the creek beds and head uphill to a flat part of the trail. At an intersection, turn right for a short detour to the Brazos River. The trail goes slightly uphill and affords a good view of, as well as access to, the river. Parts of this short detour (about 70 yards) can be overgrown with tall weeds, but it's well worth it. After enjoying the river view, turn back and retrace to the Brazos Bend Trail. Head right onto the Brazos Bend Trail.

At a fork where the trail opens, bear left. Around noon, this part of the trail may be sunny. At the next Brazos Bend Trail sign and the intersection, go left. Pass the sign to the Raccoon Bend Trail on your left. Shortly after the Raccoon Bend Trail sign, look for a yellow streamer in the trees on the right side of the trail. At the streamer, go right onto a new section of trail. (This small loop may not be on state park maps. Ask the rangers at headquarters and they will draw the loop on the park map.) Take the next fork left and continue along the primitive and, in places, overgrown trail. Look for the streamers in trees and on small stakes on the forest floor. At the intersection, take the trail to the left and follow it into a more open area with tall grasses. At times the trail can be challenging to follow, but just look for the trail markers.

Continue until you reach a fence that marks the park's boundary. Turn left, away from the fence. The trail, while not well defined here, is navigable by walking straight and watching for trail markers. Go right at each of the next two forks. A large tree may block the trail here, but continue around the tree and you will see the trail on its other side. Once past the tree, head uphill and then left, entering an area that the park uses to dispose of its fallen trees. Walk through this area heading left, then turn right on the Cottonwood Trail.

The Cottonwood Trail now becomes roadlike. There is even a trace of asphalt on some sections of it. Continue on the trail past the Possum Loop and Raccoon Bend trails, both left. Take the next fork to the right. A pileated woodpecker stand is set up for viewing, with benches and a viewing wall containing cutouts at varying levels. Just past the stand is a small amphitheater on the right. Before you get to the amphitheater, turn left onto the park road to walk back to the parking lot and the Sycamore Trail trailhead. Continue down the road past the Group Camp road and you should see your car, less than 100 yards away.

Note: The first mile of the trail is very primitive, so wear long pants. Be aware of numerous spider webs on the first mile of the trail: anywhere there are two trees flanking the path, look for webs and active spiders.

NEARBY ACTIVITIES

Included in the Stephen F. Austin State Park system is the San Felipe State Historic Site. San Felipe is where Stephen F. Austin brought the first 297 families to
colonize Texas in 1824. It was the capital of the American colonies in Texas and
is called the "Cradle of Texas Liberty," as the conventions of 1832 and 1833 and
the Consultation of 1835 were held here. These meetings led to the Texas Declaration of Independence. San Felipe is home to the first settler newspaper (the
Texas Gazette), the home of the Texas postal system, and the original home of the
Texas Rangers. Historical tours are given every Saturday and Sunday at 1 p.m.
Also nearby is the Stephen F. Austin Golf Course, an 18-hole golf course, at the
entrance to the park. The San Felipe Trail, a 21-mile trail running through post
oak savannah and coastal prairie ecosystems is part of the Sam Houston Trail &
Wilderness Preserve. Starting at the San Felipe de Austin State Historic Site, the
trail heads north through Stephen F. Austin State Park, Katy Prairie Conservancy
Preserve System, and the Cypress Creek Trail.

18 TERRY HERSHEY PARK:
Quail Trail

 **KEY AT-A-GLANCE
INFORMATION**

LENGTH: 10.2 miles

CONFIGURATION: Out-and-back

DIFFICULTY: Moderate

**SCENERY: Bayou, open fields, urban
scenery, maple trees**

**EXPOSURE: Sunny with some shady
areas**

**TRAIL TRAFFIC: Moderate with bik-
ers weekdays, heavy weekends**

TRAIL SURFACE: Asphalt

HIKING TIME: 4 hours

**DRIVING DISTANCE: At the intersec-
tion of Beltway 8 and Boheme Drive
(this is where you park)**

ACCESS: Free; open dawn to dusk

**MAPS: USGS Hedwig Village; trail
signs**

WHEELCHAIR ACCESS: Yes

**FACILITIES: Restrooms (at Eldridge
Pkwy. end of the trail), parking,
water fountains, dog fountains,
benches, exercise stations**

**SPECIAL COMMENTS: Although
an urban hike, this is a very nice,
serene trail to walk in the morning or late afternoon. Pets, which
must be leashed at all times, are
welcome; dog fountains are located
wherever you see human water
fountains.**

GPS TRAILHEAD
COORDINATES

LATITUDE: N 29° 45.792'
LONGITUDE: W 95° 33.490'

IN BRIEF

Terry Hershey Park encompasses approximately 12.5 miles of trails from TX 6 west to
Beltway 8 east. Quail Trail is currently the longest of the park's trails at 5.1 miles, making for
a 10.2-mile out-and-back hike (unless you can
arrange a pickup or car shuttle). Thus, length
and the unusually hilly terrain along Buffalo
Bayou earn this hike its moderate rating.

DESCRIPTION

Find the trail on the northwest side of the
parking lot. Turn left and follow an asphalt
trail to the trail map. Take a right at the map
to get on the Quail Trail. Hiking and biking
trails are the main attractions in Terry Hershey Park, but there are other fun features too,
including picnic sites, a playground, gazebos,
a lighted walking trail, and a walk-in sundial
near Memorial Drive and Eldridge Parkway.
At the sundial, if you stand on the appropriate
stone and the sun is shining, you cast a shadow
on the correct time.

As you hike along Buffalo Bayou, take
note of the riparian landscape that includes
plants such as yaupon holly, roughleaf dogwood, black willow, sunflowers, and sedges.
In spring look for passionflower, lantana,
Turk's cap, and *Bidens*. The Quail Trail runs
along Buffalo Bayou with the bayou entirely
on the left and detention areas on the right to
control flooding.

Directions ⟶

**From the intersection of Beltway 8 and I-10,
head south on the access road of Beltway 8 for
1.2 miles. At Boheme Drive, turn right into the
Terry Hershey Park parking lot. The lot is
located under Beltway 8.**

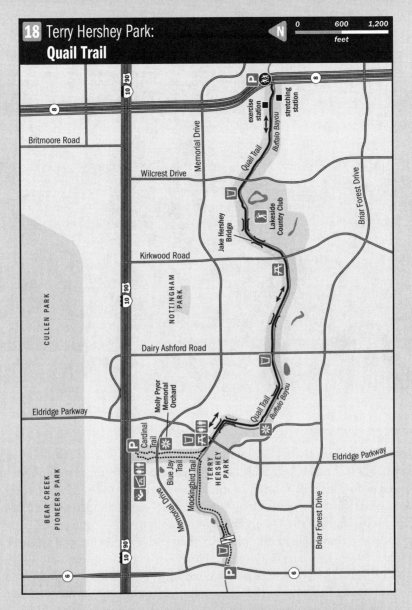

N

0   600   1,200
feet

Britmoore Road

Memorial Drive

Wilcrest Drive

Quail Trail

Buffalo Bayou

exercise station

stretching station

Lakeside Country Club

Jake Hershey Bridge

Kirkwood Road

NOTTINGHAM PARK

CULLEN PARK

Dairy Ashford Road

Molly Pryor Memorial Orchard

Eldridge Parkway

Cardinal Trail

Blue Jay Trail

Mockingbird Trail

Memorial Drive

TERRY HERSHEY PARK

Quail Trail

Buffalo Bayou

Eldridge Parkway

Briar Forest Drive

BEAR CREEK PIONEERS PARK

Briar Forest Drive

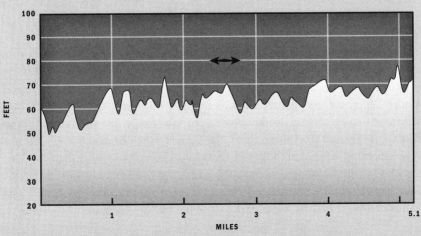

FEET

MILES

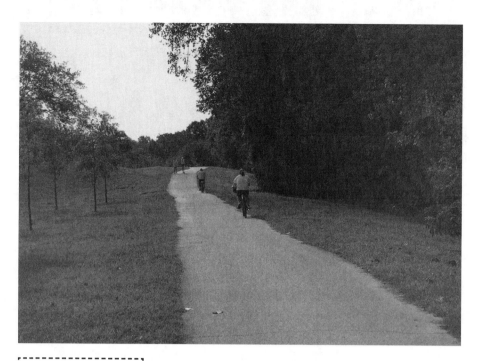

Cyclists on the Quail Trail

Continue past a stretching station, hiking past a fence on the left that was constructed to keep hikers and bikers from falling into the bayou. The sandy soil makes for unstable footing on the edges of the bayou, so stay on the trail. The trails along the bayous often contain more elevation change than is typical in Houston, and the Quail Trail is no exception. It is quite a workout for flatlanders accustomed to the pitch in their driveway being the steepest hill they encounter. This part of the trail, which is overgrown and shady, masks the sound of Beltway 8. Continue past a pond on the right until you reach one of the trail's many benches. Beyond the pond, the right side opens up with large greenways built to detain water. These greenways are mowed and maintained as open spaces, so it is permissible to walk on them. There are houses about 100 yards from the trail, on the right.

The trail becomes more open, with vegetation growing only along the bayou. Continue past some exercise stations to a very steep and curvy section: be wary of cyclists coming around blind spots here. Once through the curves, the trail takes you under Wilcrest Drive, where there is another trailhead. At a fork, bear left and continue to a bench and drinking fountains (one for people and one for dogs). Cross two bridges and stop at the third, the Jake Hershey Bridge.

Jake Hershey is the late husband of Terese "Terry" Hershey, the conservationist who led the campaign to stop the paving of the banks of Buffalo Bayou and was instrumental in convincing Harris County to set aside 500 acres along the banks of Buffalo Bayou for a park. The Hersheys are founders of the Bayou

Preservation Association, and Terry Hershey is a former member of the Texas Parks and Wildlife Commission.

A path down to the banks of Buffalo Bayou is located just past the Jake Hershey Bridge. Pass several more benches as you continue along the trail and under the Kirkwood Road bridge. Bear left, passing another trail map, some benches, two water fountains, and a shower. Kirkwood Road is also an access point to the trail. While hiking, look for great blue herons, loggerhead turtles, and an occasional alligator. Other birds here include ospreys, cardinals, herons, hawks, and killdeer, along with wood ducks, warblers, cedar waxwings, and sparrows.

The trail continues to be open on the right with houses along the fence line. When you reach a bench, an exercise station, and a picnic table on the right, look left for a bat house. Houston is home to one of the few nonmigratory bat populations in the world, which consists of the Mexican free-tailed bat. More than 150,000 bats fly into the sky at dusk to feed on mosquitoes and other insects. Hike past several more exercise stations and benches until you cross under Dairy Ashford, the last major street before Eldridge Parkway. Along with a trailhead, the Dairy Ashford section of the trail has a water fountain and an exercise station. Look left and you can see some rapids in the bayou. Continue straight, over a bridge and past several benches. This part of the trail is exposed and can be hot during the summer.

Cross a creek on a small bridge and then cross Buffalo Bayou to Eldridge Parkway and the end of the hike. A restroom is right and uphill, before you get to Eldridge Parkway. From here, retrace your route to the parking lot at Beltway 8 to complete the 10.16-mile hike.

Note: This trail is popular with cyclists in black, so be watchful; bike speed limit is 10 mph, but some riders may have left their speedometers at home. In-line skaters love the trail as well, with no streets to cross and a smooth asphalt surface. The trail is wide enough, though, to accommodate both hikers and people on wheels. Although the bikers and skaters are supposed to yield to hikers, try to hike on the right side of the trail and give them room on the left.

NEARBY ACTIVITIES

Bear Creek Park, George Bush Park, and Cullen Park are just a short drive away.

19 TERRY HERSHEY PARK:
Cardinal, Mockingbird, and Blue Jay Trails

KEY AT-A-GLANCE INFORMATION

LENGTH: 4.8 miles

CONFIGURATION: Out-and-back and loop

DIFFICULTY: Easy

SCENERY: Bayou, creek, open fields, woodlands, urban scenery

EXPOSURE: Sunny with some shade

TRAIL TRAFFIC: Light weekdays, moderate weekends

TRAIL SURFACE: Asphalt

HIKING TIME: 1.5 hours

DRIVING DISTANCE: 3.51 miles from the intersection of Beltway 8 and I-10

ACCESS: Free; open dawn to dusk

MAPS: USGS Hedwig Village and Addicks; trail signs

WHEELCHAIR ACCESS: Yes

FACILITIES: Restrooms (at the beginning of the Cardinal Trail and at the Eldridge Pkwy. end of the Blue Jay Trail), parking, water fountains, dog fountains, benches, exercise stations, playground, showers

SPECIAL COMMENTS: Pets, which must be leashed at all times, are welcome; dog water fountains are located wherever you see human water fountains.

GPS TRAILHEAD COORDINATES

LATITUDE: N 29° 47.000'
LONGITUDE: W 95° 37.391'

IN BRIEF

Terry Hershey Park encompasses approximately 12.5 miles of trails, from TX 6 west to Beltway 8 east. The Cardinal, Mockingbird, and Blue Jay trails run from I-10 south and then west to TX 6. These three trails join to make one continuous asphalt hiking and biking trail; however, there are no trail signs to indicate when you have left one trail and started another. Make sure you look at the trail map at the parking lot to get your bearings.

DESCRIPTION

Once parked, go east toward a trail map sign on the southeast corner of the parking lot. The trailhead for the Cardinal Trail starts just past the sign. The hike and bike trails are the main attractions in Terry Hershey Park, but there are other fun features including picnic sites, a playground, gazebos, a lighted walking trail along the Cardinal and Blue Jay trails, and a walk-in sundial near Memorial Drive and Eldridge Parkway. At the sundial, if you stand on the appropriate stone and the sun is shining, you cast a shadow on the correct time.

As you hike along South Mayde Creek and Buffalo Bayou, take note of the riparian landscape that includes plants such as yaupon holly, roughleaf dogwood, black willow, sunflowers, and sedges. In the spring look for passionflower, lantana, Turk's cap, and *Bidens*.

Directions ⟶

From the intersection of Beltway 8 and I-10, head west 4.84 miles on I-10 to the TX 6 exit. U-turn left by going under the freeway, and then go 1.33 miles after the U-turn on the access road to the entrance and parking lot of Terry Hershey Park, on the left.

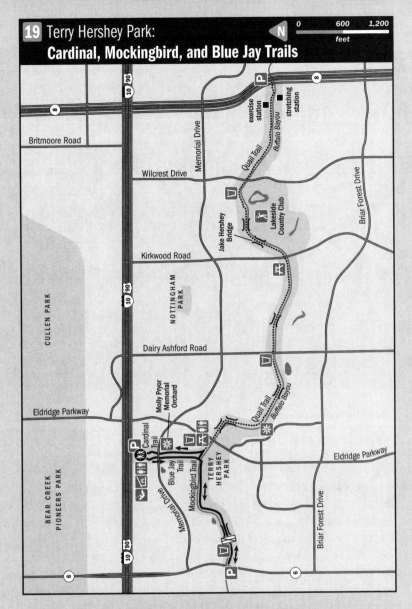

19 Terry Hershey Park:
Cardinal, Mockingbird, and Blue Jay Trails

N

0   600   1,200
feet

Britmoore Road

Memorial Drive

Wilcrest Drive

Quail Trail

Buffalo Bayou

exercise station

stretching station

Briar Forest Drive

Jake Hershey Bridge

Lakeside Country Club

Kirkwood Road

NOTTINGHAM PARK

CULLEN PARK

10 90

Dairy Ashford Road

Quail Trail

Buffalo Bayou

Eldridge Parkway

Molly Pryor Memorial Orchard

Cardinal Trail

Blue Jay Trail

Mockingbird Trail

Memorial Drive

TERRY HERSHEY PARK

Eldridge Parkway

BEAR CREEK PIONEERS PARK

Briar Forest Drive

6

6

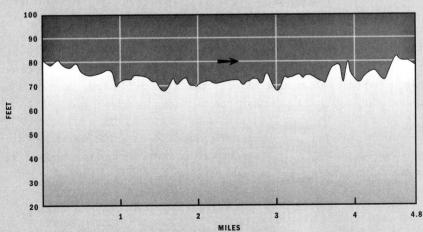

FEET

100
90
80
70
60
50
40
30
20

1   2   3   4   4.8

MILES

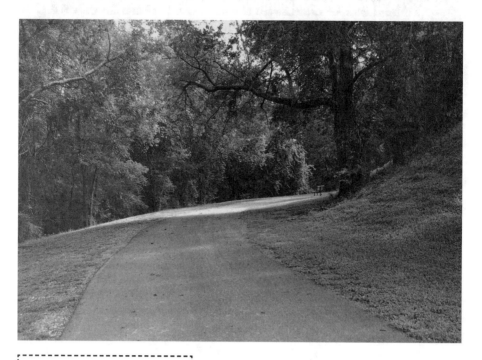

The wide trail in Terry Hershey Park

This hike runs entirely along either South Mayde Creek or Buffalo Bayou and includes three different trails—Cardinal, Mockingbird, and Blue Jay.

Once on the trail, take the first fork right to get on the Cardinal Trail. Cross South Mayde Creek on a small bridge and take the next fork left, heading away from the freeway. Continue past a playground on the left and restrooms on your right. Behind the restrooms is a small pond with a fishing pier. There are several benches, a gazebo, water fountains, a runner's shower, and a parking lot to accommodate hikers, bikers, and picnickers. Take the left fork in front of the parking lot and follow the trail along South Mayde Creek, on your left. This part of the hike, as well as the Blue Jay Trail, has lights for walking safely at dusk.

Continue along the trail to Memorial Drive. The creek can be quite deep here, with swift currents, so stay out of the water. Go under Memorial Drive and up the embankment to view one of the more urban parts of the trail. Once past Memorial Drive, the trail becomes the Blue Jay Trail. Just past several office buildings on the right, you eventually enter a more rural green space.

Stay away from the edge of the creeks and bayous, as the embankments are very steep and the sandy soil makes for unstable footing. The trails along the bayous often contain more elevation change than is typical in Houston, and the trails here are no exception. Continue past two benches and through a gated fence. The creek is left and there are houses on your right. This part of the trail is exposed, so take precaution with sunscreen, hats, and plenty of water.

Soon the trees start to overarch the trail, creating needed shade. The most prevalent animal on this part of the hike is definitely the squirrel. They are in the trees, on the ground, everywhere. Go past several benches and follow the trail left over a bridge. At the other end of the bridge is the trailhead for the Mockingbird Trail; turn right and begin the out-and-back part of the hike. Once on the Mockingbird Trail, Buffalo Bayou is on your right and open fields, or retention areas, are on your left.

Lights continue on this part of the trail but only for a short distance. At a fork, bear right, past a bench on the left. A high embankment on the left and the bayou on the right creates a tunnel, with trees as the roof. Continue over a bridge, walking beside an unofficial bike trail. Beyond a bench, the trail bends left. After a long straight-away, the trail swings right to cross a bridge. Cross two more bridges and go through a gate (closed and locked at night). The bayou is to the right, and if you look long enough you may see an alligator swimming below.

Continue past a water fountain and under TX 6 and through parts of Barker Dam. Once up the other side of the dam, turn around and retrace 1.3 miles on the Mockingbird Trail. Where the Blue Jay and Mockingbird trails join, go straight. The Mockingbird and Blue Jay trails overlap for 0.3 miles.

While hiking, look for great blue herons, loggerhead turtles, and an occasional alligator. Other birds include ospreys, cardinals, herons, hawks, and kill-deer along with wood ducks, warblers, cedar waxwings, and sparrows.

With Eldridge Parkway on your right, cross the bridge over Buffalo Bayou. (To find restrooms, follow the trail left and downhill, and then, at a fork, go left. Do not cross Eldridge Parkway.) To continue on the hike, take the right fork instead of the left. There is a trail map at this intersection, along with a bench. Go past a water fountain, bench, and runner's shower, noting the urban feel to this part of the hike. There are townhomes to the right, with the bayou on the left. Ahead, a straight part of the trail has benches and picnic tables. Continue through this parklike area to an exercise station and nature sign on the right. The sign includes information on the trees found in the park, including cotton-wood, green ash, pecan, live oak, sycamore, burr oak, and crepe myrtle. Just past the sign is a parking lot and benches on the right.

At a fork, bear left to cross under Memorial Drive, and transition from the Cardinal Trail to the Blue Jay Trail. Look as you cross under Memorial Drive for the trail you were on at the start of the hike. Continue past the Molly Pryor Memorial Orchard (an orchard dedicated to a late Harris County clerk) on the left, a bench overlooking South Mayde Creek on the left, and two birdhouses on the right. Once past the last bench on the right, take the right fork back to the parking lot and the trailhead.

Note: This trail is popular with cyclists, so be watchful; bike speed limit is 10 mph but some riders may have left their speedometers at home. In-line skaters love the trail as well, with no streets to cross and a smooth asphalt surface. The trail is wide enough, though, to accommodate both hikers and people on wheels.

20 BEAR CREEK PIONEERS PARK:
Equestrian and Nature Trail

KEY AT-A-GLANCE INFORMATION

LENGTH: 1.9 miles

CONFIGURATION: Loop

DIFFICULTY: Easy

SCENERY: Creeks, woods, ponds, nature signs, open fields, equestrian center

EXPOSURE: Shady with some sunny areas

TRAIL TRAFFIC: Light

TRAIL SURFACE: Dirt

HIKING TIME: 1 hour

DRIVING DISTANCE: 4 miles from Beltway 8 and Clay Road

ACCESS: Free; open 7 a.m. to dusk

MAPS: USGS Addicks

WHEELCHAIR ACCESS: None

FACILITIES: Restrooms, parking, nature signs, picnic areas, pavilions

SPECIAL COMMENTS: Due to the location of the park (part of the Addicks Reservoir), parts of the trails may be under water after heavy rains. Stay on the Nature Trail to avoid most of the low-lying areas. Pets are not allowed on the trails; bikes and motorized vehicles are also prohibited.

GPS TRAILHEAD COORDINATES

LATITUDE: N 29° 49.429'
LONGITUDE: W 95° 38.028'

IN BRIEF

Part of the Addicks Reservoir, Bear Creek Pioneers Park was created in the 1940s by the Army Corps of Engineers to prevent a repetition of a flood that occurred in the area in 1935. In 1965, Harris County leased 2,154 acres of the reservoir to develop a park that now includes a lighted walking trail, an equestrian trail, a small zoo, soccer fields, tennis courts, little league and softball fields, picnic pavilions, horseshoe courts, and picnic tables. The park is named after one of the creeks that flows through the area. Although the area is subject to flooding, the majority of the land is dry most of the time.

DESCRIPTION

The Equestrian and Nature Trail starts out as a single trail but then splits, creating the 1.9-mile Nature Trail and the 3.5-mile Equestrian Trail. Before starting the hike, take a moment to study the two signs at the trailhead, one about park rules, the other about the area's poisonous snakes. Go past the signs, through an open field, and head straight for the trail.

The trail is about 12 feet wide, with visibility into the woods being very good. As you approach the Tall Pine Trail sign, high in a tree, take the right fork and head along the mowed trail. Although the trail is well maintained, be aware that after heavy rain it could be under water in some places. At the Nature

---

Directions

From Beltway 8 and Clay Road, head west 4 miles to the entrance of Bear Creek Pioneers Park on the left. Drive 0.68 miles to the entrance of the Equestrian and Nature Trail on the left.

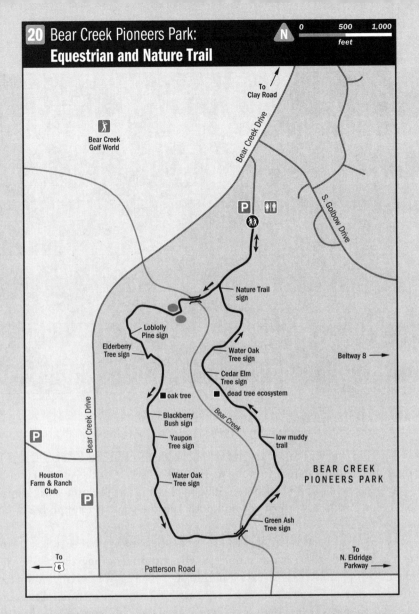

N

0   500   1,000
feet

To
Clay Road

Bear Creek Drive

S. Golbow Drive

Bear Creek
Golf World

P

Nature Trail
sign

Loblolly
Pine sign

Elderberry
Tree sign

Water Oak
Tree sign

Cedar Elm
Tree sign

Bear Creek Drive

oak tree

dead tree ecosystem

Bear Creek

Blackberry
Bush sign

Yaupon
Tree sign

low muddy
trail

Beltway 8 →

P

Houston
Farm & Ranch
Club

P

Water Oak
Tree sign

BEAR CREEK
PIONEERS PARK

Green Ash
Tree sign

To
6

Patterson Road

To
N. Eldridge
Parkway →

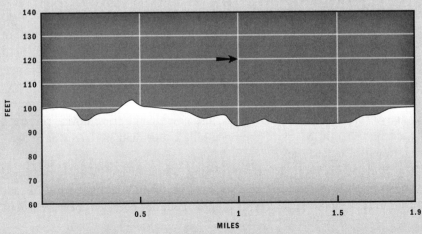

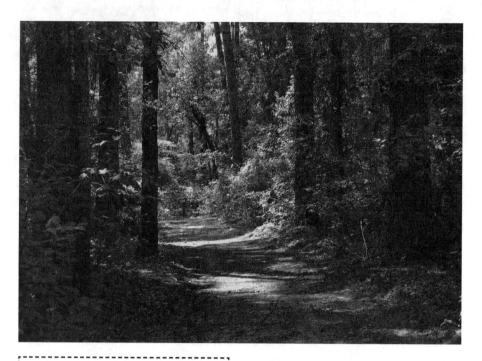

The dense woods of Bear Creek Pioneers Park

Trail sign, go right, into a clearing with two benches and a bridge. Cross the bridge and head to a nature sign for willow oak. Just left of the sign is Pond 2A; on your right is an unnamed pond. Stay on the trail, as the ponds are popular habitats for both the western cottonmouth and the southern copperhead, both poisonous snakes.

As the trail curves left, any noise from the park and the area suburban homes is quieted by trees and undergrowth. Continue along the trail, where evidence of horse use exists. Pass a nature sign for sugarberry tree, a lowland, fruit-bearing tree. Go straight; there is a small pond on the right, and the forest undergrowth starts to get denser. A nature sign for loblolly pine tells how it is the fastest growing pine in the Southeast and can reach heights of more than 100 feet. As you continue, the trail gets grassier but remains easy to follow. A nature sign for elderberry describes it as having one of the brightest purple berries in the area. At an intersection, go straight; the trail to the right leads to the Houston Farm and Ranch Club, where rodeo and equestrian events are held.

Continue into a clearing and past several nature signs describing beautyberry, greenbriar, and trifoliate orange. Just past this clearing notice the trees to the left of the trail. Many of the once-tall, 2-foot-diameter trees have been reduced to mulch by termites.

The trail curves right, briefly traversing a sunny, open area. Once back under the trees, hike past an oak tree standing in the middle of the trail. Ahead, a nature sign describes blackberry as one of the more prevalent berry vines in the Houston area. Where the underbrush clears, you come to a nature sign for the yaupon tree. About 250 yards to the right, you can see the Houston Farm and Ranch Club and its parking lot. Continue along the trail to a clearing with a nature sign for water oak. Head straight past a pond on your right and then through a grassy stretch of trail. Look low for white-tailed deer and high for hawks, as both are common in the park. Parts of the trail here may be muddy, so watch your step.

Enter another clearing with nature signs on willow oak, hawthorn, slippery elm, and cedar elm. All of these trees are present on the edges of the clearing. Cross a bridge and continue straight. There are banana spider webs across some parts of the trail from spring to late fall, so be aware while you hike. Once past a nature sign for green ash, go straight, as directed by a Nature Trail sign. (Turning left here puts you on the equestrian trail that can be very wet and messy in places.) The Nature Trail passes through low-lying, possibly muddy areas, and crosses a small culvert. As the trail gains elevation it dries out and becomes easier to hike. Continue past a nature sign for dead tree ecosystems on the right, and a sign for cedar elm and water oak on the left. Beyond these signs, look left to see the bridge you crossed at the start of the hike. Take a right at another Nature Trail sign, then go left through a clearing and into the parking lot.

NEARBY ACTIVITIES

Bear Creek Golf World, a 54-hole golf course, is adjacent to the park. George Bush Park, Cullen Park, and Terry Hershey Park are just a short drive away. For more information on park activities, go to **pct3.hctx.net.**

21 CULLEN PARK HIKE AND BIKE TRAIL

KEY AT-A-GLANCE INFORMATION

LENGTH: 7.6 miles

CONFIGURATION: Out-and-back

DIFFICULTY: Easy

SCENERY: Woodlands, picnic areas, open fields, Chinese tallow trees, marshes, cemetery

EXPOSURE: Sunny with some shade

TRAIL TRAFFIC: Light weekdays, moderate weekends

TRAIL SURFACE: Asphalt

HIKING TIME: 2.5 hours

DRIVING DISTANCE: 9.17 miles from intersection of Beltway 8 and I-10

ACCESS: Free; open dawn to dusk

MAPS: USGS Addicks

WHEELCHAIR ACCESS: Yes

FACILITIES: Restrooms, parking, picnic areas, baseball fields, soccer fields, benches, exercise stations, playgrounds, Alkek Velodrome

SPECIAL COMMENTS: This trail is popular with bikers, so be watchful and hike on the right to give them room. Beware of poisonous snakes such as copperheads and water moccasins on the trail after a heavy rain: they blend with the trail and can be hard to detect until you are right on them.

GPS TRAILHEAD COORDINATES

LATITUDE: N 29° 48.231'
LONGITUDE: W 95° 41.981'

IN BRIEF

Cullen Park, which was leased to the City of Houston in 1983, encompasses more than 10,500 acres of land just west of Addicks Reservoir. The hike and bike trail and picnic areas are on the north side of Saums Road, whereas the soccer fields and Velodrome are on the south side.

DESCRIPTION

Start the hike at the first parking lot on your right, as there seems to be more availability here on weekends. Park near the restrooms and head east to get on the asphalt trail. There are a playground and picnic areas on your right and the parking lot on your left. At the first fork head left, into the trees. At a street, go right, heading back into the trees and through picnic areas. Continue along the trail past soccer and baseball fields on your left and picnic tables on your right. Watch for low spots on the trail as these could be under water after a heavy rain.

The foliage in Cullen Park includes the Chinese tallow, pecan, oak, elderberry, and honeysuckle. You may occasionally see a deer but are most likely to see rabbits, birds, snakes, and an occasional squirrel. Many of the snakes are of a poisonous variety, so stay clear.

Continue past one more picnic and playground area and go through an intersection to a T-intersection. Turn left, heading toward

Directions

From the intersection of Beltway 8 and I-10, head west 7.68 miles on I-10 and exit at Barker Cypress Road. Turn right, go 1.06 miles to Saums Road, and turn left. Cullen Park is 0.69 miles on the right. The parking area is immediately on your right.

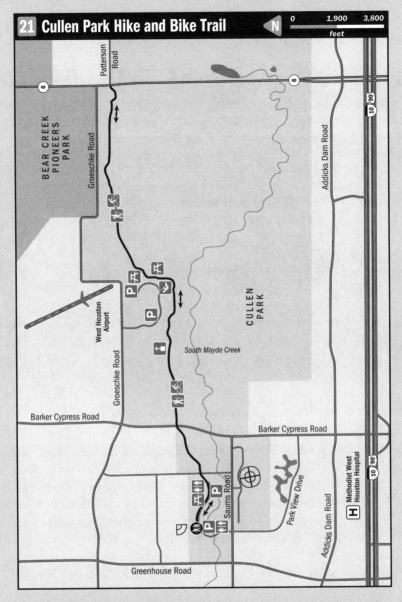

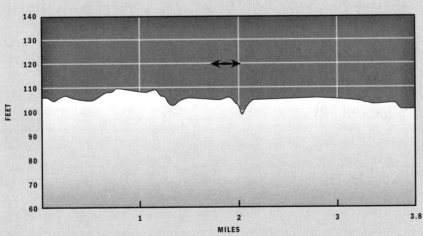

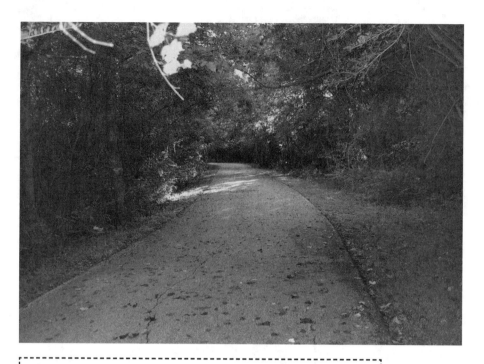

The hike and bike trail at Cullen Park is wide enough to accomodate everyone.

an open field with a parking lot on your left. At the next intersection, bear right and go through a gate to get on the official beginning of the Cullen Park Hike and Bike Trail. The trail's mile markers are being measured from this point, which is about 0.5 miles from the parking area. Follow the Cullen Park Hike and Bike Trail past an open field on the left and into a marshy area. Cross Groeschke Road, watching for traffic. Once across, follow the 12-foot-wide trail, which accommodates both hikers and bikers comfortably. As the trail bends right it becomes more open, with low-lying plants on each side. Go past a bench and the 0.25-mile marker. Continue past another bench where the trees arch over the trail and provide much-needed shade. Go past two benches on the left, under an ancient oak. At a fork, bear left to the stoplight at Barker Cypress Road. This is a very busy four-lane road, so be careful: push the button on the light pole and the light will change, allowing you to cross. (And yes, these buttons actually work.) Once across, at the 0.5-mile marker, a gated community is on the left. The neighborhood is only visible for a few hundred feet before you are once again on a tree-canopied trail. Cross a bridge and drainage spillway and continue past several benches and the 0.75-mile marker, on the right. This part of the trail is shady and pleasant, even during Houston summers. Continue past a bench on the left and curve left.

Two benches on the right appear just before the 1-mile marker, on the right. Go past several more benches as the underbrush opens on both sides. The 1.25-mile marker is on the right, followed by an entrance on the left to another

Cullen Park picnic area. This picnic area is closed weekdays and open on weekends only by reservation. Note the small cemetery to the left of the trail. At the 1.5-mile marker, cross a bridge that includes open side rails to allow flowing water to wash over the top during heavy rains. Just past the bridge is a baseball field on the right; other fields and a picnic area with restrooms, playgrounds, and tables are on the left. This part of the park is also closed on weekdays but the restrooms are open.

Continue past the 1.75-mile marker and look left for West Houston Airport, a small suburban airport for private planes. The foliage beside the trail is dense and visibility off the trail is poor. Go past several benches to the 2-mile marker.

A large stand of Chinese tallow is on your left, with a bench under another venerable oak tree to your right. Continue to the 3-mile marker, where you approach TX 6. The trail winds between a large stand of Chinese tallow on the left and a marsh on the right. The Chinese tallow tree is one of the more beautiful trees in Houston, providing crimson foliage in fall.

At the 3.25-mile marker, the undergrowth has opened somewhat, allowing you to look deeper into the woods. While it seems tempting to explore, stay on the trail for your own safety. Continue past benches on both sides of the trail until you reach TX 6. Turn around and retrace your steps to complete the hike.

Note: There are several parking lots along the trail, but only the ones at the start of the trail are open during the week. The picnic area and parking lot just past the 1.25-mile marker are closed unless you have a reservation. Although the picnic areas at the entrance can be crowded on weekends, the trail is only moderately used.

NEARBY ACTIVITIES

Bear Creek Park, George Bush Park, Terry Hershey Park, and West Houston Airport are just a short drive away. Also located in Cullen Park, the Alkek Velodrome is a 333-meter outdoor banked concrete track built in 1983 to accommodate the bike races in the 1986 U.S. Olympic Festival. It is now open to the public, but you must have a track bike to ride. Rentals are available. Go to **houstoncycling.org** for more information on schedule and hours.

22 GEORGE BUSH PARK:
Fry Road to Barker Clodine Trail

KEY AT-A-GLANCE INFORMATION

LENGTH: 10.8 miles

CONFIGURATION: Out-and-back

DIFFICULTY: Moderate

SCENERY: Woodlands, flood-control channel, bayou, wetlands, boardwalk

EXPOSURE: Sunny; some shade

TRAIL TRAFFIC: Light

TRAIL SURFACE: Asphalt

HIKING TIME: 4 hours

DRIVING DISTANCE: 10.62 miles from the intersection of Beltway 8 and I-10

ACCESS: Free; open 7 a.m to dusk

MAPS: USGS Addicks and Clodine

WHEELCHAIR ACCESS: Yes

FACILITIES: Parking, benches

SPECIAL COMMENTS: This is a hike and bike trail, so be aware of bikers and stay to the right. Keep pets on leash.

GPS TRAILHEAD COORDINATES

LATITUDE: N 29° 45.600'
LONGITUDE: W 95° 43.784'

IN BRIEF

This long hike takes you from a neighborhood park into a reservoir teeming with wildlife. Because it is part of Barker Reservoir, which was created in the 1940s to control flooding, parts of the trail are extremely low and may flood after heavy rains. The Army Corps of Engineers impounds water when necessary in George Bush Park. The George Bush Park trails connect to the trails in Terry Hershey Park near TX 6, allowing you to hike from Fry Road to Beltway 8 on fully paved and traffic-free trails.

DESCRIPTION

Start this hike at Greenbelt Park off Highland Knolls Road and Norwalk Drive. Park in the Epiphany of the Lord Catholic Church parking lot and go across Norwalk Drive to the trailhead for Greenbelt Park. Take the right fork to get on a concrete walkway and head south toward Highland Knolls Road. Take the left fork just before getting to the street and head east along the trail, crossing first Cobble Springs and then Fry Road. When crossing at the light, wait for the "walk" sign, as this is a very busy four-lane road. The George Bush Park Hike and Bike Trail begins in a residential area, just inside a gate. There is a trail map on the left. Follow the straight asphalt trail past a park-rules sign on the right.

Directions ⟶

From the intersection of Beltway 8 and I-10, head west 9.32 miles and exit at Fry Road. Turn left, go 2.3 miles to Highland Knolls Road, and turn right. Go 0.59 miles to Epiphany of the Lord Catholic Church and park. (There is no parking lot at the trailhead on Fry Road.) The hike from the church to the trailhead is through Greenbelt Park and is 0.59 miles.

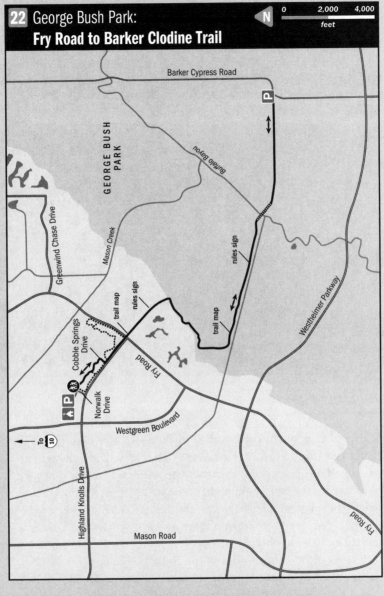

0   2,000   4,000
feet

N

Barker Cypress Road

P

GEORGE BUSH PARK

Buffalo Bayou

Greenwind Chase Drive

Mason Creek

rules sign

rules sign

trail map

trail map

Cobble Springs Drive

Fry Road

Norwalk Drive

P

To 10

Westgreen Boulevard

Highland Knolls Drive

Mason Road

Westheimer Parkway

Fry Road

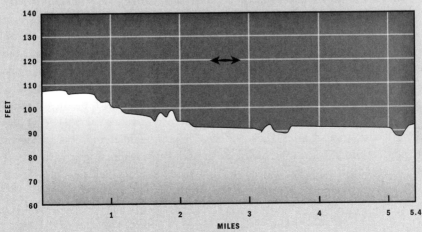

FEET

140
130
120
110
100
90
80
70
60

1   2   3   4   5   5.4

MILES

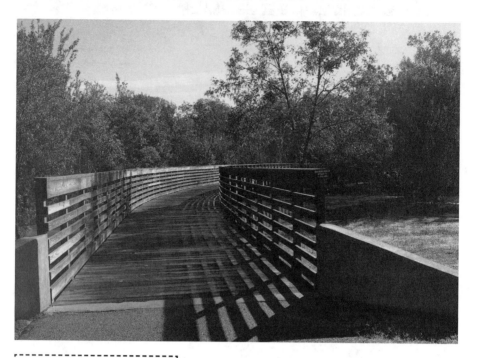

A long bridge over Buffalo Bayou

This trail is popular with cyclists so be watchful; bike speed limit is 10 mph, but some riders travel a bit faster. The trail is wide enough, though, to accommodate both hikers and cyclists. Although cyclists are supposed to yield to hikers, hike on the right to give them room. The trail makes a sweeping bend to the right as you pass a garbage can on the left. This is a very exposed trail, so make sure you wear sunscreen and bring plenty of water. Continue into the trees and away from the houses behind you. There are numerous tall pine trees and thick vegetation on both sides of the trail.

George Bush Park encompasses about half of the 13,500 acres of Barker Reservoir. Originally it was called the Cullen-Barker Park, but with Cullen Park just across I-10 there was confusion with the similar names. The name was officially changed to George Bush Park on January 28, 1997, creating the largest park in Harris County. Most of the area was used for growing rice and raising cattle until the creation of Barker Reservoir in the 1940s. Other sections of the park include picnic pavilions, restrooms, soccer fields, baseball fields, a fishing lake, and a playground designed to accommodate children with physical limitations. Besides hiking and biking trails, the park also includes the Scobee Model Airplane Fields, named after Dick Scobee, the commander of the Challenger spacecraft lost in 1986; and the Millie Bush Bark Park, where dogs can be let off their leashes. Millie Bush was the name of former President George and Barbara Bush's springer spaniel.

The trail, which moves out from under the canopy of the trees and back into the sun, crosses a small creek over a culvert. The 7-foot-wide trail has a clearance of about 15 feet on both sides before the vegetation starts. There are low spots in the trail, so watch your step after heavy rains. Look for rabbits, squirrels, large turtles, snakes (some poisonous), waterfowl, and songbirds while hiking. Continue past a park-boundary fence and a flood-control channel, both on the right. There are few benches on this hike, so take your time on hot days and enjoy the scenery.

As the trail bends left, away from the flood-control channel, there are two large birdhouses to the right. The trail goes gently uphill until you come to a trail map on the left. There is a large bridge on the right that leads to restrooms and soccer fields. Go straight past the trail map and uphill. Cross several small culverts. The flood-control channel is still on your right and may be quite full after heavy rains. You are now heading due east, and during a morning hike the sun may be directly in your eyes. Go past newly planted trees on both sides of the trail: a future shade canopy but for now too small to offer much cover.

This is a quiet and serene trail with little noise from traffic, people, or planes. Continue past a park-rules sign on the right and then more birdhouses by the flood-control channel. Cross several more small creeks using small bridges before reaching a 200-yard boardwalk that spans Buffalo Bayou. The flood-control channel on the right feeds into Buffalo Bayou, creating a large expanse of water where they meet. The boardwalk is high above the forest floor, which after a heavy rain may be completely under water. Go past two benches and a viewing area on the boardwalk, then leave the boardwalk heading slightly left. Now pass large open fields to the left of the trail. Continue along the trail to the equestrian and trail parking lot. Once at the parking lot, turn around and retrace your route.

Note: Be aware that after heavy rains parts of this trail near the flood-control channel and Buffalo Bayou may be under water.

NEARBY ACTIVITIES

Terry Hershey Park, Cullen Park, Bear Creek Pioneers Park are close; other facilities in George Bush Park include the Scobee Model Airplane Fields, Millie Bush Bark Park, and the American Shooting Center. Another hike in George Bush Park is a 7.8-mile out-and-back hike along old Barker Clodine Road. This very straight and paved trail is ideal for cyclists.

23 ATTWATER PRAIRIE CHICKEN NWR:
Auto Tour and Pipit Trail

(i) KEY AT-A-GLANCE INFORMATION

LENGTH: 6.5 miles

CONFIGURATION: Two loops

DIFFICULTY: Moderate

SCENERY: Texas prairie, prairie marsh, wetlands, ponds, riparian area

EXPOSURE: Sunny

TRAIL TRAFFIC: Light

TRAIL SURFACE: Dirt and sand

HIKING TIME: 3 hours

DRIVING DISTANCE: 47 miles from the intersection of Beltway 8 and I-10

ACCESS: Free; open year-round daily, sunrise to sunset

MAPS: USGS Eagle Lake NE; trail maps available

WHEELCHAIR ACCESS: None

FACILITIES: Visitor center, restrooms, driving tour, hiking trails, bird-watching, picnic tables

SPECIAL COMMENTS: Pets on leash no longer than 6 feet at all times. This is an open trail with no shade, so make sure you wear sunscreen and bring plenty of water. The refuge is busiest during spring, when wildflowers are abundant.

GPS TRAILHEAD COORDINATES

LATITUDE: N 29° 40.116'
LONGITUDE: W 96° 15.992'

IN BRIEF

The Attwater Prairie Chicken National Wildlife Refuge was established in 1972 to preserve habitat for the declining population of Attwater prairie chickens. Despite numbering approximately 1 million at the turn of the 1900s, they now total fewer than 100 and can be found only in two geographic regions in Texas. The 10,339-acre refuge is made up of marshes, ponds, native prairies, croplands, woodlots, and riparian areas along the San Bernard River. The auto tour, which goes along Winterman Prairie, Lafitte Prairie, and Foster Prairie, is a 5-mile rectangular loop that can be hiked as well as driven. The Pipit Trail is a small 1.5-mile hiking loop off the auto tour that takes you closer to the riparian vegetation and past several small ponds.

DESCRIPTION

Start the hike at the visitor center parking lot. Head out of the parking lot toward the Auto Tour sign and take a left to get on the grass trail. Go past an information sign on your right to get on the dirt trail. Continue as the trail heads uphill, curves left, and then goes back downhill. Vegetation on both sides of the trail is predominantly prairie grasses with no trees or shrubs. The refuge performs periodic burns to control encroaching vegetation, such as the Chinese tallow, and to keep the

---

Directions ————————————→

From Beltway 8 and I-10, head west 35.8 miles on I-10 to the FM 36 exit in Sealy. Head south on FM 36 for 1 mile to TX 3013 and turn right. Go 10 miles to County Road 291 and the entrance to the refuge and turn right. The visitor center is 2 miles from the entrance.

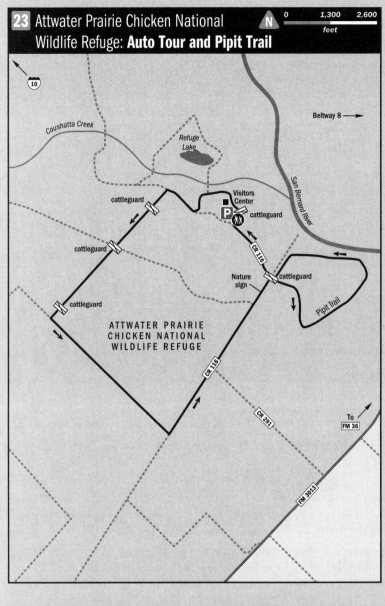

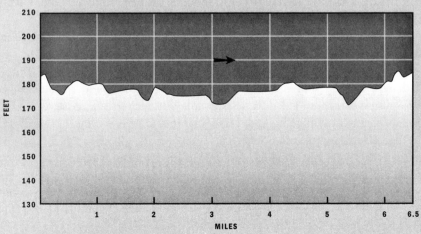

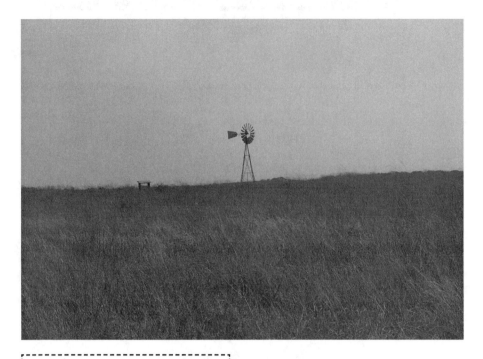

A rare view of a prairie west of Houston

fire-adapted prairie healthy. Burning also invigorates grass growth by removing dead stems.

Cross a cattle guard and follow the trail as it winds and climbs. There is a fence on your left and maybe some cows in a field on your right. Farther to your right is the San Bernard River and the riparian landscape that borders it. Now there is a fence on your right and the refuge headquarters is on your left. Go through the next intersection; the road on the right is closed. After heading downhill, take the right fork and then follow the trail as it stretches out ahead of you. After the trail bends left and uphill, take the left fork and continue on the Auto Tour. The trail narrows to only about 8 feet here, making it a one-way road at best.

While hiking, take note of the birds, since there are more than 250 species besides the Attwater prairie chicken. Listen for the whistle of fulvous and black-bellied whistling ducks, which inhabit the marshes, and look above to see white-tailed hawks as they soar over the prairies. Other birds found in the refuge include crested caracaras, vultures, scissor-tailed flycatchers, dickcissels, roseate spoonbills, geese, sandhill cranes, Sprague's pipit, and several types of sparrows. The refuge also supports about 50 species of mammals, mostly nocturnal. They include bobcats, coyotes, nine-banded armadillos, and on a good day, bison. Reptiles and amphibians include the Texas coral snake, western cottonmouth, and southern copperhead—all poisonous. The American alligator is also present in the ponds, so be watchful and stay on the road at all times. If you see a snake or alligator, stay clear of the area.

Cross another cattle guard and continue down the road as it stretches west for quite some distance. If it has rained recently, there will be water on both sides of the road. Go through the next intersection and continue straight. Soon there is a creek on your left and Teal Marsh on your right. This part of the road is elevated as it cuts between Teal Marsh and Pintail Marsh, on the left. Cross a small drainage bridge with culverts and go through a gate. At an intersection, bear left; the area to the right is closed to visitors.

Continue through the next intersection; the roads going left and right are closed. Look far to your left for refuge headquarters and the visitor center in the distance. Go through the next three intersections, continuing straight. At the fourth, take the left fork to stay on route. Cross another bridge over culverts and go by a trail marker on the left side of the trail. The ground on the right is higher than the trail and there are short shrubs growing among the grasses. Cross another small bridge as you hike by a stream on your right and higher vegetation on your left. Go through the next intersection. The road to your right is the one you drove in on. Cross a cattle guard and follow the signs to the visitor center.

Go by a nature sign on your left that explains why the refuge has controlled burns. There is a windmill in the prairie on your right and the refuge headquarters is on your left.

Just to the right of an informational sign, go right to get on the Pipit Trail. This is a 5-foot-wide, mowed-grass trail through the prairie. The trail bends right and passes a small weather station on the right and a small pond on the left. This part of the hike is just as exposed as the Auto Tour, as there are no trees. The trail heads uphill and winds left past the pond, which is still on your left. Continue along a long straight stretch before the trail curves left. You are headed past stands of cactus toward the San Bernard River. Just before reaching the riparian zone, the trail bends left, toward the visitor center. You are hiking in Foster Prairie, past trees and much thicker vegetation on your right. The trail surface changes from grass to a mixture of grass and sand and narrows to about 2 feet wide.

Continue straight, then bend left to head back toward the start of the Pipit Trail. There is a fence and a sandy area, both on your right: stay left for better footing. Head toward an information sign and then turn right to get back on the Auto Tour. Cross a cattle guard and go through the next intersection. The trail bends left and uphill before coming to the parking lot.

Note: Every second weekend in April, the refuge hosts the Attwater Prairie Chicken Festival. If Easter falls on this weekend, the festival is held during the first weekend in April. Due to the low number of Attwater prairie chickens, the chances of seeing one while hiking are low, but you can increase your chances by visiting in the spring.

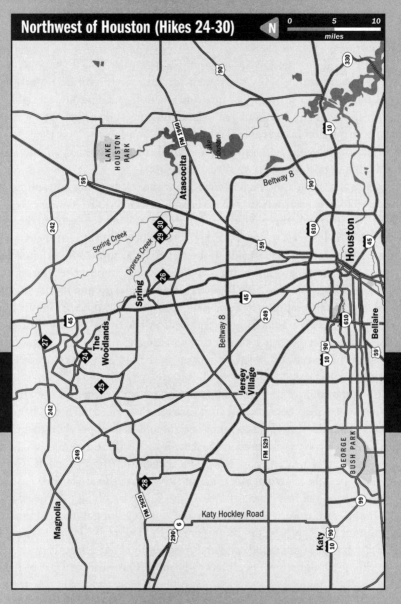

N

0   5   10
miles

330

90

10

FM 1960

LAKE
HOUSTON
PARK

Lake
Houston

Atascocita

Beltway 8

90

59

242

610

Spring Creek

29 30

Cypress Creek

59

Houston

45

26

Spring

45

249

45

The
Woodlands

27

24

Beltway 8

610

610

25

Jersey
Village

10 90

Bellaire

59

242

249

GEORGE
BUSH PARK

28

FM 529

FM 2920

99

Magnolia

Katy Hockley Road

290   6

Katy

10 90

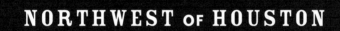

NORTHWEST OF HOUSTON

24 GEORGE MITCHELL NATURE PRESERVE: Nature Loop

KEY AT-A-GLANCE INFORMATION

LENGTH: 1.7 miles

CONFIGURATION: Loop

DIFFICULTY: Easy

SCENERY: Forestland, creek, lake

EXPOSURE: Shady

TRAIL TRAFFIC: Moderate

HIKING TIME: 45 minutes

DRIVING DISTANCE: 20 miles from the intersection of Beltway 8 and I-45

ACCESS: Free

MAPS: USGS Tamina

WHEELCHAIR ACCESS: No

FACILITIES: None

SPECIAL COMMENTS: There are no restrooms or water on the trail, so take plenty of water with you. While the trail is a bit secluded, many locals take their dogs on the trail, so you are rarely alone. Be cautious of poisonous snakes and stay on the trail at all times.

GPS TRAILHEAD COORDINATES

LATITUDE: N 30° 9.757'
LONGITUDE: W 95° 31.072'

IN BRIEF

The George Mitchell Nature Preserve is in The Woodlands, a community just north of Houston. It is located close to one of the newer neighborhoods, which are all known for excellent running trails. Across Flintridge Drive is one of the cement trails accessible to bikes, wheelchairs, strollers, and of course runners and hikers. National Tails awarded The Woodlands the 2010 Developer Award to recognize high-quality, well-designed, multi-use trail systems that are integrated into private developments. With more than 125 miles of trails, The Woodlands is one of the more trail-oriented communities in Texas. While most of the trails wind throughout the neighborhood, the George Mitchell trail is a wooded trail offering a good glimpse of native Texas flora and fauna.

DESCRIPTION

Part of the Spring Creek Greenway, which will connect 12,000 acres of forestland on both sides of Spring Creek, the George Mitchell Nature Preserve is located in The Woodlands. This 1,700-acre preserve opened in 2007 to provide trails for both hikers and cyclists. To begin the hike, park in the small parking lot on Flintridge Drive.

Head toward the bench and a sign indicating that the preserve is open from dawn

----

Directions ——————————————➤

From Beltway 8 and I-45 head north 15.3 miles to The Woodlands Parkway and take the flyover to the left. Drive 4 miles to Gosling Road, turn left, and drive .5 miles to Flintridge Drive. Turn right and drive .5 miles to George Mitchell Nature Preserve on the left.

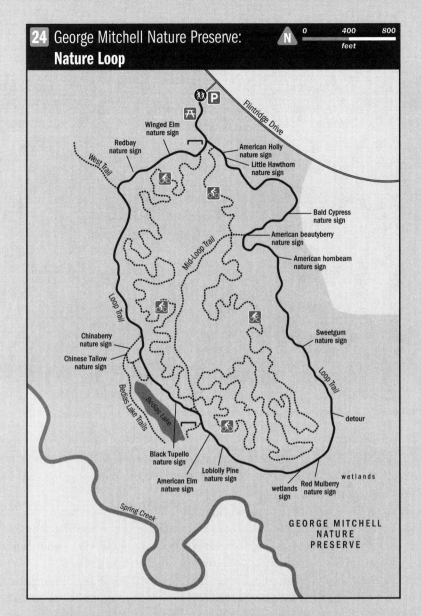

0   400   800
feet

N

Flintridge Drive

West Trail

Redbay
nature sign

Winged Elm
nature sign

American Holly
nature sign

Little Hawthorn
nature sign

Bald Cypress
nature sign

American beautyberry
nature sign

American hornbeam
nature sign

Mid-Loop Trail

Loop Trail

Sweetgum
nature sign

Chinaberry
nature sign

Chinese Tallow
nature sign

Loop Trail

detour

Bedias Lake Trails

Bedias Lake

Black Tupelo
nature sign

American Elm
nature sign

Loblolly Pine
nature sign

wetlands
sign

Red Mulberry
nature sign

wetlands

Spring Creek

GEORGE MITCHELL
NATURE
PRESERVE

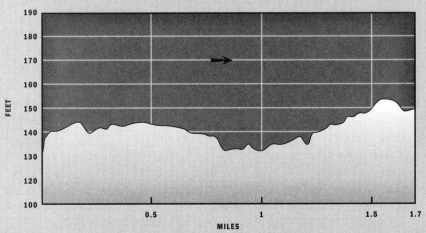

FEET

190
180
170
160
150
140
130
120
110
100

0.5   1   1.5   1.7

MILES

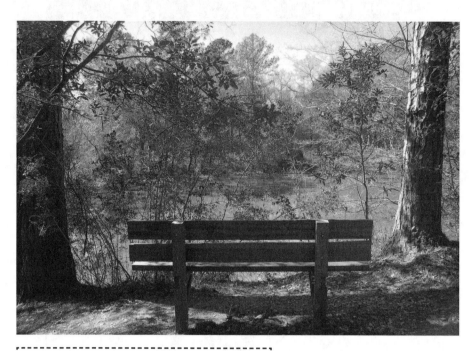

Bench overlooking Cypress Creek on the Creek View Trail

until dusk. Hike past a trail-map sign on a 4-to-5-foot-wide dirt trail away from the road and civilization. At the trail-loop sign and the Y intersection, head left to get on the loop.

Hike past a bike-trail sign on your right. While the bike trails, which are much narrower than the hiking trails, wind throughout the preserve, the hiking trail is a loop. Continue straight over exposed tree roots and watch your footing. The trail surface is not conducive to either wheelchairs or strollers.

Continue past a nature sign on the American holly and one on the little hip hawthorne before the trail winds downhill and to the right. The vegetation is quite thick, offering considerable shade. As it winds to the left, you can hear the traffic off to your left. Much of the vegetation opens up giving you some views into the thick canopy.

Follow the trail-loop sign as the path heads away from the road and past a nature sign on the bald cypress. Continue onto a slight rise with a very low area to your left. This low spot could have water after rain so stay on the rise. As you step off the rise, the trail winds past a nature sign on the American beautyberry. Hike past the Mid Loop Trail sign and continue on the main loop. The trail heads uphill slightly under a beautiful canopy of trees.

Hike past a nature sign on the American hornbeam. Poison ivy is very prevalent, so stay on the trail and away from any vines. Continue past a nature sign on the sweetgum and head downhill past a number of bike trails that cross the main hiking trail. Spring Creek, which is now on your left, also has a number of trails that head toward the creek. Stay on the trail as it winds through the trees and past a sign that says NO LEFT TURN.

Head past a nature sign on the red mulberry and another sign directing you toward a wetlands area. As you head downhill, the trail winds to the right. There is a fairly steep drop-off into the creek on your left, so use caution. At the Creek View Trail sign, head left toward the creek to "get a view." This trail is very short and quite narrow as it winds toward an overlook. Once at the overlook, head back the same way you came until you get back to the main loop. Turn left to continue the hike.

Hike past nature signs on the loblolly pine and American elm before getting to another Creek View Trail sign. Head left down this short spur toward a bench and a great view of the creek. While this trail is a small spur that connects to the first Creek View Trail, it does not seem well maintained. Turn around and head back up the trail toward the main loop and take a left.

At the next Y intersection, head left following the EXIT SIGN. Heading right puts you on the bike trail. Continue past another Mid Loop Trail sign and go straight. Hike past a nature sign on the black tupello and toward a sign for Bedias Lake. Take this trail to the left as it heads downhill. The lake is off to your left. Turn around and take the trail on the left uphill past a nature sign on the Chinese tallow and one on the chinaberry.

At the next intersection, get back on the main loop and head toward a nature sign on the water oak. The trail winds for quite some distance before going by signs on the redbay tree and winged elm. Follow all signs that point toward the exit until you get to the bench at the start of the hike. Head left toward the parking lot and to the end of the hike.

NEARBY ACTIVITIES

The Woodlands is just south of Lake Conroe and Huntsville State Park. Parts of the Lone Star Hiking Trail in the Sam Houston National Forest are less than 30 minutes north, along with Stubblefield Recreation Area, Cagle Lake Recreation Area, and Big Creek Scenic Recreation Area. Spring Creek runs along the southwest side of the trail and offers paddlers an opportunity to put in or take out in the area.

25 BURROUGHS PARK

KEY AT-A-GLANCE INFORMATION

LENGTH: 1.2 miles

CONFIGURATION: Loop

DIFFICULTY: Easy

SCENERY: Dense forest with short-leaf pines, stands of hickory, and holly bushes

EXPOSURE: Shady all day

TRAIL TRAFFIC: Light

TRAIL SURFACE: Crushed granite, dirt, sand, and pine needles

HIKING TIME: 30 minutes

DRIVING DISTANCE: 21 miles from SH249 and Beltway 8

ACCESS: Free; open dawn to dusk

MAPS: Trailhead map posted

WHEELCHAIR ACCESS: No, because of loose dirt and sand and steps

FACILITIES: Parking, restrooms, picnic tables, fishing pond, soccer fields

SPECIAL COMMENTS: Dogs are welcome but must be leashed at all times.

GPS TRAILHEAD COORDINATES

LATITUDE: N 30° 8.199'
LONGITUDE: W 95° 34.588'

IN BRIEF

Burroughs Park is a 320-acre county park that offers 8 miles of hiking trails, a stocked fishing pond, picnic facilities, a playground accessible to disabled children, soccer and softball fields, and an elevated boardwalk. Most of the foot and bike traffic is on the paved walkways that wind through the playgrounds and picnic areas. The hiking trails have very little activity, making them a quiet retreat, away from the hustle and bustle of the other park facilities.

DESCRIPTION

From the Burroughs Park trailhead sign head left onto a crushed granite trail. The trail is soon bordered by towering pines and Big Thicket underbrush. The noise of the park is quickly diminished by the dense forest of tall pines. Less than 50 feet from the trailhead is the only bench on the trail. Continue along the trail, passing a primitive path on the right.

Follow the trail to the 0.25-mile marker and a fork. Bear left, past hickory trees, short-leaf pines, blackjack, and farkleberry bushes. The trail is comfortably wide, allowing for easy walking without having to brush aside vines or tree limbs. Stay on the trail to minimize contact with poison ivy or poison sumac.

The underbrush is dense but with openings that allow for wildlife viewing. Small

----

Directions

From Beltway 8 in Houston, take TX 249 west 15 miles to FM 2920 and turn right. Go 3 miles to FM 2978 (Hufsmith–Kohrville Road) and turn left. Go 1.7 miles and turn right on West Hufsmith Road. The park entrance is 1.3 miles on the left. Follow the park road to the last parking lot. The signed trailhead is on your left.

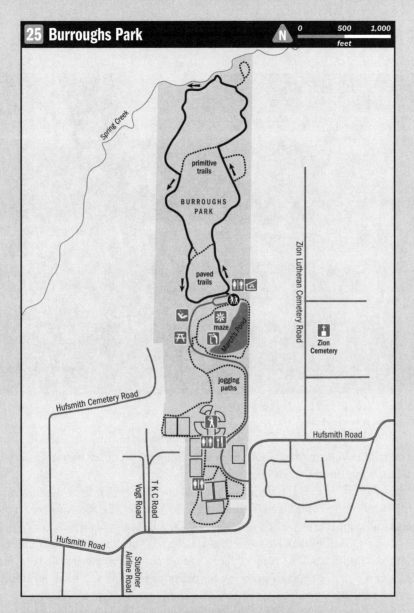

0   500   1,000
feet

N

Spring Creek

primitive
trails

BURROUGHS
PARK

paved
trails

maze

March's Pond

Zion Lutheran Cemetery Road

Zion
Cemetery

jogging
paths

Hufsmith Cemetery Road

Hufsmith Road

Vogt Road

T K C Road

Hufsmith Road

Stuebner
Airline Road

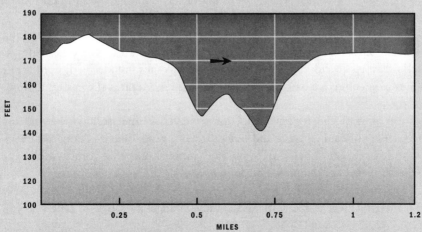

FEET

190
180
170
160
150
140
130
120
110
100

0.25   0.5   0.75   1   1.2

MILES

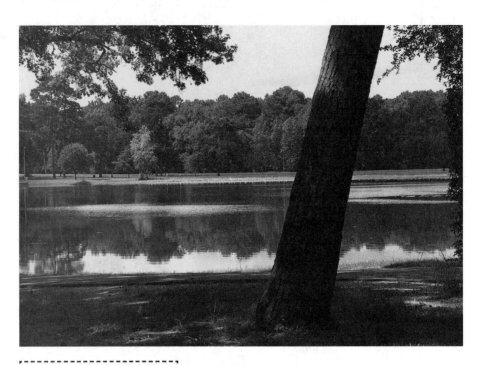

A view of the stocked fishing lake

white-tailed deer are often seen in the area, along with other native Texas mammals such as armadillos and opossums.

The birds you might see include the American robin, brown-headed cowbird, Northern cardinal, cedar waxwing, and blue jay. Be aware of water moccasins and copperheads when near the lake and in low-lying areas.

After a trail merges from the right, bear left into deeper woods and more primitive conditions. The trail surface changes from crushed granite to dirt and rock, with patches of moss growing on many of the rocks. The moss indicates that the trail stays shady most of the year and is not heavily traveled.

Wind gently downhill via the trail and a series of steps. At the bottom of the hill is a dry streambed that may flood in heavy rains.

Head up the other side of the streambed, gaining back the slight elevation you lost earlier. Cross an access road and pick up the trail on the other side. As the foliage starts to close in, the trail surface becomes less defined. Follow the trail until you come to a barbed-wire fence. This fence marks the eastern boundary of the park.

Turn right at the fence. Walk along the fence line, following pink and orange streamers tied to trees and fence posts to guide hikers. Along the fence line, the tree canopy opens up, dappling sunlight onto the forest floor. The underbrush is less dense and visibility improves greatly into the forest.

Cross the access road again, staying close to the fence. Go left at the next fork in the trail, where the trail surface now changes to a bed of pine needles.

In less than 200 feet you will be at the end of the hiking trail and facing the fishing lake.

The lake is stocked with largemouth bass and catfish. Any largemouth bass must be released if caught, and there is a limit of three catfish more than 12 inches. In January of each year, the Texas Parks & Wildlife Department stocks the lake with rainbow trout; however, as temperatures rise above 70°F, these fish die out. If you want to catch trout (a rarity in this part of Texas), fish from January to March.

At the lake, turn right and walk past the picnic pavilion and restrooms to reach the parking area.

NEARBY ACTIVITIES

Burroughs Park is less than 5 miles from Tomball, a historic Texas town with abundant shopping and eating possibilities. In the 1960s, Tomball had the distinction of being named in Ripley's Believe It or Not as the only town with free water and gas and no cemetery. This is no longer the case. The Spring Creek Greenway, which runs from Burroughs Park to Jesse H. Jones Park, is part of the Sam Houston Trail & Wilderness Preserve. It will eventually connect these parks running along Spring Creek through the George Mitchell Nature Preserve, Montgomery County Preserve, Old Riley Fuzzel Road Preserve, Peckinpaugh Preserve, and Pundt Park.

26 MERCER ARBORETUM AND BOTANIC GARDENS: West Trails

KEY AT-A-GLANCE INFORMATION

LENGTH: 2.5 miles

CONFIGURATION: Loop

DIFFICULTY: Easy

SCENERY: Woodlands, bald cypress stands, bog, creeks, wetlands, boardwalks, maple-tree collection

EXPOSURE: Shady with some sun

TRAIL TRAFFIC: Light

TRAIL SURFACE: Asphalt and boardwalk

HIKING TIME: 1 hour

DRIVING DISTANCE: 9.89 miles from the intersection of Beltway 8 and I-45

ACCESS: Free; in summer, Monday–Saturday, 8 a.m.–7 p.m. ; Sunday, 10 a.m.–7 p.m.; in winter, daily, 8 a.m.–5 p.m.

MAPS: USGS Spring; trail maps available

WHEELCHAIR ACCESS: Yes

FACILITIES: Restrooms, arboretum, visitor center, parking, picnic areas, playgrounds, library, water fountains, trail markers

SPECIAL COMMENTS: Although most of the garden areas are accessible to wheelchairs and strollers, officials here ask that you call ahead for any special accommodations.

GPS TRAILHEAD COORDINATES

LATITUDE: N 30° 2.298'
LONGITUDE: W 95° 22.981'

IN BRIEF

Mercer, which is a nationally recognized arboretum and botanic garden, was preserved as a Harris County Precinct Park in 1974. Thelma and Charles Mercer presented the 250 acres along Cypress Creek to the county to create the region's largest collection of native and cultivated plants. This hike is located on the west side of Aldine Westfield Road and includes many different trails and loops—all well marked. Look for deer and other wildlife, and be aware of poisonous snakes.

DESCRIPTION

Start the hike at the trailhead adjacent to the dining pavilion on the north side of the west parking lot. There are restrooms on the left and the trail begins on a wooden boardwalk. Beyond the boardwalk, the trail surface changes to crushed granite and asphalt for the remainder of the hike. Before starting, use bug spray for protection against both mosquitoes and horseflies, which can bite through clothing. Continue onto the granite walkway and past elderberry bushes on your left. Bear left at a fork, away from the parking lot and into the woods. A creek-bank erosion area is now on your right: due to loose, sandy soil, you are advised to stay on the trail.

Directions ⟶

From the intersection of Beltway 8 and I-45, head north 5.69 miles on I-45 to FM 1960 and turn right. Go 3 miles to Aldine Westfield Road and turn left. Go 1.2 miles to the entrance to Mercer Arboretum and Botanic Gardens. Turn left into the west side of the park to reach the trailhead. Take the first right and park in the Cypress parking lot on your immediate left, close to the dining pavilion on the north side of the lot.

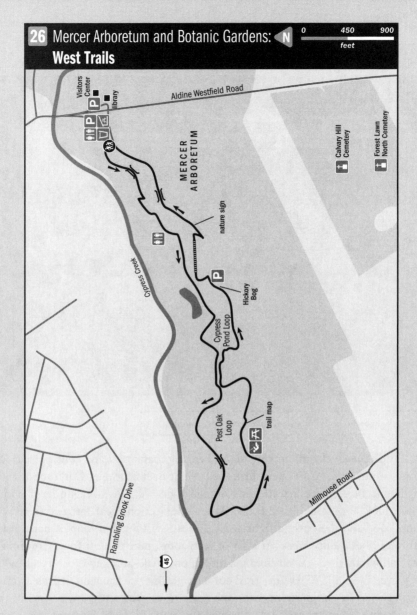

26 Mercer Arboretum and Botanic Gardens: **West Trails**

N

0   450   900
feet

Visitors Center

library

Aldine Westfield Road

M E R C E R   A R B O R E T U M

Calvary Hill Cemetery

Forest Lawn North Cemetery

nature sign

Cypress Creek

Hickory Bog

Cypress Pond Loop

trail map

Post Oak Loop

Rambling Brook Drive

Millhouse Road

45

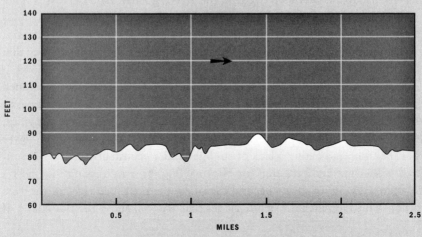

140				
130				
120		→		
110				
100				
90				
80				
70				
60				

FEET

0.5   1   1.5   2   2.5

MILES

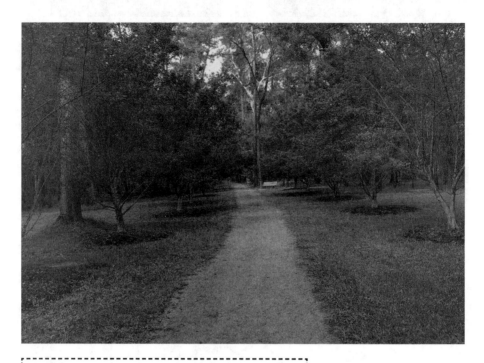

The Jake Roberts Maple Collection, a stand of Trident maples

With the creek still on your right, bear right at a fork and continue through dense woodlands. At the next fork, bear right over a bridge. Continue through an intersection where a trail joins on the right. As you walk under a natural arbor, look left to see other trails. At an intersection, bear left to the Cypress Pond Loop and then take a right at a trailhead sign for that loop. A nature sign, left, describes quince trees. At a set of restrooms, take the left fork. Continue as the trail winds through Virginia magnolia, post oak, and hawthorn trees, which arch over the trail. Where the trail curves right, notice the bald cypresses growing in the creek on the right. Although these trees need a wet environment, they can survive droughts, which do occur in the area regularly. Bald cypress is not a true cypress but is more closely related to the coast redwood of California. They can grow to more than 90 feet tall and can live up to 1,000 years. Go past a bench on the right and head up the oxbow, an old channel of Cypress Creek that was left when the main channel moved farther north, perhaps during a flood.

Continue along the trail and take the next fork right. Keep your eyes open for deer, which are frequently seen in this area. As the trail curves left, you pass a grassy clearing on the right. The forest consists of tall trees and numerous vines, which are killing many of the trees. There is green moss on many of the lower parts of the trees, indicating a lack of sunlight and a persistently damp environment. At a fork marked by a sign for Hickory Bog, bear right. Continue past a bench and trail map on the right, and then take the next fork right to the Post Oak Loop. This loop includes gentle ridges that are well above the floodplain of

Cypress Creek. These uplands are home to hardwood trees such as post oak and red oak. The trail is more shaded here, beneath a canopy of trees. Cross over a large bridge that curves right and continue to the next trailhead and trail map. Continue straight to the Hawthorn Loop, where the trees get denser. Look for the cream-colored flowers of parsley hawthorn and pasture haw.

Continue straight through the next intersection. The Post Oak parking lot is now on your right, with another dining pavilion on the left. Take the next fork left at a trail sign and continue past a playground, restrooms, and picnic areas. Go through the next intersection, where a trail joins on the right. At the end of the picnic area, continue straight past a trail map on the left and an intersection with a trail on the right. Immediately after leaving the picnic area, you are back in the woods. Swing left and slightly downhill to the next trailhead and map on the left. Go straight until you come to a sign for Hickory Bog and then take the right fork. A mowed clearing is left, with the forest 30 yards or more away. Continue past more clearings until you get to a boardwalk and Hickory Bog. This bog is home to water hickory and water elm, which have adapted to grow in seasonal wetlands. Also growing in the bog are water oak and Louisiana iris. Stay on the boardwalk, as snakes are more likely in wetlands. As you leave the boardwalk, the trail curves right. Go past a water fountain on the right and take the right fork at the next trailhead. Bald Cypress Swamp is straight ahead with a long boardwalk, an observation stand, benches, and nature signs.

Follow the boardwalk to its end and exit left and back onto a crushed-granite surface. There is a parking lot across the swamp and a road to your right. Take the next fork right and cross a bridge which has benches at both ends. Ahead is the Jake Roberts Maple Collection, a stand of Trident maples that produce a tunnel effect. In the fall, these maples change color brilliantly creating beautiful autumn foliage of reds and oranges. Continue through the maple collection, past several benches, and take the next fork left. There is a water fountain and several benches on your right, just this side of the parking lot. At the next intersection, fork right to get to the parking lot.

Note: All plants are protected and are not to be removed from the trails or gardens. The arboretum and botanic gardens are located on both sides of Aldine Westfield Road, with the hiking trails located on the west side. The visitor center, botanic gardens, and library are all located on the east side. Pets on leash may visit the park on the west side only. Bikes are allowed on the asphalt trails of the west side. Swimming, ball playing, and other team sports are not permitted. For more information, go to **hcp4.net/mercer.**

NEARBY ACTIVITIES

The Spring Creek Greenway, which runs from Burroughs Park to Jesse H. Jones Park, is part of the Sam Houston Trail & Wilderness Preserve. It will eventually connect these parks running along Spring Creek through the George Mitchell Nature Preserve, Montgomery County Preserve, Old Riley Fuzzel Road Preserve, Peckinpaugh Preserve, and Pundt Park.

27 W. GOODRICH JONES STATE FOREST:
Middle Lake Trail

KEY AT-A-GLANCE INFORMATION

LENGTH: 1.5 miles

CONFIGURATION: Out-and-back

DIFFICULTY: Easy

SCENERY: Woodlands, lake, red-cockaded woodpecker viewing area

EXPOSURE: Shady

TRAIL TRAFFIC: Light

TRAIL SURFACE: Dirt

HIKING TIME: 1 hour

DRIVING DISTANCE: 23 miles from the intersection of Beltway 8 and I-45

ACCESS: Free; open Monday–Friday, 8 a.m.–5 p.m.

MAPS: USGS Tamina

WHEELCHAIR ACCESS: None

FACILITIES: Parking, equestrian parking and trails, fishing, picnic areas, benches

SPECIAL COMMENTS: There is no drinking water available on the trails. Keep pets on leash.

GPS TRAILHEAD COORDINATES

LATITUDE: N 30° 13.781'
LONGITUDE: W 95° 29.832'

IN BRIEF

Named after W. Goodrich Jones, the founder of the Texas Forestry Association, the W. Goodrich Jones State Forest was purchased by the state in 1926. The 1,733-acre forest operates as a demonstration and working forest. The park includes nature trails, two small fishing ponds, picnic areas, and parking for horse trailers. There are service roads and horse trails that run throughout the park: stay on the marked trail so as not to get lost; don't take shortcuts, as these may cause erosion. The Middle Lake Trail, although short, is one of the few places in the Houston area where you might get a glimpse of the endangered red-cockaded woodpecker.

DESCRIPTION

From the parking lot, go toward the brown sign in the trees heading away from a small lake. Continue to the Middle Lake picnic sign and go through traffic barriers used to prevent motorized traffic. While there are many horse trails throughout the park, horses are not allowed on this trail. The trail surface is dirt with some exposed tree roots. Although the forest on the left is very dense, the vegetation on the right is only about 2 or 3 feet high, scattered beneath the tall loblolly and shortleaf pines. Many of the pines are more than 50 years old, with a few 100 years old. It appears that the area on the right had been cleared at one time but is now left to grow back to its native state.

Directions ⟶

From the intersection of Beltway 8 and I-45, head north 20.63 miles on I-45 to FM 1488 and go left on the overpass. Go 2.45 miles to the forest entrance on the left.

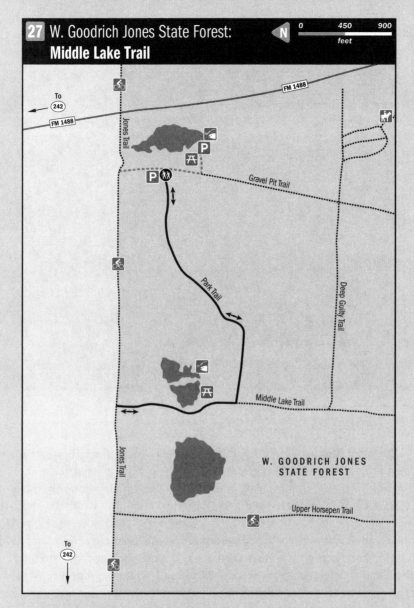

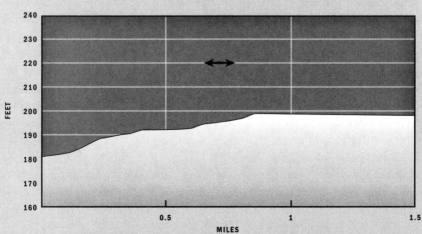

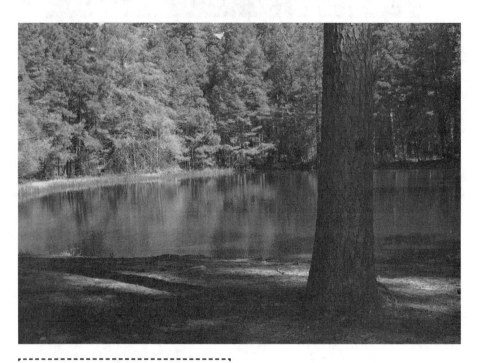

A view of Middle Lake near the end of the trail

Continue slightly uphill. Go past a trail marker on the left, where the trail curves left. Look through the trees on your right for an old barn and other farm buildings next to a clearing. This hike is very shady with only short open stretches. Go through an intersection where a trail joins on your left. The 7-foot-wide trail heads slightly downhill as you go by a trail marker on the right. Home to the endangered red-cockaded woodpecker, W. Goodrich Jones State Forest is one of only two state forests with a significant population of the bird. The red-cockaded woodpecker is a small black and white woodpecker with a red streak on each side of its black cape called a cockade. It is the only woodpecker that build nests in cavities in living pine trees. All other woodpeckers bore out the cavities of dead trees. Periodic burning of the underbrush is used to protect the bird's habitat from predators such as the flying squirrel, which is able to get to nests easier with a dense hardwood midstory under the pines. There were 15 clusters of red-cockaded woodpeckers spotted in the forest in 2003, making W. Goodrich Jones State Forest one of the easiest sites in Texas to spot the endangered species. (A cluster is an aggregate of cavity trees that may include from 1 to 20 cavity trees on 3 to 60 acres.) Early mornings and late afternoons are the best times of day to spot them.

The trail passes through an open field with a sign indicating a picnic area ahead and to the right. A nature sign describing the red-cockaded woodpecker is on your right. The picnic area and Middle Lake are both right. Continue along the trail until it ends, then turn right onto a service road.

Designated a "demonstration forest," W. Goodrich Jones State Forest is used for testing and researching many forest-management techniques, forest genetics, and forest-product utilization. Areas of the forest have been set aside to demonstrate ways to protect water from pollution during normal forestry operations. The forest was established as a resource for educating the public on forest-management practices to protect native flora and fauna. Run by the Texas Forest Service, the W. Goodrich Jones State Forest offers demonstrations and nature study for groups by appointment.

Continue along the service road with picnic tables on both sides of the road and the lake still on your right. Pass by the lake and continue past another nature sign, left, for the red-cockaded woodpecker. Just past the nature sign is a red-cockaded woodpecker viewing area, one of the better spots to see the rare bird. Be aware of horses crossing in this area and give them plenty of room to get by. When you reach Jones Road, the park entrance road, turn around and retrace your route.

NEARBY ACTIVITIES

Sam Houston Memorial and Park Complex (**samhouston.org**), The Texas Prison Museum (**txprisonmuseum.org**), H.E.A.R.T.S. Veterans Museum (**heartsmuseum .com**), Sam Houston National Forest, Lake Conroe, Huntsville State Park, The Woodlands.

28 KLEB WOODS NATURE PRESERVE TRAILS

KEY AT-A-GLANCE INFORMATION

LENGTH: 2.3 miles

CONFIGURATION: 2 loops

DIFFICULTY: Easy

SCENERY: Woodlands, wetlands, homestead, marsh

EXPOSURE: Shady

TRAIL TRAFFIC: Light

TRAIL SURFACE: Dirt and crushed granite

HIKING TIME: 1 hour

DRIVING DISTANCE: 19 miles from the intersection of Beltway 8 and I-290

ACCESS: Free; trails are open daily 7 a.m. to dusk, but the nature center is only open Monday–Friday, 8 a.m.–5 p.m.

MAPS: USGS Rose Hill

WHEELCHAIR ACCESS: None

FACILITIES: Restrooms, picnicking, nature center, campsites, old homestead

SPECIAL COMMENTS: Some parts of the trail can be under water after heavy rains, so call ahead for trail conditions. Mosquitoes, which are bad anywhere around Houston, are very bad here, even in late fall. Bring insect repellent all year. Pets on leash are permitted.

GPS TRAILHEAD COORDINATES

LATITUDE: N 30° 4.323'
LONGITUDE: W 95° 44.387'

IN BRIEF

Kleb Woods was part of a family farm owned by one of the original German descendants to the area in 1840. Conrad Kleb's son Edward ran the farm between 1904 and 1933 on a total of 132 acres, but his son Elmer stopped farming and let the land go back to its natural state. Elmer Kleb planted trees to encourage the birds and animals to stay on the land, but due to his inability to pay his taxes, he accrued a large tax bill and was taken to court. The Texas Parks and Wildlife Department and The Trust for Public Lands worked with County Commissioner Steve Radack to buy the land and turn it into a nature preserve, allowing Elmer to live here until his death in 1999 at age 90. The original section of the nature preserve opened in 1994 and included picnic areas, restrooms, paved parking, a hiking trail, and campsites.

DESCRIPTION

Start the hike by walking out of the parking lot, turning left, and following Draper Road south to two gates. There is farmland to your right and dense forest on your left. Go through the gate on the right, as the left gate is on private property. Beyond the gate, go left of a barrier and stop sign. Head down the old roadlike trail for about 40 yards until you see a trail in the trees to your right.

Directions ⟶

From Beltway 8 and I-290, head west 12.3 miles on I-290 to the Muschke Road exit and turn right. Go 6.8 miles to Draper Road and turn left. There is a sign for Kleb Woods on Muschke Road. The parking lot is 0.24 miles on the left.

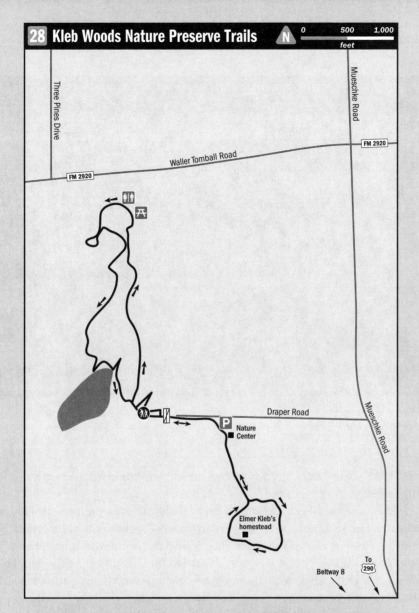

28 Kleb Woods Nature Preserve Trails

N

0   500   1,000
feet

Three Pines Drive

Mueschke Road

FM 2920

Waller Tomball Road

FM 2920

Draper Road

Mueschke Road

P Nature Center

Elmer Kleb's homestead

To 290

Beltway 8

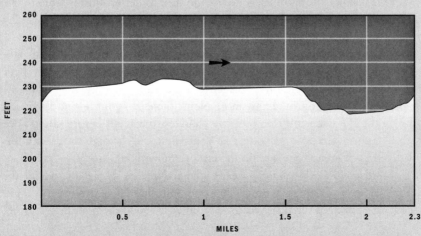

FEET

260
250
240
230
220
210
200
190
180

0.5   1   1.5   2   2.3

MILES

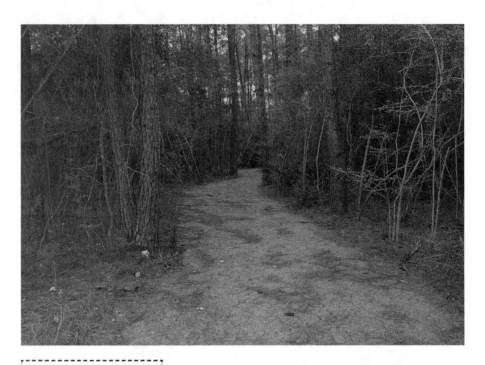

The dirt trail in Kleb Woods

Follow the shady trail as it winds amid thick vegetation and beneath tall lob-lolly pines.

There are small pink trail markers on the sides of the trail to help you navigate. The wide trail is mostly dirt with some pine needles. Continue past a trail marker on the left to a clearing. Farmland lies beyond the trees to the right. At a fork, bear right, past some very tall loblolly pines. As the trail heads downhill slightly, the forest floor opens up considerably on both sides. This part of the trail is prone to flooding after heavy rains. If there is water on the trail, there is usually room on the sides of the trail to get around it. Due to the presence of standing water, mosquitoes in this area are particularly bad. Bring bug repellent and use it.

Continue through the open area and head uphill. Now the trail widens, but with thicker vegetation on both sides. Go past a marker on the left, then bear right at an intersection to get on a crushed-granite trail that wanders past picnic tables and campsites. Continue past more picnic tables on your left and a marsh on your right. The wide trail temporarily changes to asphalt before going back to crushed granite. Go past restrooms on your right and through the next inter-section. There is a water fountain on the left, along with additional picnic tables and a covered pavilion. At a fork, bear right and pass a garbage can and the pavilion, both on your left. Go down the short spur and circle around a fire pit. Exit the loop back onto the trail you used to enter it and at the next intersection, go right. Continue past more picnic tables until you come to the next intersection. Take the right fork to get back onto the dirt trail. Fork right again, staying in the trees and on the dirt trail.

The trail is now more open. At a yellow marker, the trail turns left. Continue past another marker on the left as the trail curves left. At a fork, bear right, then curve left. A wetlands area, on the right, has many Chinese tallow trees. Continue through an overgrown area where trees hanging over the trail make progress a bit more difficult, causing you to have to duck in some areas. At a fork, bear right, now in a tunnel of trees. Soon you reach the roadlike trail that you started on. Head left to go back through the gate and onto Draper Road. Once back at the parking lot, turn right to head toward the nature center. Follow the Nature Trail sign.

Continue through a gate at the Nature Trail sign to get onto a crushed-granite trail. The vegetation is greener here, indicating increased sunlight reaching the forest floor. Hike past several lights on the left side of the trail and a road-runner-crossing sign on the right. The trail is about 10 feet wide here with the appearance of a road. There are several nature signs pointing out different trees and bushes, including American beautyberry, yaupon, sugarberry, lantana, dewberry, and loblolly pine. Go past a sign on the left describing the importance of brush piles in the forest to protect insects from winter freezes. Continue past the nature center on the left and go left around the building. Go to the right through two marked gardens to get on the trail heading away from the nature center. The trail here is very wide, with thick vegetation on both sides. It winds past nature signs on Schumard's oak, bladderpod, and water oak. Notice the lichen and moss growing on the base of many of the trees, indicating a damp environment. As the trail takes a big bend right, it gets more open and less overgrown. Continue past nature signs on water oak and pecan trees. As you reach the nature sign on the muscadine, left, you can see Elmer Kleb's old homestead ahead.

Go around the homestead to the right and then right again around the cornfield. Head back to the nature center and go left to retrace the trail you used originally. Just across from the nature center is a sign describing Elmer's hardware supply. Mr. Kleb was apparently frugal and allowed his neighbors to dump their trash here, so that he could use parts to fix things of his that broke. You can see cages, farm implements, car parts, and just garbage in his hardware-supply pile. Continue along the trail to the parking lot.

NEARBY ACTIVITIES

Tomball, a small town specializing in antiques stores, is just north of the preserve; Cullen Park, Bear Creek Pioneers Park, and George Bush Park are just a few minutes south and east. For information on overnight camping, call (281) 496-2177.

29 JESSE H. JONES PARK:
East Trails

KEY AT-A-GLANCE INFORMATION

LENGTH: 2.2 miles

CONFIGURATION: Loop with short out-and-back

DIFFICULTY: Easy

SCENERY: Woodlands, drainage channel, wetlands, Akokisa Indian Village

EXPOSURE: Shady

TRAIL TRAFFIC: Light weekdays, moderate weekends

TRAIL SURFACE: Asphalt

HIKING TIME: 1 hour

DRIVING DISTANCE: 12.36 miles from the intersection of Beltway 8 and I-59

ACCESS: Free; March to October, 8 a.m.–7 p.m.; November and February, 8 a.m.–6 p.m.; December and January, 8 a.m.–5 p.m.

MAPS: USGS Maedan; trail maps available

WHEELCHAIR ACCESS: Yes, on most trails

FACILITIES: Restrooms, nature center, parking, picnic areas, playgrounds, fishing on Spring Creek, historical sites

GPS TRAILHEAD COORDINATES

LATITUDE: N 30° 1.445'
LONGITUDE: W 95° 17.607'

IN BRIEF

The East Trails hike at Jesse H. Jones Park uses the Jones Bender and Homestead trails. The Jones Bender Trail is a rectangular loop that starts and ends at the first parking lot on the right as you enter the park. The Homestead Trail is in the middle of the Jones Bender Trail and is an out-and-back trail that takes you to the Redbud Hill Homestead and the Akokisa Indian Village. The homestead is a re-creation of an 1820–1830 East Texas homestead, and the Akokisa Indian Village sits adjacent to the homestead. Both are open for self-guided touring on Wednesdays and Saturdays, 1–4 p.m.

DESCRIPTION

The East Trails hike starts from the first parking lot on your right as you enter the park. Hike toward the Homestead Trail sign and head left to the trailhead for the Jones Bender Trail. This trail is part of the Spring Creek Greenway project that has extended trails throughout the park and is the only trail in Jesse H. Jones Park open to bikes on weekdays only. The trail surface is asphalt and runs along a riparian floodplain ecosystem. Continue on the trail to the first nature sign pointing out the Texas sugarberry tree, which is noted for the corky warts found on the bark. Go through an intersection, where a trail joins on the left.

Directions ⟶

From the intersection of Beltway 8 and I-59, head north 4.66 miles on I-59 to FM 1960 and turn left. Go 1.7 miles to Kenswick Drive and turn right. Go 1 mile to the end of the road and the entrance to the park. Park headquarters are immediately on your left as you enter. The parking lot is on your right.

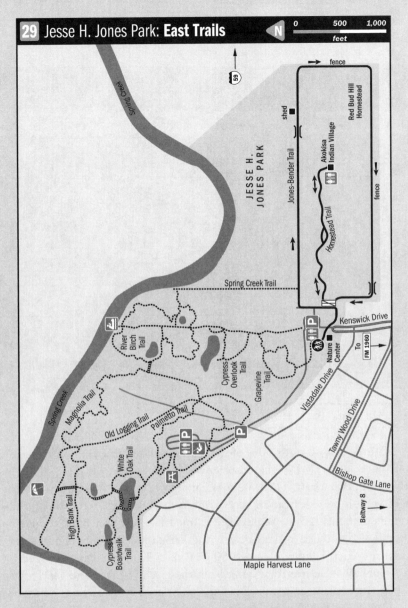

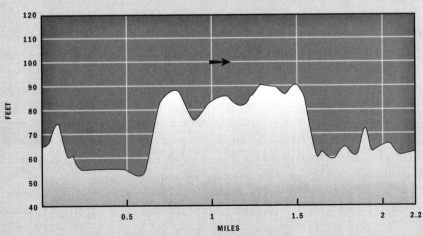

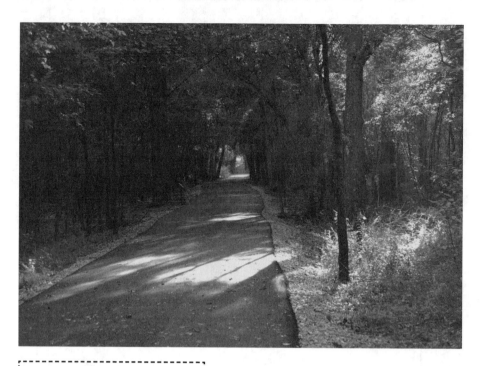

The asphalt surface of the east trails

Nature signs on both sides of the trail supply information on the trees and plants in the area. One of the first signs is on water oak, the most common oak in the floodplain forest. The water oaks and pines are the main trees that canopy over the 10-foot-wide trail. There is more than enough room on the trail to accommodate hikers and cyclists at the same time. Just remember to hike on the right, allowing cyclists room to pass. Another nature sign points out sweetgum, which can reach heights of up to 80–150 feet. They are characterized by the spiny gumball structures that hang from the tree until ripe and then fall to the ground. Other plants in the park include cedar elm, water hickory, yaupon holly, American holly, and red oak.

Continue past a small creek on the left and up a steep incline, as the trail heads for a flood-control channel. Go through an intersection with a trail on the right; there is a bench on the left. The flood-control channel, which was built as a flood-control channel for the area neighborhoods, is a good spot to look for some of the area's native mammals, including opossum, raccoons, armadillos, swamp rabbits, squirrels, coyotes, bobcats, deer, and beavers. Birds include the pileated woodpecker, red-bellied woodpecker, red-shouldered hawk, barred owl, cardinal, crow, mockingbird, blue jay, wood duck, egret, and heron. There are more than 30 kinds of snakes in Jesse H. Jones Park, but only the copperhead, coral snake, and cottonmouth are poisonous.

The bridge over the drainage channel is the only open part of the hike; otherwise, the trail is almost exclusively under the canopy of trees. Once across the bridge, there is a nature-viewing blind to the left, which has small slits in the wall facing the water and the wetlands below. Continue hiking uphill to where the forest floor gets denser on both sides of the trail. The trail nears the park-boundary fence, which is now on your left. The fence continues to the left of the trail, with dense forest on your right. As the trail starts downhill, the forest floor on the right opens considerably, with young trees. Soon the trail curves right, taking you back west. The fence, which continues to be on the left, is now the boundary for the south side of the park. The forest floor gets denser and the trail continues to head downhill.

Continue down the hill past a bench and into another section of the flood-control channel, where there is a large birdhouse and a wetlands on the right. The drainage channel, although artificial, has created a wetlands that attracts egrets, herons, ibis, plovers, and sandpipers. Several species of dragonflies may also be found hovering nearby. Hike up the other side of the drainage channel and back onto the shaded trail, past very dense undergrowth on the right. There is a nature sign for post oak, a member of the white oak family, on the right. Now go through an intersection where a trail joins on the right. The vegetation on the left is now very thick, but the right side has opened, allowing better visibility into the woods. Cross a small bridge and continue down the trail.

The trail curves past a neighborhood swimming pool and tennis courts, both left. The park-boundary fence is still on the left but it is now marking the west side of the park. Continue as the trail descends and curves left, allowing you to see the parking lot up ahead. Exit the Jones Bender Trail and bear right through the parking lot to the trailhead for the Homestead Trail. Take a right out of the parking lot to get on the 0.6-mile out-and-back trail and go through a wooden gate. The trail surface is now crushed granite and continues to be very wide. There is a bench on the right where the trail swings right. The forest floor is very open, as the understory vegetation does not get enough sunlight to allow for much growth. Continue past a nature sign on greenbriar, a root food source for Native Americans. There is considerable moss on the trees, indicating that the area stays moist.

Bear left at an intersection and then go straight through the next one. Park maintenance buildings are on the right about 75 yards. Continue past a nature sign describing Hercules club, a tree better known as the toothache tree due to its numbing effects when applied to an afflicted area. Go past a bench on the right and an old wood fence on the left. The trail curves right and into the Red-bud Hill Homestead and Akokisa Indian Village. The homestead has a log cabin, smokehouse, root cellar, chicken house, garden, bread oven, privy, woodworking shop, blacksmith shop, barn, and corral. The Akokisa were encountered by early 18th-century explorers, and a large Akokisa village was located just across Spring Creek from the present-day park. By the 1850s, the Akokisas had either merged with other tribes in the area or had died from European diseases. This village represents their way of life, showing that they were skilled at making dugout canoes from cypress logs and tanning hides from bearskins. The village also features a hut, chickee, lean-to, sweat lodge, and council lodge.

At the homestead and village, turn around and retrace the Homestead Trail. At a fork, bear left; a nearby nature sign describes Alabama supplejack and sassafras. Sassafras, used by Native Americans for medicinal purposes, now flavors root beer. Take the next left fork, past a bench on your right. The hike soon ends at the Homestead Trail trailhead and the parking lot.

Note: Children under 12 must be supervised at all times and no pets are allowed in the park. Venomous snakes, fire ants, and poison ivy are found along the trails, so stay alert and stay on the trail: park rules prohibit hiking off the developed trails. Fishing is allowed in Spring Creek only; bicycles are allowed on most hiking trails only on Sundays, 8 a.m.–noon, except on the Jones Bender Trail, where they are permitted also during the week (but not on Saturday).

NEARBY ACTIVITIES

Guided nature and pioneer tours for school groups are available at the park. The nature center is open year-round, 8 a.m.–4:30 p.m., except when the park is closed. Call ahead to ensure that it is open. Lake Houston Park is just a few miles north, off I-59. The Spring Creek Greenway, which runs from Burroughs Park to Jesse H. Jones Park, is part of the Sam Houston Trail & Wilderness Preserve. It will eventually connect these parks running along Spring Creek through the George Mitchell Nature Preserve, Montgomery County Preserve, Old Riley Fuzzel Road Preserve, Peckinpaugh Preserve, and Pundt Park.

JESSE H. JONES PARK:
West Trails

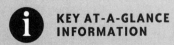

IN BRIEF

This hike uses parts of the Palmetto, High Bank, White Oak, Old Logging, Cypress Boardwalk, and Picnic Loop trails. These trails are open to bikes on Sunday mornings only. The High Bank and Old Logging trails both lead directly to the beaches at Spring Creek.

DESCRIPTION

Start the West Trails hike at the Palmetto Trail. All of these trails have trailhead signs, making it very easy to follow this hike. At the Palmetto Trail trailhead, take the left fork heading northwest. The trail surface is asphalt and is about 4 or 5 feet wide. The trail winds into the trees; the forest floor is dense with pine needles hanging down from trees creating an eerie sensation.

Soon you gain better visibility into the woods, because the tall, moss-covered trees have kept most vegetation, other than fan palms, from taking root on the forest floor. At a trailhead sign, go straight on the Cypress Boardwalk Trail. As with the East Trails hike, there are nature signs along the way. Plants in the park include the cedar elm, water hickory,

KEY AT-A-GLANCE INFORMATION

LENGTH: 2.1 miles

CONFIGURATION: Loop

DIFFICULTY: Easy

SCENERY: Woodlands, bald cypress stands, drainage channel, creeks, wetlands, boardwalks, beach

EXPOSURE: Shady

TRAIL TRAFFIC: Light

TRAIL SURFACE: Asphalt and boardwalk

HIKING TIME: 1 hour

DRIVING DISTANCE: 12.36 miles from the intersection of Beltway 8 and I-59

ACCESS: Free; March to October, 8 a.m.–7 p.m.; November and February, 8 a.m.–6 p.m.; December and January, 8 a.m.–5 p.m.

MAPS: USGS Maedan; trail maps available

WHEELCHAIR ACCESS: Yes, on most trails

FACILITIES: Restrooms, nature center, parking, picnic areas, playgrounds, fishing on Spring Creek, historical sites

---

Directions ➝

From the intersection of Beltway 8 and I-59, head north 4.66 miles on I-59 to FM 1960 and turn left. Go 1.7 miles to Kenswick Drive and turn right. Go 1 mile to the end of the road and the entrance to the park. To get to the West Trails hike, park in the lot in the back of the park. Once you enter the park, drive past the nature center and take a left after the restrooms. Follow the park road to the first parking lot on your right and park just adjacent to a swing and benches. The trailhead for the Palmetto Trail is just right of the lot.

GPS TRAILHEAD COORDINATES

LATITUDE: N 30° 1.682'
LONGITUDE: W 95° 17.928'

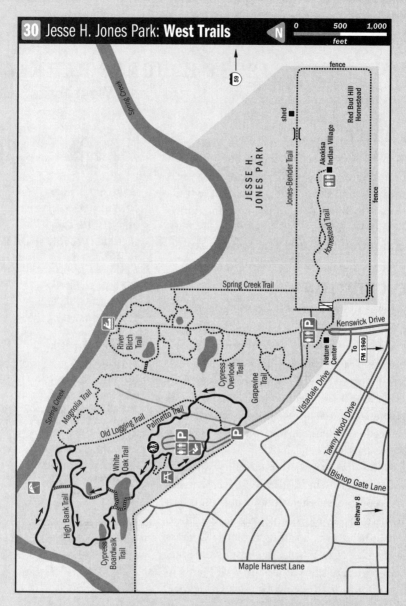

0   500   1,000
feet

N

Spring Creek

59

JESSE H. JONES PARK

fence

shed

Red Bud Hill Homestead

Jones-Bender Trail

Akokisa Indian Village

Homestead Trail

fence

Spring Creek Trail

Kenswick Drive

River Birch Trail

Cypress Overlook Trail

Grapevine Trail

Nature Center

To FM 1960

Spring Creek

Magnolia Trail

Old Logging Trail

Palmetto Trail

Vistadale Drive

Tawny Wood Drive

White Oak Trail

Bishop Gate Lane

Beltway 8

High Bank Trail

Cypress Boardwalk Trail

Maple Harvest Lane

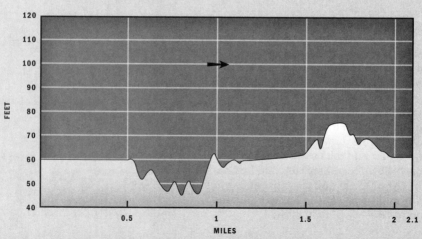

120
110
100
90
80
70
60
50
40

FEET

0.5   1   1.5   2   2.1

MILES

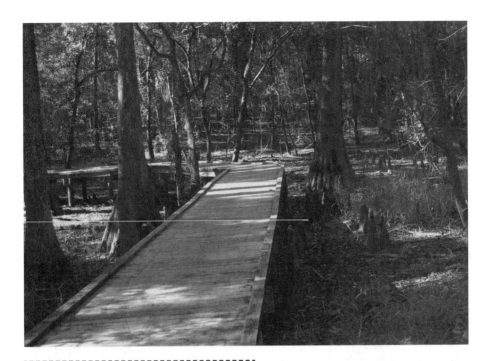

The Cypress Boardwalk Trail over a cypress bog

yaupon holly, American holly, Southern red oak, and, in this area, bald cypress, which is characterized by "cypress knees," parts of the root system that stick up out of the water, at some distance from the trunk.

Bear right at the next intersection. Go past a bench and a nature sign for hip hawthorn, a tree that produces red berries in fall, providing food for many birds. At the next trailhead sign, take the right fork to get on the White Oak Trail. The trail curves left, taking you farther away from the park road behind you. To the left and through the trees is a marshy area. Continue on the White Oak Trail by turning right at the next intersection. (The sign also points the way to Spring Creek, which you can visit by going right a little past the White Oak Trail.) Now traverse an elevated boardwalk with bald cypresses lining both sides. This area can be quite wet, so stay on the boardwalk and do not let small children wander off it. Snakes are much more likely to be found in wet areas. A fallen magnolia, which is left and just off the trail, has actually taken root on the forest floor and supports several magnolias growing out of its trunk. Exit the boardwalk as the trail goes downhill and left to an intersection with the High Bank Trail. Turn right on the High Bank Trail and cross a bridge to your left.

Now there is a small creek to your left and forest on your right. As you head downhill, the trail winds to an area that is more open and possibly sunny. The trees are no longer so dense, allowing for more weeds and wildflowers. Continue past a bench on the right and take the left fork toward Spring Creek. Go straight through some low spots that may be muddy to get on the Old Logging Trail. The trail swings left as you hike between embankments. This part of the trail could be under water after heavy rains. A boggy marsh is on your left, about 40 yards off the trail. Stay on the trail as directed by park rules.

Soon the trail goes left and crosses an access road. Go straight through the next intersection, where a trail joins on the left. At the end of the Old Logging Trail, go right if you wish to visit the beaches of Spring Creek. The beach trail is dirt- and weed-covered but easy to follow. If you visited the beach, turn around and head back to the trail to continue the hike. Back on the trail, bear left, passing a garbage can on the right. At the next intersection, bear right onto an asphalt trail. Cross a wide bridge over a field of wildflowers and other low-lying vegetation. At the next intersection, bear right to rejoin the High Bank Trail. The trails swings sharply right and then winds to the next trailhead sign and a bench on the right.

Angle left, toward the Cypress Boardwalk Trail. Continue uphill as the trail curves left. The forest floor here is very dense and overgrown, with Spring Creek in the distance to your right. Stay on the Cypress Boardwalk Trail, ignoring the angler-access paths to Spring Creek. Go past a bench on the left and cross a bridge to get on a boardwalk ahead. Beyond the boardwalk, the forest floor opens, allowing better visibility. Veer slightly right to get on the next section of boardwalk. This is an extensive boardwalk system through the bald cypress trees, with the trail going right and then left. At a trailhead sign, bear left on the Cypress Boardwalk Loop. Bald cypress trees are on both sides of the boardwalk, creating an eerie and beautiful scene with the cypress knees sticking up out of the dark boggy water. Be aware of snakes in this part of the park. Once off the boardwalk, you get on an asphalt trail. At a trailhead sign, bear right to get back on the Cypress Boardwalk Trail. At the next trailhead sign, angle left. Go to the next intersection and turn right. Stay on the trail and do not take the shortcut that has been created by thoughtless hikers. Respect the park by staying on the trail.

At a fork veer right, then go right again on the Picnic Loop Trail, which takes you through a picnic area, past a playground and restrooms on your left. Just before you reach the parking lot, turn right at an intersection and walk past a dining hall on the right. Cross the park road and continue straight to get back on the Palmetto Trail. The trail winds between the park road, right, and a small creek, left. Go downhill to a grassy area on your right at the start of a flood-control channel that runs through the park. The flood-control channel, which was built for the area neighborhoods, is a good spot to look for some of the area's native mammals, including opossums, raccoons, armadillos, swamp rabbits, squirrels, coyotes, bobcats, deer, and beavers. Birds include the pileated woodpecker, red-bellied woodpecker, red-shouldered hawk, barred owl, cardinal, crow, mockingbird, blue jay, wood duck, egret, and heron. There are more than 30 kinds of snakes in Jesse H. Jones Park, but only the copperhead, coral snake, and cottonmouth are poisonous.

Continue past a bench on the left and through an intersection. Go straight at a trailhead sign, which points in the direction of the parking lot. As the trail curves right, continue until you reach the parking lot.

Note: Children under 12 must be supervised at all times and no pets are allowed in the park. Venomous snakes, fire ants, and poison ivy are found along the trails, so stay alert and stay on the trail: park rules prohibit hiking off the developed trails. Fishing is allowed in Spring Creek only; bicycles are allowed on most hiking trails only on Sundays, 8 a.m.–noon, except on the Jones Bender Trail, where they are permitted also during the week (but not on Saturday).

NEARBY ACTIVITIES

Guided nature and pioneer tours for school groups are available at the park. The nature center is open year-round, 8 a.m.–4:30 p.m., except when the park is closed. Call ahead to make sure the nature center is open. Lake Houston Park is just a few miles north, off I-59. The Spring Creek Greenway, which runs from Burroughs Park to Jesse H. Jones Park, is part of the Sam Houston Trail & Wilderness Preserve. It will eventually connect these parks running along Spring Creek through the George Mitchell Nature Preserve, Montgomery County Preserve, Old Riley Fuzzel Road Preserve, Peckinpaugh Preserve, and Pundt Park.

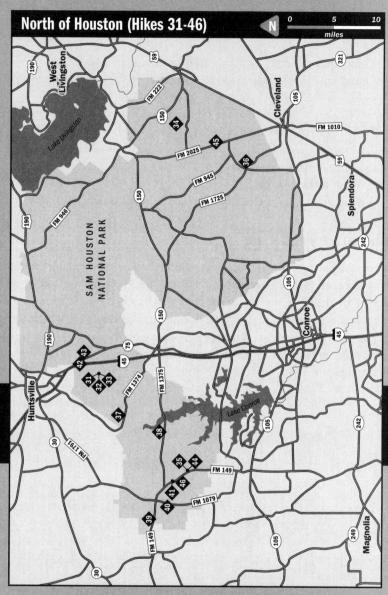

West
Livingston

190

59

FM 222

Lake Livingston

150

34

45

FM 2025

36

Cleveland

105

321

FM 1010

59

Splendora

242

FM 945

FM 1725

190

FM 946

150

SAM HOUSTON
NATIONAL PARK

150

105

Conroe

45

190

75

45

42 43

FM 1374

FM 1375

Lake Conroe

105

242

Huntsville

31
32 33

37

38

30

FM 1791

35 44

46

FM 149

41

40

105

249

39

FM 149

30

FM 1079

Magnolia

NORTH of HOUSTON
(INCLUDING HUNTSVILLE)

31 HUNTSVILLE STATE PARK:
Outer Loop

KEY AT-A-GLANCE INFORMATION

LENGTH: 8.6 miles

CONFIGURATION: Loop

DIFFICULTY: Moderate to difficult

SCENERY: Woodlands, marsh, lake, wetlands, spillway, boardwalks

EXPOSURE: Shady

TRAIL TRAFFIC: Light weekdays, moderate weekends

TRAIL SURFACE: Dirt and sand

HIKING TIME: 4 hours

DRIVING DISTANCE: 49 miles from the junction of Beltway 8 and I-45

ACCESS: $4 per person age 13 and older, or buy a yearly Texas State Parks Pass; open 8 a.m.–10 p.m.

MAPS: USGS Huntsville and Moore Grove; trail maps available

WHEELCHAIR ACCESS: None

FACILITIES: Restrooms, bathhouse, nature center, parking, picnic areas, camping, fishing piers, bike trails, park store, boat rentals, playground. There is no drinking water available on the trails. There are no restrooms on this hike except at the very beginning.

SPECIAL COMMENTS: Be cautious of bikers—the terrain is hilly and the trail is narrow. Boating on the lake is restricted to boats under 19 feet long, and water skiing is prohibited.

GPS TRAILHEAD COORDINATES

LATITUDE: N 30° 37.599'
LONGITUDE: W 95° 31.639'

IN BRIEF

Huntsville State Park is a 2,083-acre recreational area that was opened in 1938 but later closed in 1940 for ten years after a flood caused the dam spillway to collapse. It was officially reopened to the public in 1956. The park adjoins the Sam Houston National Forest and encloses Lake Raven. White-tailed deer, raccoon, opossum, armadillo, migratory waterfowl, and fox squirrel are just some of the wildlife found in the area. Located near the western edge of the Southern Pine Belt, the park is dominated by loblolly pines and shortleaf pines. The Outer Loop hike is long and has (for the Houston area) considerable elevation changes. Know your limits before starting on this hike and make sure you bring plenty of water, snacks, sunscreen, and a first-aid kit.

DESCRIPTION

The Outer Loop trail at Huntsville State Park includes parts of the Chinquapin and the Triple C trails. Start the hike at the trailhead behind the nature center, located just inside the park. There are restrooms, parking, picnic tables, and water fountains in this area. From the trailhead, follow the dirt- and pineneedle–covered surface across an access road and back into the trees. The trail is very well maintained and easy to follow, but has considerable elevation changes throughout, making the 8.6-mile hike difficult for many. Although you can still

Directions

From the intersection of Beltway 8 and I-45, head north 49 miles on I-45 to Park Road 40 and turn left. The park entrance is approximately 2 miles ahead. Park on the right just past the park entrance at the nature center.

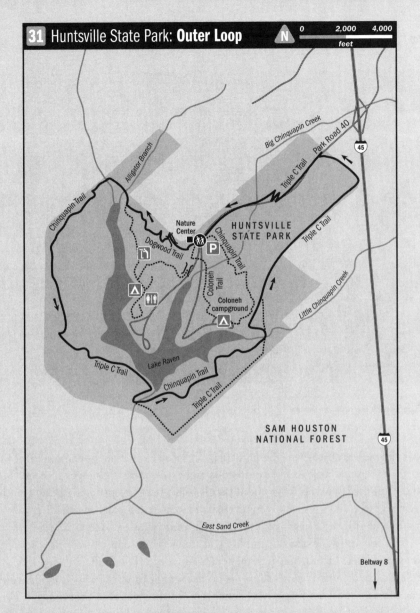

N

0   2,000   4,000

feet

Big Chinquapin Creek

Park Road 40

45

Chinquapin Trail

Alligator Branch

Triple C Trail

Nature Center

HUNTSVILLE STATE PARK

Dogwood Trail

Chinquapin Trail

P

Triple C Trail

Coloneh Trail

Coloneh campground

Little Chinquapin Creek

Triple C Trail

Lake Raven

Chinquapin Trail

Chinquapin Trail

Triple C Trail

SAM HOUSTON NATIONAL FOREST

45

East Sand Creek

Beltway 8

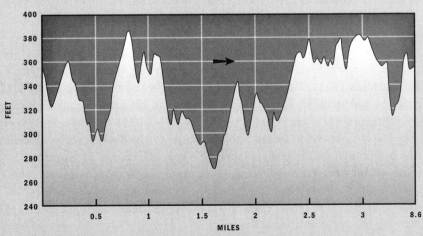

FEET							
	0.5	1	1.5	2	2.5	3	8.6

MILES

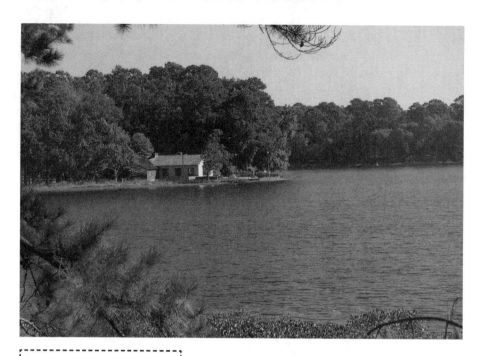

The boathouse on Lake Raven

hear the park traffic off to the left, you cannot see any evidence of a road, camp-sites, or picnic tables. As the trail bends right, the surface changes to more loose sand than dirt, making for some difficult hiking and even more difficult biking. Because the trail is also used by cyclists, stay alert. Also be aware of poisonous snakes and alligators near Lake Raven and some of the wetlands areas.

As the trail goes right it takes you deeper into the woods, past towering pines and oaks. Continue past a bench on the left and then curve left. The underbrush, although quite dense, is open enough to walk into, as evidenced by geocachers (GPS-wielding treasure hunters) in the park. Go past another bench on the right and continue across another access road. As you reenter the woods, the forest floor slopes considerably on your left. Cross a wooden bridge marked by a metal marker with the number 1. The trail goes uphill to the next intersection, where you go straight. Continue winding uphill for quite some time before descending. The trail here is about 3 feet wide, allowing for easy hiking, but if cyclists approach, step to the side as there is not enough room for both you and a bicycle. As you continue downhill, the footing can become tenuous, with the loose sand and exposed tree roots.

The forest floor opens on the right as you reach the bottom of the descent. Head back uphill on the other side of an embankment. The trail narrows here but is still easy to follow and consists more of pine needles than sand. At the next trail-head, bear right. Go past a bench on the right and continue straight through the next intersection to a bridge over a wetlands. Continue to a boardwalk, watching for snakes and other wildlife in the wetlands. Beyond the boardwalk, the root-crossed trail gets quite steep. Look left for the beginning of a marsh you will soon cross. Head left to get onto another boardwalk and continue past a large marsh on the left. Exit left to get back in the shade of the trees. Cross over a bridge marked number 5 and then over two small bridges marked number 6. The trail quickly becomes steep enough to have a few switchbacks before heading back uphill.

Continue uphill at a fairly steep incline and onto a part of the trail that is narrower and a bit overgrown. Although easy to follow, it seems this part of the trail is not used as much. Go past a bench on the right and then downhill on a long, straight section of trail. Once past the straight-away, the trail heads back uphill very steeply over loose, sandy soil. Cyclists have a particularly hard time traversing this section but hikers do just fine. On the next downhill, the surface becomes packed dirt. At the next bridge, cross a creek bed and then go back uphill on the other side. Swing right and across another bridge. You are now walking on the south side of the park heading east toward the spillway for Lake Raven. At the number 9 sign, cross a bridge and continue to the number 10 sign and another bridge. You can see Lake Raven to the left as the trail again goes uphill. At a fork, bear right, up a steep embankment and then back down the other side.

Now you are on an elevated section of trail, with the forest sloping steeply right. At the next intersection, go straight to the spillway. There is a bench immediately on the right, and the campgrounds and park headquarters are to the left, on the other side of Lake Raven. Go straight across the top of the spillway. This is a very open part of the hike, with a number of felled trees stacked on both sides of the trail to help control erosion along the spillway. Before you get to the end of the spillway, bear right down a steep embankment and back into the trees. There are a considerable number of small dead pines in this area, but there are enough tall trees for shade. As the trail bends left, cross a deep creek via a bridge with no railings—stay to the center for a safe crossing. Once you cross a bridge marked 12, the spillway is now on your left with a marsh on the right side of the spillway and Lake Raven on the left. Fork left up the spillway and then fork right when you are at the top. The trail here is about 10 to 12 feet wide.

Continue past a viewing stand on the left as the trail swings right. This part of the trail is part of the spillway access road, so watch for maintenance vehicles. At the next fork, bear left past a bench to get back on the trail. Go uphill over roots and continue straight through the next intersection, beyond which the trail narrows. Head downhill, turn sharply right, and then cross a bridge marked 13. Bear left and then over a bridge marked 14. You can still see Lake Raven on your left, but you are now on the east side of the park headed north. Cross the number 15 bridge and then curve right. At the road bear left and go past a bench on the right. At a trail sign, take the left fork. Continue over bridge 16 and then take a right. Take the next fork left to get on the Triple C Trail. A fence marking the park boundary is immediately to the right. Just to the right of the fence is noisy I-45. Once past a park exit gate, the trail heads left, back into the trees. Continue past an observation stand on the right to a trail map ahead. The trail map is on Park Road 40, the park entrance road. Bear to the left to hike up the park road. Go past parking on the left and continue through the park gate. Cross Big Chinquapin Creek and head uphill on the road, past park headquarters. Head straight past a small parking lot on the right to the larger lot next to the nature center, where you parked.

Note: Alligators and poisonous snakes are occasionally observed in the park. Keep pets on leash. Stay on the trail at all times to protect you, the wildlife, and the vegetation.

NEARBY ACTIVITIES

Sam Houston Memorial and Park Complex (**samhouston.org**), the Texas Prison Museum (**txprisonmuseum.org**), H.E.A.R.T.S. Veterans Museum (**heartsmuseum .com**), Sam Houston National Forest, Lake Conroe.

HUNTSVILLE STATE PARK:
Chinquapin Trail

IN BRIEF

Huntsville State Park is a 2,083-acre recreational area that was opened in 1938 but later closed in 1940 for ten years after a flood caused the dam spillway to collapse. It was officially reopened to the public in 1956. The park adjoins the Sam Houston National Forest and encloses Lake Raven. White-tailed deer, raccoon, opossum, armadillo, migratory waterfowl, and fox squirrel are just some of the wildlife found in the area. Located near the western edge of the Southern Pine Belt, the park is dominated by loblolly pines and short-leaf pines. This hike includes part of the Coloneh Trail along with part of the Chinquapin Trail. It is an easy hike if you only have an hour and is accessible from the Coloneh Campground and the nature center parking lot.

DESCRIPTION

Start the hike by parking at the nature center and walking across Park Road 40 to the trailhead marked CHINQUAPIN TRAIL AND BICYCLE TRAIL. Once on the trail, fork left and then cross a sidewalk that connects the road to a parking lot on your right. Continue over the road into the parking lot, and then into the woods straight ahead. The trail surface is dirt with some loose sand and tree roots. It is about 3 feet wide with dense woodlands on both sides of the trail. Although this is an easy hike, watch your footing on the loose sand.

Directions

From the intersection of Beltway 8 and I-45, head north 49 miles on I-45 to Park Road 40 and turn left. The park entrance is approximately 2 miles ahead. Park on the right just past the park entrance at the nature center.

KEY AT-A-GLANCE INFORMATION

LENGTH: 2.2 miles

CONFIGURATION: Loop

DIFFICULTY: Easy

SCENERY: Woodlands, marsh, lake, boardwalk, campsites

EXPOSURE: Shady

TRAIL TRAFFIC: Light weekdays, moderate weekends

TRAIL SURFACE: Dirt and sand

HIKING TIME: 1 hour

DRIVING DISTANCE: 49 miles from the intersection of Beltway 8 and I-45

ACCESS: $4 per person age 13 and older, or buy a yearly Texas State Parks Pass; open 8 a.m.–10 p.m.

MAPS: USGS Huntsville and Moore Grove; trail maps available

WHEELCHAIR ACCESS: None

FACILITIES: Restrooms, bathhouse, nature center, parking, picnic areas, camping, fishing piers, bike trails, park store, boat rentals, playground. There are no restrooms on this hike except at the very beginning.

SPECIAL COMMENTS: Be cautious of bikers—the terrain is hilly and the trail is narrow. Boating on the lake is restricted to boats under 19 feet long, and water skiing is prohibited.

GPS TRAILHEAD COORDINATES

LATITUDE: N 30° 37.599'
LONGITUDE: W 95° 31.639'

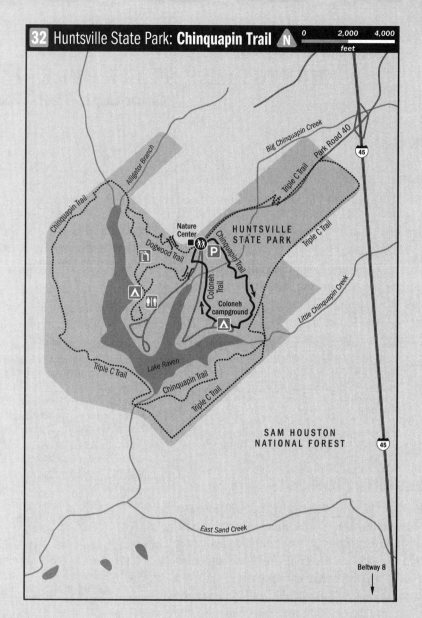

Big Chinquapin Creek

Park Road 40

45

Triple C Trail

Triple C Trail

Alligator Branch

Chinquapin Trail

Nature Center

Dogwood Trail

P

HUNTSVILLE STATE PARK

Chinquapin Trail

Coloneh Trail

Coloneh campground

Little Chinquapin Creek

Triple C Trail

Lake Raven

Chinquapin Trail

Triple C Trail

SAM HOUSTON NATIONAL FOREST

East Sand Creek

Beltway 8

45

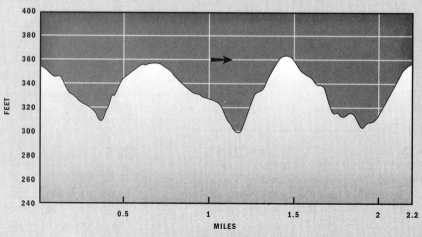

FEET

400
380
360
340
320
300
280
260
240

0.5   1   1.5   2   2.2

MILES

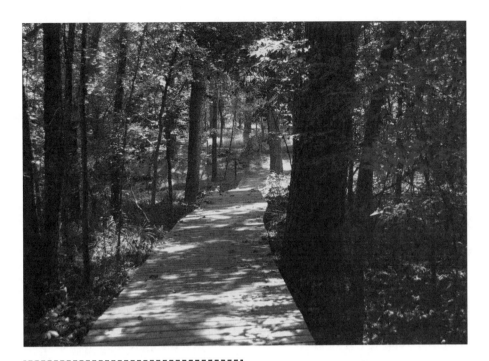

A boardwalk crossing Big Chinquapin Creek

Cross an elevated boardwalk, then step off the boardwalk and bear right on a shady, well-used trail.

Be aware of spider webs across the trail from spring to early fall. The leaf-cluttered trail bends sharply left and then right, heading downhill. At a fork marked by a green metal marker, angle right. The trail is mostly sand but with some indications that this is also an equestrian trail. Take a left toward a board-walk ahead. The boardwalk crosses Big Chinquapin Creek and heads downhill and to the right. Go left off the boardwalk and uphill. There are many fan palms growing among the pines and oaks, making the forest floor here more lush and green than in other areas of the park.

Swing right and uphill again as the trail surface is once again more loose sand than dirt, making for difficult hiking and even more difficult biking. Because the trail is also used by bikers, stay alert. Hike down into a small creek bed and then head uphill and out of the creek bed. The trail narrows to only a few feet wide but is still easy to follow. As it widens, the trail heads downhill steeply over large tree roots and then goes right. Continue via wooden steps that aid the steep descent. The trail continues winding downhill toward a park road, picnic tables, and campsites.

At the next intersection, fork right, past a bench on the right, to head toward the park road and past a trail map. At the map, head straight and then right to get on the park road. You are in the middle of the Coloneh camp-sites, with a restroom just across the road to the left. Continue until you reach campsite 116. Head right, into the trees, onto the Coloneh Trail. Although there is no trailhead marker, the trail is easily seen from the park road. During fall and spring, there could be a number of Scout groups in the area. The Coloneh Trail is about 4–5 feet wide with dense forest on both sides. At a fork marked by a Loblolly Pine Trail sign, bear right onto an access road. The trail heads uphill and left, with a water treatment station on the right. At the next intersection, veer left on the well-shaded trail.

At a park road, cross and head right, hiking on the road. There is a trailer dumping station to your right, campsites behind you, and a trail behind the trees on your left. Although you can see the trail through the trees, stay on the road until you get to a designated trailhead. Continue past parking spaces on the left and then veer left into the trees. Take the next fork right, putting the park road now on your right and the forest on your left. At a creek, head right to get back to the road to cross the creek via a bridge. Once off the bridge, go left to get back on the trail. Continue straight to the trail bearing right. Now you are hiking between two park roads. Cross a small bridge and then the park road, heading back into the trees and to the trail. Bear right and cross another bridge. The park road you crossed is now on your right, with parking straight ahead. The trail heads uphill and left. Go past a bench on the right and hike across an access road. Just past the road is the nature center, near where you parked. Here there are restrooms, picnic tables, and benches. Continue past the nature center in the parking lot to your car and the end of the hike.

Note: Keep pets on leash. Stay on the trail at all times to protect you, the wildlife, and the vegetation.

NEARBY ACTIVITIES

Sam Houston Memorial and Park Complex (**samhouston.org**), the Texas Prison Museum (**txprisonmuseum.org**), H.E.A.R.T.S. Veterans Museum (**heartsmuseum .com**), Sam Houston National Forest, Lake Conroe.

HUNTSVILLE STATE PARK:
Dogwood Trail

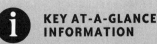

IN BRIEF

Huntsville State Park is a 2,083-acre recreational area that was opened in 1938 but later closed in 1940 for ten years after a flood caused the dam spillway to collapse. It was officially reopened to the public in 1956. The park adjoins the Sam Houston National Forest and encloses Lake Raven. White-tailed deer, raccoon, opossum, armadillo, migratory waterfowl, and fox squirrel are just some of the wildlife found in the area. Located near the western edge of the Southern Pine Belt, the park is dominated by loblolly pines and shortleaf pines. The Dogwood Trail to Prairie Branch Trail is a moderate hike with some elevation changes. It is not long but can be a challenge for hikers who have limited physical abilities.

DESCRIPTION

The Dogwood Trail hike includes parts of the Dogwood Trail, the Prairie Branch Trail, and the Chinquapin Trail. Start the hike at the trailhead to the left of the nature center, located just inside the park. There are restrooms, parking, picnic tables, and water fountains at the nature center. Head toward the Dogwood Trail sign and go left to start the hike. The trail surface is mostly dirt with old pieces of asphalt. The park road is on your left, with dense woodlands on your right. Hike across an access road and go straight to get back on

KEY AT-A-GLANCE INFORMATION

LENGTH: 3.2 miles

CONFIGURATION: Loop

DIFFICULTY: Moderate

SCENERY: Woodlands, marsh, lake

EXPOSURE: Shady

TRAIL TRAFFIC: Light weekdays, moderate weekends

TRAIL SURFACE: Dirt and sand

HIKING TIME: 1.5 hours

DRIVING DISTANCE: 49 miles from the intersection of Beltway 8 and I-45

ACCESS: $4 per person age 13 and older, or buy a yearly Texas State Parks Pass; open 8 a.m.–10 p.m.

MAPS: USGS Huntsville and Moore Grove; trail maps available

WHEELCHAIR ACCESS: None

FACILITIES: Restrooms, bathhouse, nature center, parking, picnic areas, camping, fishing piers, bike trails, park store, boat rentals, playground

SPECIAL COMMENTS: Be cautious of bikers—the terrain is hilly and the trail is narrow. Boating on the lake is restricted to boats under 19 feet long, and water skiing is prohibited. There is no drinking water available on the trails, and the only restrooms are at the very beginning of the hike.

GPS TRAILHEAD COORDINATES

LATITUDE: N 30° 37.599'
LONGITUDE: W 95° 31.639'

Directions ———————————————➤

From the intersection of Beltway 8 and I-45, head north on I-45 49 miles to Park Road 40 and turn left. The park entrance is approximately 2 miles ahead. Park on the right just past the park entrance at the nature center.

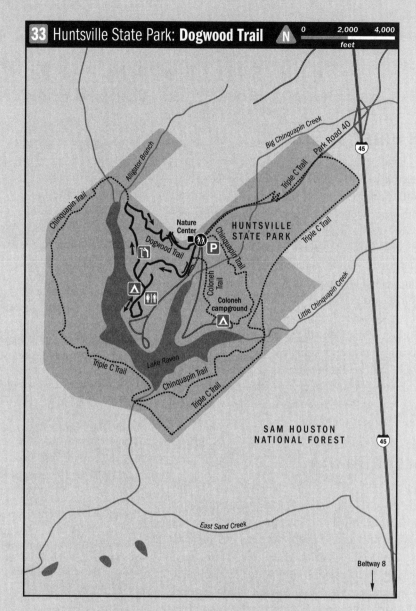

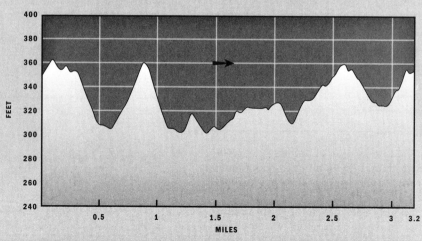

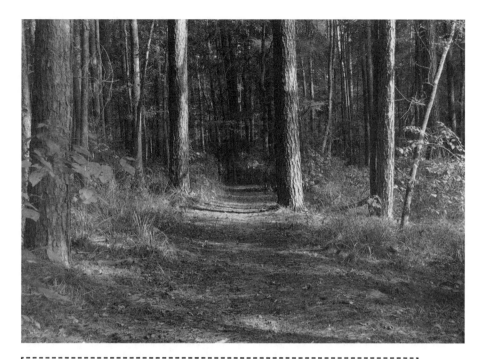

The wide, well-groomed trails of Huntsville State Park are used by hikers and cyclists.

the trail. The vegetation here consists of tall loblolly pines, oaks, and thick shrubs such as elderberry and holly.

The trail winds steeply downhill. Continue past a bench on the left as the trail zigzags toward the park road. Go past some parking spaces, left, before crossing a bridge marked 20. Once off the bridge, the trail heads uphill. Continue through an intersection and look ahead for Lake Raven in the distance through the trees. Take a right fork to stay on the Dogwood Trail. There is a trail sign ahead but it is for hikers coming the other way. The trail heads uphill and away from the road, narrowing to only about 4 feet wide. A large clearing with many fallen trees—evidence of storms such as Hurricane Rita—is to the right and in other parts of the park.

Cross a service road and go straight to stay on the trail. Especially from late spring to early fall, be aware of spider webs across the trail and try to hike under them. Continue across another service road and head straight and downhill. There are loose rocks here: be careful and go slow until the trail levels.

Parts of the trail have been washed out, and the center of it is a good foot below the sides. Either hike down the middle or hike on either side of the recessed area. The trail continues downhill with a peek at Lake Raven up ahead. Although you can see the lake from this route, you don't ever get close to it. The trail narrows to about a foot wide and then widens again as you reach an intersection. Take the left fork going downhill. Campsites are now visible on your right, with restrooms and a playground up ahead. These are the last available restrooms until the end of the hike. At a HIKE AND BIKE TRAIL sign on your left, turn around and retrace to the previous intersection. Now bear left and then immediately right to get on the signed Prairie Branch Trail. The ascending trail has exposed tree roots, so be careful and watch your footing. This is a wide dirt trail of 5 feet or more that heads away from the campgrounds and back into the woods. Pass by a viewing stand on the left and head downhill as the trail bends left. As you go by a trail marker on your left, the trail heads downhill and left. Roller-coaster past several more trail markers. Look to your left for a marsh through the trees. At the signed Chinquapin Trail, bear right and then wind uphill. Go straight at an intersection marked by a HIKING TRAIL sign. The trail descends steeply to a bridge, then ascends just beyond. Continue across an access road and past a viewing stand on your right. Cross a service road and go slightly right to get back on the trail. The trail heads uphill slightly before you come to the end of the hike and the nature center. At the trail map on the left, go right to get to the parking lot.

Note: Alligators and poisonous snakes are occasionally observed in the park. Keep pets on leash. Stay on the trail at all times to protect you, the wildlife, and the vegetation.

NEARBY ACTIVITIES

Sam Houston Memorial and Park Complex (**samhouston.org**), the Texas Prison Museum (**txprisonmuseum.org**), H.E.A.R.T.S. Veterans Museum (**heartsmuseum .com**), Sam Houston National Forest, Lake Conroe.

BIG CREEK SCENIC RECREATION AREA: Big Creek Loops

IN BRIEF

The Big Creek Loops consist of four short loops just inside the Big Creek Scenic Recreation Area. This is the only hike on the Lone Star Hiking Trail that is part of the recreation area.

The Sam Houston National Forest is one of four national forests in Texas. It contains more than 163,000 acres and is located between Huntsville, Conroe, Cleveland, and Richards. The district ranger's office is located on FM 1375, 3 miles west of New Waverly. Archeological evidence that dates back 7,000 years has been found in a number of sites in the national forest. Any artifacts found must not be disturbed, as they are protected by federal and state regulations. Hiking, fishing, and hunting are allowed in most of the national forest. Check the website for the Sam Houston National Forest at **www .fs.fed.us** for more information.

DESCRIPTION

The Big Creek Scenic Recreation Area loops, which include parts of the Lone Star Hiking Trail, consist of four loops that are all accessed from the parking lot on Forest Service Road 217. Start the hike at the HIKER TRAIL sign and head into the woods past an information sign on the left and a bench on the right. There is a creek on the left as you head uphill on the

---

Directions

From the intersection of Beltway 8 and I-59, head north 31 miles. On I-59 exit at FM 2025, and turn left. Go 10 miles to FM 2666 and turn right. Go 2.5 miles to FS Road 221 and turn left. Drive 0.5 miles to FS 217, turn right, and go 0.9 miles to the trailhead, on the left.

KEY AT-A-GLANCE INFORMATION

LENGTH: 2.7 miles

CONFIGURATION: Loops

DIFFICULTY: Easy

SCENERY: Woodlands, creeks

EXPOSURE: Shady

TRAIL TRAFFIC: Light

TRAIL SURFACE: Dirt

HIKING TIME: 2.5 hours

DRIVING DISTANCE: 45 miles from the intersection of Beltway 8 and I-59

ACCESS: Free

MAPS: USGS Camilla; trail map available at the Lone Star Hiking Trail Club website, lshtclub.com

WHEELCHAIR ACCESS: None

FACILITIES: Parking, trail markers

SPECIAL COMMENTS: There are no facilities on many of the trails in the Sam Houston National Forest except for parking, so make sure you bring sunscreen, bug repellent, water, and food. Pets must remain on a leash at all times. Motorized vehicles and bicycles are not allowed on the trails in the national forest. Wear appropriate footwear and long pants whenever hiking in the Sam Houston National Forest.

GPS TRAILHEAD COORDINATES

LATITUDE: N 30° 30.296'

LONGITUDE: W 95° 5.339'

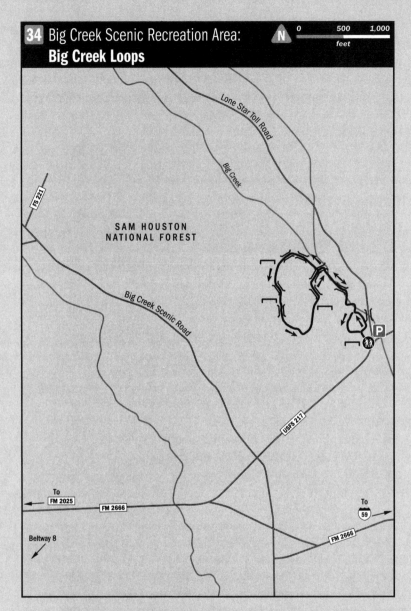

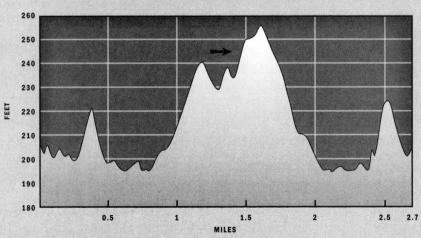

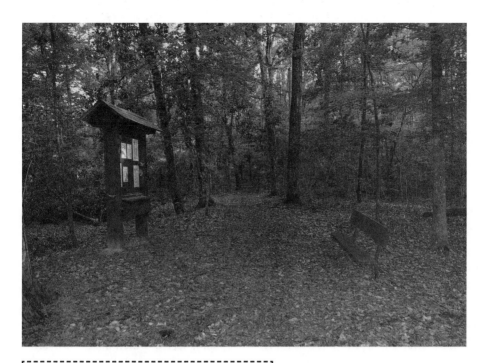

An information sign at the trailhead for Big Creek Loops

wide dirt trail. The vegetation on the forest floor is very thick with tall oak trees towering above. Continue on the trail as it heads steeply uphill via steps. At an intersection there is a sign about the local wildlife, which includes wood ducks, armadillos, copperheads, river otters, red-shouldered hawks, bobcats, green anoles, and Carolina wrens. A map of the Big Creek trails is on the right. Bear right, and look for silver markers in the trees to help guide you. If during any hike on the Lone Star Hiking Trail you have not seen a nearby marker in a few minutes, stop and get your bearings: look ahead and to both sides and you should be able to see a marker in the distance.

At the double trail markers on a post straight ahead, fork left and head downhill. Cross a small bridge and follow the trail markers as the trail winds through the trees, with a deep creek bed on your right. The foliage is close to the trail, so wear long pants to help protect you from poison ivy, poison sumac, and poison oak. The trail now heads uphill with a boggy area on your right. There are considerable lichen and moss growing on the rocks and roots in this area, indicating a very damp environment.

At the next intersection, follow trail signs and bear right to get on a board-walk over a creek. This bridge can be quite bouncy so take your time. Once off the bridge, watch your footing as there are numerous exposed tree roots. The trail heads uphill and bends left, away from the creek. Watch for spider webs across the trail when hiking from early spring to late fall, and try to duck under them. Go past a trail marker on the left as the trail curves left and then heads downhill. Go slightly left to cross a bridge. There is a deep creek bed on your left as the trail heads uphill and out of a low area. The woods are very dense and dark here. Cross a small creek bed and head uphill out of the creek bed. The trail widens, crosses a sunken bridge, and then swings left.

Go past a sign for the Magnolia Trail on the right. This loop is closed due to unsafe conditions and excessive erosion. Continue past another Magnolia Loop sign on the right, then cross two small bridges. The trail narrows to only a small footpath past the second bridge. At the next intersection, there is a trail sign for the Big Creek Loops. Turn right to get on the Big Creek Trail and hike past an M marker and a number 74 marker in the tree on the left. These markers indicate that you are on the Lone Star Hiking Trail at mile 74 from the start of the trail. The trail heads uphill slightly. Cross another bridge and amble along a very straight stretch. The trail widens to 3–4 feet before reaching a bridge; cross it and then head uphill, out of the creek bed.

Now go straight through an intersection. The trail heads uphill and bends left. There are orange trail markers along the trail and orange blazes on the trees. Go across a bridge and head up the other side of the embankment over steps. Continue uphill past a bench on the left and an old log bench on the right. After a long straight ascent, the trail bends left and then heads downhill. Continue downhill and cross a creek via a bridge. Hike uphill steeply following the trail as it swings right and narrows. Go gently downhill, pass two more benches, and cross a bridge. Now head uphill and left. At the top of the hill, the trail curves right.

At a White Oak Trail sign, bear left. The trail markers are now green. As you go downhill, the vegetation gets thicker and there is less sunlight filtering through the trees. The trail bends to the right after a long straight section, narrows, and again heads downhill. Go past two more benches and through a very overgrown area. The trail heads downhill to a creek bed, which you cross via a bridge. The trail crests a hill, then heads back down to another bridge. At the next intersection, bear right to head back to the parking lot. Go past the Magnolia Loop Trail sign you hiked past at the beginning of the hike and head back in the direction you came earlier. Once off the bouncing bridge, take the right fork to gain the Pine Trail, marked with yellow, and the parking lot, which is 0.3 miles away. At the next intersection, angle left. As you come up to the wildlife sign at the beginning of the hike, take the right fork to head back to the parking lot.

Note: The Big Creek Scenic Recreation Area loops are part of the Lone Star Hiking Trail, a 128-mile trail that has gained National Recreation Trail recognition. The trail winds through the Sam Houston National Forest and consists of three major sections: a 40-mile Lake Conroe section, the Central section, and the Winters Bayou/Tarkington Creek section. The trails were developed and are now maintained by the Lone Star Hiking Trail Club.

SAM HOUSTON NATIONAL FOREST:
Palmetto Trail

35

IN BRIEF

The Palmetto Trail, while straight and easy to follow, is a demanding hike that requires patience and perseverance. The palmetto stand that you reach is a beautiful site not often seen around the Houston area, but it can be wet, muddy, and dark. Make sure you start the hike early in the day so that the sun is high above when you come to the palmettos. The Sam Houston National Forest is one of four national forests in Texas. It contains more than 163,000 acres and is located between Huntsville, Conroe, Cleveland, and Richards. The district ranger's office is located on FM 1375, 3 miles west of New Waverly. Archeological evidence that dates back 7,000 years has been found in a number of sites in the national forest. Any artifacts found must not be disturbed as they are protected by federal and state regulations. Hiking, fishing, and hunting are allowed in most of the national forest. Check the website for the Sam Houston National Forest at **www.fs.fed.us** for more information.

DESCRIPTION

This hike ends at a large stand of palmetto fan palms just west of Lake Conroe. The area beyond the fan palms is very low and can be under water so it is best to end the hike once you get into this very different part of the forest. To start the hike, head toward a hiker trail

KEY AT-A-GLANCE INFORMATION

LENGTH: 7 miles

CONFIGURATION: Out-and-back

DIFFICULTY: Moderate to difficult

SCENERY: Woodlands, creeks, ponds, palmetto bog

EXPOSURE: Shady with some sun

TRAIL TRAFFIC: Light

TRAIL SURFACE: Dirt and grass

HIKING TIME: 4 hours

DRIVING DISTANCE: 62 miles from the intersection of Beltway 8 and I-45

ACCESS: Free

MAPS: USGS Montgomery; trail map available at the Lone Star Hiking Trail Club website, lshtclub.com

WHEELCHAIR ACCESS: None

FACILITIES: Parking, trail markers

SPECIAL COMMENTS: There are no facilities on many of the trails in the Sam Houston National Forest except for parking, so make sure you bring sunscreen, bug repellent, water, and food. Pets must remain on a leash at all times. Motorized vehicles and bicycles are not allowed on the trails in the national forest. Wear appropriate footwear and long pants whenever hiking in the Sam Houston National Forest.

GPS TRAILHEAD COORDINATES

LATITUDE: N 30° 28.959'
LONGITUDE: W 95° 41.838'

Directions ⟶

From the intersection of Beltway 8 and I-45, head north 41.5 miles on I-45, exit at FM 1375, turn left, and go 14 miles to FM 149. Turn left and go 3.5 miles to the first Lone Star Hiking Trail parking lot, on the left.

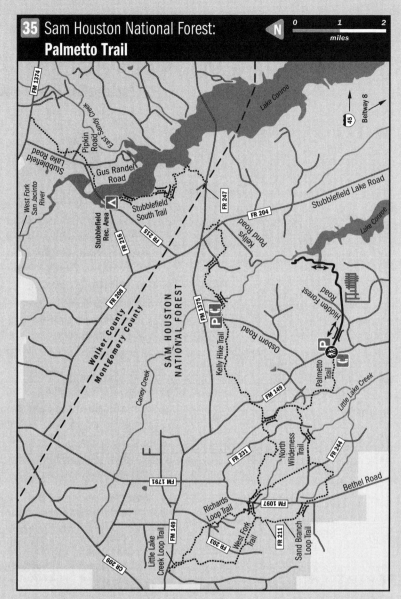

N

0   1   2
miles

FM 1374

East Sandy Creek

Pipkin Road

Stubblefield Lake Road

Gus Randel Road

West Fork San Jacinto River

Lake Conroe

45

Beltway 8

FR 247

FR 204

Stubblefield Lake Road

Lake Conroe

Stubblefield Rec. Area

Stubblefield South Trail

FR 216

FR 215

Kelly's Pond Road

Hidden Forest Road

FR 208

Walker County
Montgomery County

SAM HOUSTON
NATIONAL FOREST

FM 1375

P

Caney Creek

Kelly Hike Trail

Osborn Road

Palmetto Trail

Little Lake Creek

FM 149

North Wilderness Trail

FR 244

FR 231

Bethel Road

FM 1791

Richards Loop Trail

FM 1097

West Fork Trail

FR 203

FR 211

Sand Branch Loop Trail

Little Lake Creek Loop Trail

FM 149

CR 209

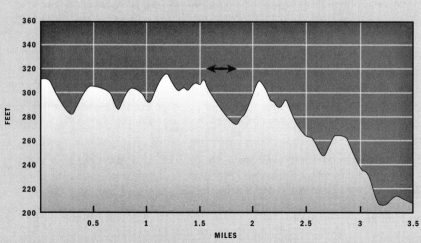

FEET

360
340
320
300
280
260
240
220
200

0.5   1   1.5   2   2.5   3   3.5

MILES

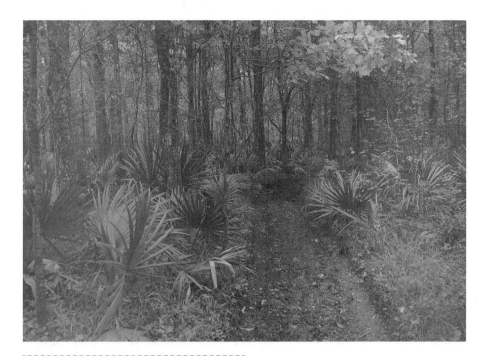

A view of a large stand of palmetto fan palms

sign and enter the woods. At a telephone easement, turn right and go about 1 mile. The trail markers are orange and are located 6–7 feet high in the trees or on the telephone poles. If during any hike on the Lone Star Trail you have not seen a marker in a few minutes, stop and get your bearings. Look ahead and to both sides and you should be able to see a marker in the distance. Many of the markers on this part of the hike are located on the telephone poles in the middle of the easement. Make sure you watch for the orange markers at all times on this hike. Wear proper footwear and watch your footing at all times. Follow the grassy easement as it heads downhill. Hike over a creek using a small bridge and head uphill. The vegetation on both sides of the easement is thick and impenetrable. Go by a number 13 trail marker and then a bench on the left.

Follow the trail downhill into a creek bed and up the other side. This part of the route is very sunny, so wear a hat and sunscreen at all times. At a dirt road, cross and continue straight and head toward the trail marker on a telephone pole ahead. At the pole, the trail heads downhill and bends left before going uphill and over some hilly sections. At Hidden Forest Road, cross and get back on the trail at the hiker trail sign. Continue hiking down the easement and cross another section of Hidden Forest Road, heading toward the hiker trail sign and a sign for the Little Lake Creek Loop. Enter the woods, head right, and then back to the left, getting back on the easement. The trail heads downhill directly under the telephone lines before coming to another hiker trail sign to the left.

Leave the easement and enter the woods at the hiker trail sign. The foliage is very thick and dense. The trail goes downhill and through a small creek bed. Once out of the creek bed, there is a deep creek bed on your right as the trail heads downhill steeply. Cross another creek and head up the other side. Step over a fallen tree. The trail heads uphill over more fallen trees. Although the vegetation closes in on the trail, it is still 4–5 feet wide. At the double trail markers on a tree on the right, go straight and then slightly left. The trail heads downhill under some low-hanging trees and shrubs and then through an alley of thick vegetation. After the trail bends right, it heads downhill for a very long distance.

Now look for the blue blazes on the trees ahead. Make sure you stay on the designated trail and do not wander off onto other paths. The trail goes uphill and through a cut log before heading back downhill over numerous roots and ruts. Continue hiking downhill for a long stretch. The trail then curves right. At a junction, take the right fork; the trail narrows and heads uphill. Go through a dense area that canopies over the trail, causing you to duck in some instances. Step over a large fallen tree and hike past a trail marker in a tree on the right.

After the fallen tree, the trail opens, with less foliage brushing up against your legs. The trail heads downhill slightly. Take the left fork following the orange markers in a tree on the left. At an intersection, go straight, stepping over a fallen tree. Now enter a more tropical area, with palmettos and very low but thick vegetation. Hike through a creek bed, looking for the trail marker on the other side. This part of the trail is not easy to see so make sure you look for trail markers at all times. The trail narrows and gets very overgrown with grass and weeds. Go through a very low muddy area with a large bog on your right. Hike toward a tree on the right with a trail marker to get back on higher ground. The trail here is obscured by grass and weeds, so make sure you follow the trail markers to the next and last palmetto area. This area is wet and muddy most of the year, so you may not want to go this far before ending the hike. Turn around and retrace your route to the parking area.

Note: The Palmetto Trail hike is part of the Lone Star Hiking Trail, a 128-mile trail that has gained National Recreation Trail recognition. The trail winds through the Sam Houston National Forest and consists of three major sections: a 40-mile Lake Conroe section, the Central section, and the Winters Bayou/Tarkington Creek section. The trails were developed and are now maintained by the Lone Star Hiking Trail Club.

NEARBY ACTIVITIES

Sam Houston Memorial and Park Complex (**samhouston.org**), the Texas Prison Museum (**txprisonmuseum.org**), H.E.A.R.T.S. Veterans Museum (**heartsmuseum .com**), Sam Houston National Forest, Lake Conroe.

SAM HOUSTON NATIONAL FOREST:
Winters Bayou Hike

36

IN BRIEF

The Winters Bayou Hike is a long but beautiful hike. It ends at Rivers Creek 4.3 miles from the trailhead at a nice spot for a picnic. After heavy rains this creek can be flowing swiftly, so be cautious. The Sam Houston National Forest is one of four national forests in Texas. It contains more than 163,000 acres and is located between Huntsville, Conroe, Cleveland, and Richards. The district ranger's office is located on FM 1375, 3 miles west of New Waverly. Archeological evidence that dates back 7,000 years has been found in a number of sites in the national forest. Any artifacts found must not be disturbed, as they are protected by federal and state regulations. Hiking, fishing, and hunting are allowed in most of the national forest.

DESCRIPTION

Start the hike by going through the motorized-vehicle barriers by the Lone Star Hiking Trail signs. Once on the trail, go left and toward a white trail marker in the trees. Go through another set of barriers, hiking parallel to FM 1725. The trail surface is dirt and pine needles with thick vegetation on both sides of the trail. Look left for an old cemetery across the road. The trail heads slightly uphill before turning away from FM 175. The trail markers on this entire hike are white and located 6–7 feet high on trees along the trail. If during any hike on the Lone Star Trail you have not seen a marker

KEY AT-A-GLANCE INFORMATION

LENGTH: 8.6 miles

CONFIGURATION: Out-and-back

DIFFICULTY: Moderate to difficult

SCENERY: Woodlands, creeks, bayous, ponds, old fire-tower base

EXPOSURE: Shady

TRAIL TRAFFIC: Light

TRAIL SURFACE: Dirt

HIKING TIME: 5 hours

DRIVING DISTANCE: 35 miles from the intersection of Beltway 8 and I-59

ACCESS: Free

MAPS: USGS Bear Creek; trail map available at the Lone Star Hiking Trail Club website, lshtclub.com

WHEELCHAIR ACCESS: None

FACILITIES: Parking, trail markers

SPECIAL COMMENTS: There are no facilities on many of the trails in the Sam Houston National Forest except for parking, so make sure you bring sunscreen, bug repellent, water, and food. Pets must remain on a leash at all times. Motorized vehicles and bicycles are not allowed on the trails in the national forest. Wear appropriate footwear and long pants whenever hiking in the Sam Houston National Forest.

Directions ———————————————→

From the intersection of Beltway 8 and I-59, head north 30 miles on I-59, exit at TX 105, and turn left. Turn right at the stoplight onto FM 1725 and go 5.2 miles to the Winters Bayou trailhead, on the right.

GPS TRAILHEAD COORDINATES

LATITUDE: N 30° 23.473'
LONGITUDE: W 95° 9.416'

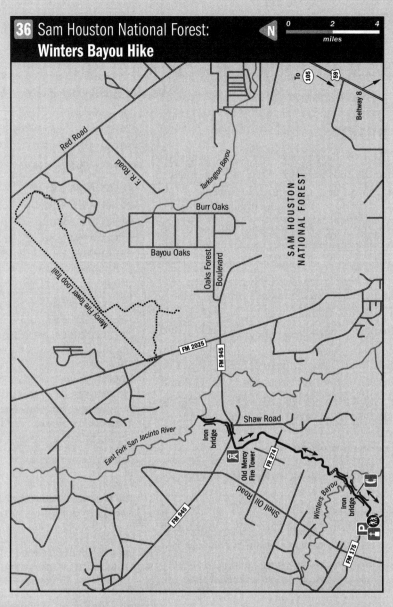

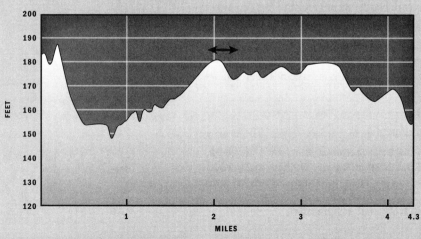

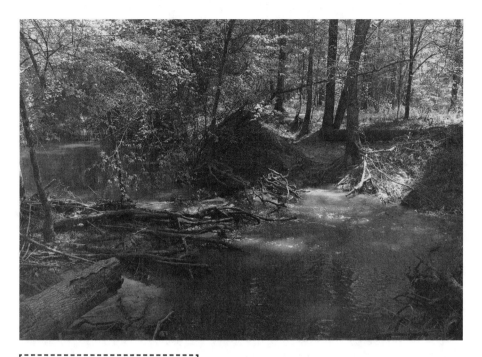

The end of the hike at Rivers Creek

in a few minutes, stop and get your bearings. Look ahead and to both sides and you should be able to see a marker in the distance.

Follow the trail as it curves right and heads downhill over some exposed roots: watch your footing here. Pass a number 96 trail marker on a tree on the right. The grassy trail narrows where the vegetation on the forest floor gets very thick and impenetrable, with only a few pines overhead. The trail bends right and downhill. As the trail swings left, it goes downhill toward taller trees and more shade. There is considerable lichen growing on the trail, indicating a lack of foot traffic and a moist environment.

Cross a small footbridge and follow the trail as it goes right. Go across a small stream heading down one side and up the other out of the creek bed. Head uphill and to the left, hiking next to a creek on your left. Cross another bridge and enter an area that contains numerous fan palms, giving it a tropical feel. Hike across a telephone easement, staying on the path through the tall grass. Cross a bridge and head left, following the trail as it runs parallel to a creek bed on the right. Hike over Winters Bayou on a very large iron bridge and then under a canopy of trees. Stay away from the water and watch for poisonous snakes at all times. Winters Bayou is now on your left. Follow the trail as it heads downhill and right, away from the bayou.

Cross another small bridge and head slightly uphill. Go past a tree with a large trail marker—make sure you go left around the tree and then turn right to stay on the trail. Parts of this trail may be muddy or wet, so wear hiking boots.

Follow the trail markers as the trail takes big bends right and then left. Continue curving left at a trail marker in the trees on the right. Go by a number 95 trail marker and an M marker in a tree on the right. Hike 30 yards or so across a boardwalk over a low, swampy area. Again, stay out of the water and stay on the boardwalk. Once off the boardwalk, cross a small creek bed and head toward a small bridge. Cross the bridge and get back on the trail. As the vegetation clears, hike across a gas-pipeline easement and then toward a hiker trail sign. The trail, which is headed uphill, is about 4–5 feet wide and very easy to follow. Hike under or over a fallen tree and follow the trail as it bends right. At the trail marker on the right, veer left, heading uphill for quite some distance. At an intersection with a dirt road, cross it and head back into the woods at the hiker trail sign. The trail goes left into the trees and through very thick vegetation.

Continue as the trail narrows and the forest floor becomes thick with small bushes and weeds. Look closely for trail markers and, in some instances, white paint, or blazes, on the trees in this area. Pass the concrete base of the Old Mercy Fire Tower, which is left. Hike through a narrow alley of trees that stretches straight ahead for several hundred yards. There is a small creek on your right as you hike on top of a low rise.

Hike through a stand of pine trees lined up on each side of the trail as if they were planted in an arbor. At two trail markers on a post on the right, bear left following the direction of the markers. Cross a small creek bed and head up the other side and to the right. The trail heads uphill slightly before going through another creek bed. The trail markers are not as easy to see here so make sure you look for the white blazes. Pass by a Lone Star Hiking Trail Recreation Trail sign on a tree on the right; watch for blazes in the upcoming stretch. Pass by another concrete base for the Old Mercy Fire Tower on your right. Go through a fence and head toward FM 945. Cross FM 945 toward the hiker trail sign on the other side. Watch for high-speed traffic and use extreme caution when crossing FM 945. Once back on the trail, hike through a motorized-vehicle barrier and get on an elevated part of the trail. The highway is now on your right as you hike through a large stand of loblolly pines. Cross a footbridge, then follow the trail as it goes left and heads downhill slightly. Hike by a very large magnolia tree on the right.

Continue past a fence on the left and cross a creek bed. The slope out of the creek bed is steep, so watch your footing. At an intersection with a dirt road, turn right. Cross a large iron bridge and wind your way to Rivers Creek. At Rivers Creek, turn around and retrace your route to the parking area.

NEARBY ACTIVITIES

Sam Houston Memorial and Park Complex (**samhouston.org**), the Texas Prison Museum (**txprisonmuseum.org**), H.E.A.R.T.S. Veterans Museum (**heartsmuseum .com**), Sam Houston National Forest, Lake Conroe.

SAM HOUSTON NATIONAL FOREST: Stubblefield North Hike

IN BRIEF

The Sam Houston National Forest is one of four national forests in Texas. It contains more than 163,000 acres and is located between Huntsville, Conroe, Cleveland, and Richards. The district ranger's office is located on FM 1375, 3 miles west of New Waverly. Archeological evidence that dates back 7,000 years has been found in a number of sites in the national forest. Any artifacts found must not be disturbed, as they are protected by federal and state regulations. Hiking, fishing, and hunting are allowed in most of the national forest. Check the website for the Sam Houston National Forest at **www.fs.fed.us** for more information.

DESCRIPTION

To start the hike, head toward the hiker trail sign and enter the woods. The trail markers are silver, since you are on the Lone Star Hiking Trail for the entire hike. They are located 6–7 feet high in the trees. If during any hike on the Lone Star Trail you have not seen a marker in a few minutes, stop and get your bearings. Look ahead and to both sides and you should be able to see a marker in the distance. This is a very densely wooded, narrow trail with thick vegetation growing close to the

---

Directions

From the intersection of Beltway 8 and I-45, head north 41.5 miles on I-45 and exit at FM 1375/1374. Continue on the feeder road to FM 1374 and turn left, driving over I-45. Drive 7 miles to the trailhead on the left. Look for a very small hiker trail sign just past the national forest sign on the left. Park beside the road, in the grass.

KEY AT-A-GLANCE INFORMATION

LENGTH: 5.6 miles

CONFIGURATION: Out-and-back

DIFFICULTY: Moderate

SCENERY: Woodlands, creeks, farms

EXPOSURE: Shady

TRAIL TRAFFIC: Light

TRAIL SURFACE: Dirt and grass

HIKING TIME: 3.5 hours

DRIVING DISTANCE: 49 miles from the intersection of Beltway 8 and I-45

ACCESS: Free

MAPS: USGS Moore Grove and San Jacinto; trail map available at the Lone Star Hiking Trail Club website, lshtclub.com

WHEELCHAIR ACCESS: None

FACILITIES: Trail markers

SPECIAL COMMENTS: There are no facilities on many of the trails in the Sam Houston National Forest except for parking, so make sure you bring sunscreen, bug repellent, water, and food. Pets must remain on a leash at all times. Motorized vehicles and bicycles are not allowed on the trails in the national forest. Wear appropriate footwear and long pants whenever hiking in the Sam Houston National Forest.

GPS TRAILHEAD COORDINATES

LATITUDE: N 30° 35.203'
LONGITUDE: W 95° 36.121'

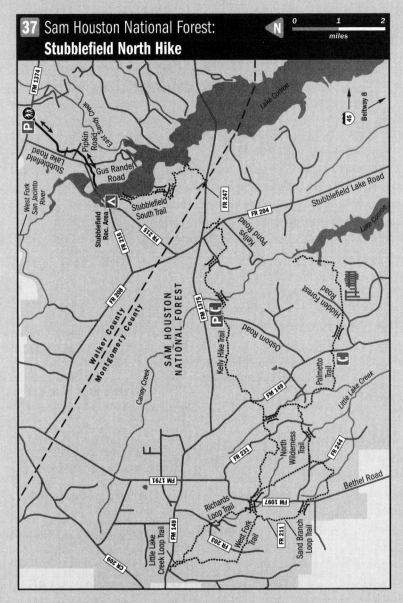

N

0   1   2
miles

FM 1374

East Sans Creek

Pipkin Road

Stubblefield Lake Road

Gus Randel Road

West Fork San Jacinto River

Stubblefield Rec. Area

Stubblefield South Trail

FR 216

FR 215

FR 247

FR 204

Stubblefield Lake Road

Lake Conroe

Kelly's Pond Road

Lake Conroe

Beltway 8

45

FR 209

Walker County
Montgomery County

SAM HOUSTON NATIONAL FOREST

FM 1375

Kelly Hike Trail

Osborn Road

Hidden Forest Road

Caney Creek

FM 149

Palmetto Trail

Little Lake Creek

FR 231

North Wilderness Trail

FR 244

FM 1791

Bethel Road

Richards Loop Trail

FM 1097

Little Lake Creek Loop Trail

FM 149

FR 203

West Fork Trail

FR 211

Sand Branch Loop Trail

CR 209

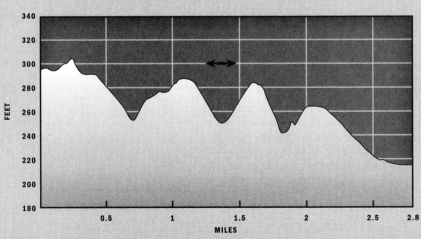

340
320
300
280
260
240
220
200
180

FEET

0.5   1   1.5   2   2.5   2.8

MILES

trail surface. Follow the trail as it heads downhill through several cut fallen trees. Hike over a rolling section with poor footing where you'll need appropriate footwear. Go past a number 26 trail marker post on the right and an M marker in a tree on the left.

Hike into and out of a creek bed over exposed tree roots, exposed by washouts. Hike by a marker on a tree on the right as the trail narrows again and the foliage encroaches: wear long pants to prevent exposure to poison ivy. Follow the trail as it bends right and then heads downhill for several hundred yards. Watch for spider webs stretching across the trail from early spring to late fall. While the spiders are not poisonous, the webs are irritating.

Watch for a trail marker in a tree on the right, and follow the trail as it goes to the right and under a canopy of trees. Go to the left following a trail marker in a tree on the right. Although the foliage is encroaching on the trail, the trail is still easy to see as it heads gradually uphill for a long, straight section. Now descend to a creek bed and hike through it. Climb the other side, hiking over exposed roots.

At an intersection, bear left and hike past a trail marker in a tree on the left. Go by a post with the number 22 on it. Cross a creek bed and climb the other side, going slightly right. The trail heads uphill steeply over roots, and then goes more moderately uphill. Hike past the bearing tree (a tree used to help your bearings while hiking the Lone Star Hiking Trail) on the right and a national forest boundary line on a tree on the right. There is a large stand of young pines on the right, past an open grassy area. Go past a hunting blind on your right and head toward a fence. Stay to the left of the fence as the trail bends left. Continue past a number 22 trail marker and a letter M in a tree on the right. There is a small creek on your right, with the trail going under a canopy of trees and around a large pine tree. Descend into a creek bed and climb the other side, putting the creek on your left.

Cross another creek bed, climbing up the other side and to the right. The trail swings left with the creek on your left. This is a very winding section of the hike but there are numerous trail markers to keep you on track. Cross an old road and head back into the trees on the other side, following the trail to the right. The trail then veers left into a creek bed. Across the creek bed, the forest is dark and shady. Go through a fallen cut tree and climb into and out of another creek bed. Hike through another fallen tree following the trail as it stretches out ahead of you. Go over a fallen tree, cross a creek bed, and climb under a very large pine tree that has fallen to the other side of the creek. Take a quick right and then a quick left to get back on the trail, which soon heads gradually uphill.

Step through a large cut tree and continue uphill on the grassy trail. Cross a paved road and head to the other side. At an intersection, go straight to stay on the trail as it heads uphill, past a deep creek bed on your left. The trail then heads steeply downhill to cross a creek bed. Climb the other side to a dark, shaded area. At an intersection marked by double trail markers on a tree to your left, bear right and uphill. At a hiker trail sign, cross the telephone easement toward the other hiker trail sign. Go past a number 21 trail marker and a letter M marker in a tree on the left, following the trail downhill. Now hike through an open area with fan palms and oak trees, beyond which the trail narrows to only about a foot wide with many exposed roots and ruts. At the double trail markers on a post on the left, bear right. Hike past the motorized-vehicle barriers and the hiker trail sign to the road. Here turn around and retrace your route to the parking area.

Note: The Stubblefield North Hike is part of the Lone Star Hiking Trail, a 128-mile trail that has gained National Recreation Trail recognition. The trail winds through the Sam Houston National Forest and consists of three major sections: a 40-mile Lake Conroe section, the Central section, and the Winters Bayou/Tarkington Creek section. The trails were developed and are now maintained by the Lone Star Hiking Trail Club.

NEARBY ACTIVITIES

Sam Houston Memorial and Park Complex (**samhouston.org**), the Texas Prison Museum (**txprisonmuseum.org**), H.E.A.R.T.S. Veterans Museum (**heartsmuseum .com**), Sam Houston National Forest, Lake Conroe.

SAM HOUSTON NATIONAL FOREST:
Stubblefield South Hike

IN BRIEF

This hike takes you east toward Lake Conroe and then heads north toward the Stubblefield Recreation Area. The Sam Houston National Forest is one of four national forests in Texas. It contains more than 163,000 acres and is located between Huntsville, Conroe, Cleveland, and Richards. The district ranger's office is located on FM 1375, 3 miles west of New Waverly. Archeological evidence that dates back 7,000 years has been found in a number of sites in the national forest. Any artifacts found must not be disturbed, as they are protected by federal and state regulations. Hiking, fishing, and hunting are allowed in most of the national forest. Check the website for the Sam Houston National Forest at **www.fs.fed.us** for more information.

DESCRIPTION

To start the hike, head east on FM 1375 for about 10 yards and turn left into the trees at the hiker trail sign. The narrow dirt trail, which is bordered by thick vegetation, quickly heads away from the highway. The white trail markers are located about 6 feet high in the trees. If during any hike on the Lone Star Trail you have not seen a marker in a few minutes, stop and get your bearings. Look ahead and to both sides and you should be able to see a marker in the distance. The trail heads downhill through

Directions ————————➤

From the intersection of Beltway 8 and I-45, head north 41.5 miles on I-45, exit at FM 1375, and turn left. Go 8.1 miles to Forest Service 247 and turn right. FS 247 is just past the Montgomery County sign. Park just as you turn onto FS 247 to begin the hike at FM 1375.

KEY AT-A-GLANCE INFORMATION

LENGTH: 8 miles
CONFIGURATION: Out-and-back
DIFFICULTY: Moderate to difficult
SCENERY: Woodlands, creeks, Lake Conroe, campground
EXPOSURE: Shady
TRAIL TRAFFIC: Light
TRAIL SURFACE: Dirt
HIKING TIME: 4 hours
DRIVING DISTANCE: 50 miles from the intersection of Beltway 8 and I-45
ACCESS: Free
MAPS: USGS San Jacinto; trail map available at the Lone Star Hiking Trail Club website, lshtclub.com
WHEELCHAIR ACCESS: None
FACILITIES: Trail markers; restrooms at turn-around point in the hike
SPECIAL COMMENTS: There are no facilities on many of the trails in the Sam Houston National Forest except for parking, so make sure you bring sunscreen, bug repellent, water, and food. Pets must remain on a leash at all times. Motorized vehicles and bicycles are not allowed on the trails in the national forest. Wear appropriate footwear and long pants whenever hiking in the Sam Houston National Forest.

GPS TRAILHEAD COORDINATES

LATITUDE: N 30° 31.556'
LONGITUDE: W 95° 37.826'

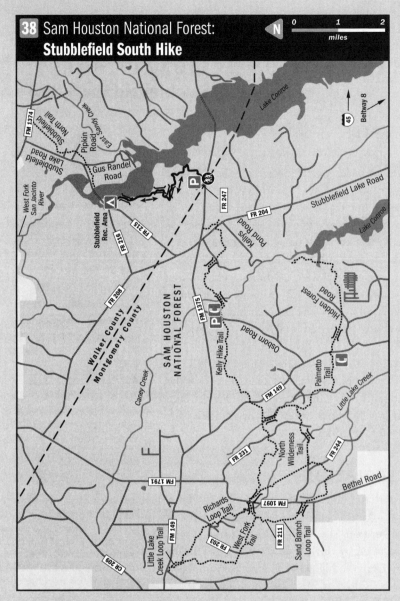

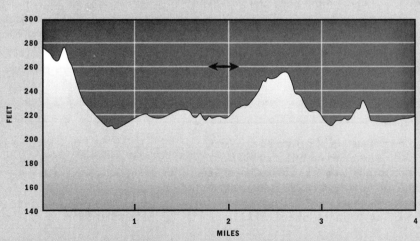

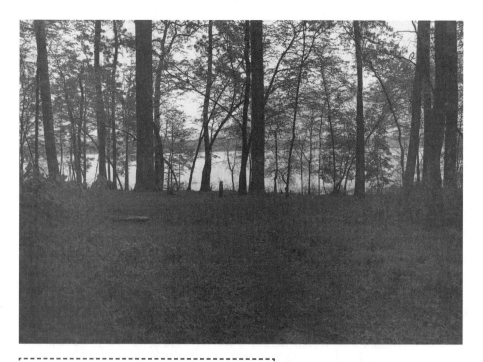

A peek at Lake Conroe on the Stubblefield South Hike

very thick foliage before entering an alley of tall trees. Look out for spider webs that may be spun across the trail trees from early spring to late fall. Continue downhill as the trail enters a large stand of loblolly pines. At an intersection, bear right, following the sign for the Lone Star Hiking Trail. The trail again heads downhill and through a small creek bed. After the creek, the trail heads uphill for several hundred yards through trees with white markers and blue paint, or blazes, on them to help guide you.

Go between two trees and follow the trail as it goes left and downhill. There are exposed tree roots on part of the trail so watch your footing. At the bottom of the hill, follow a trail marker left, as indicated. The vegetation here is thick and impenetrable. The trail widens as you head downhill and curve right, entering an area with less foliage.

Continue as the trail winds through an alley of thick foliage and exposed roots. Once out of the thick vegetation, the trail goes uphill and you can see Lake Conroe ahead. At the lake, follow a trail marker and go left. There is a primitive campsite on your left and the lake on your right. This area is open with more oaks than pines. While hiking next to Lake Conroe, stay away from the water, as there are poisonous snakes. Follow the trail uphill as you head back into the woods. Go around a big tree on the right and then veer left. Cross a small creek bed and then head up the other side over tree roots. Out of the creek bed, the trail heads right and uphill, then downhill toward the lake.

At a low area adjacent to the lake, the trail goes left. Look for a marker ahead to get your bearings. The trail narrows to about a foot wide, with grass and weeds on both sides. There is a creek on your right as the trail heads to the left and gradually uphill. Head downhill over tree roots and then parallel to the creek on your right. Go through a rolling section of the trail. When you come to double trail markers ahead and a trail marker on a tree to the right, cross the creek bed and clamber up the other side. The trail continues uphill before leveling and bending left. Go by a post on your left with a number 17 on it and an M on a tree on the right. These markers indicate that you are on the Lone Star Hiking Trail (M) and that you are 17 miles from the start of the trail. The trail then goes left and heads gradually downhill. The trail soon widens, creating a more open feel. The blazes on the trees in this area are orange, but the trail markers are still white. Follow the orange blazes and go left through thick vegetation. At the top of a ridge, the foliage opens; then the trail heads downhill and curves left. The trail heads through some low areas that may be wet, so watch your footing. As you continue downhill, you enter a more open area. There is considerable debris from storms in this area. Go to the left of the debris to see the next trail marker. Pass a sandy, swampy area on your right, making sure to stay left of it. Turn right to cross a small creek bed. There is another creek on your right that you must cross, but due to the width of the creek here, it is best to follow the orange blazes and head upstream parallel to the creek to a narrower crossing. Cross the creek and head to your right, back in the direction you came on the other side of the creek. To regain the trail, head left and back into the trees.

Cross a bridge and follow the trail as it goes left through low vegetation. There is a deep creek bed running parallel to the trail. Come out of the trees and approach the creek, then return to the trees, heading left, away from the creek. Cross another bridge and follow a narrow trail. Cross another creek bed and follow the trail as it curves right. Hike by a number 18 trail marker on the right and an M on a tree on the left. The trail heads uphill, veering left. Soon cross a dirt road and head left toward a hiker trail sign on the right. Go to the right at the sign to get back on the trail. Continue past a large stand of very narrow pine trees on the right. The trail bends right and heads downhill. The foliage in this area includes numerous fan palms, giving it a more tropical feel. Lake Conroe is again visible on your right about 75 yards away. As the trail winds in and out of the trees, you leave the fan palms and enter back into woodland vegetation of pines and oaks again. Cross two small creek beds and then follow the trail as it goes uphill. The clearing you went through earlier is now on your left. Continue as the trail winds to the right and then heads uphill. It goes to the left toward the clearing and then takes a big bend to the right and back into the thick vegetation. Follow the trail markers in the trees and go left uphill. The trail then bends to the right and heads back downhill.

Cross a bridge that is in disrepair and go left, following the trail marker in a tree on the left. Cross one last bridge and then head uphill as the trail widens.

After descending, go by a post on the left, continuing straight toward the Stubblefield Recreation Area. There is a restroom with water to the left of the trail at the campground. At the hiker trail sign in the Stubblefield Recreation Area, turn around and retrace your route to the parking area.

Note: The Stubblefield South Hike is part of the Lone Star Hiking Trail, a 128-mile trail that has gained National Recreation Trail recognition. The trail winds through the Sam Houston National Forest and consists of three major sections: a 40-mile Lake Conroe section, the Central section, and the Winters Bayou/Tarkington Creek section. The trails were developed and are now maintained by the Lone Star Hiking Trail Club.

NEARBY ACTIVITIES

Sam Houston Memorial and Park Complex (**samhouston.org**), the Texas Prison Museum (**txprisonmuseum.org**), H.E.A.R.T.S. Veterans Museum (**heartsmuseum .com**), Sam Houston National Forest, Lake Conroe.

39 SAM HOUSTON NATIONAL FOREST:
Richards Loop

KEY AT-A-GLANCE INFORMATION

LENGTH: 7.2 miles

CONFIGURATION: Loop

DIFFICULTY: Moderate to difficult

SCENERY: Woodlands, creeks, ponds

EXPOSURE: Shady with some sun

TRAIL TRAFFIC: Light weekdays, moderate weekends

TRAIL SURFACE: Dirt and grass

HIKING TIME: 3.5 hours

DRIVING DISTANCE: 60 miles from the intersection of Beltway 8 and I-45

ACCESS: Free

MAPS: USGS Richards; trail map available at the Lone Star Hiking Trail Club website, lshtclub.com

WHEELCHAIR ACCESS: None

FACILITIES: Parking, trail markers

SPECIAL COMMENTS: There are no facilities on many of the trails in the Sam Houston National Forest except for parking, so make sure you bring sunscreen, bug repellent, water, and food. Pets must remain on a leash at all times. Motorized vehicles and bicycles are not allowed on the trails in the national forest. Wear appropriate footwear and long pants whenever hiking in the Sam Houston National Forest.

GPS TRAILHEAD COORDINATES

LATITUDE: N 30° 32.361'
LONGITUDE: W 95° 47.065'

IN BRIEF

The Sam Houston National Forest is one of four national forests in Texas. It contains more than 163,000 acres and is located between Huntsville, Conroe, Cleveland, and Richards. The district ranger's office is located on FM 1375, 3 miles west of New Waverly. Archeological evidence that dates back 7,000 years has been found in a number of sites in the national forest. Any artifacts found must not be disturbed, as they are protected by federal and state regulations. Hiking, fishing, and hunting are allowed in most of the national forest. Check the website for the Sam Houston National Forest at **www.fs.fed.us** for more information.

DESCRIPTION

To start the Richards Loop hike, head toward an information sign about trail etiquette and rules and a hiking trail sign. Go through the motorized-vehicle barrier and get on a dirt trail. There are markers in the trees about 6 feet high that are color coded to the particular hike that you are on. If during any hike on the Lone Star Trail you have not seen a marker in a few minutes, stop and get your bearings. Look ahead and to both sides and you should be able to see a marker in the distance. The

----

Directions ————————————————→

From the intersection of Beltway 8 and I-45, head north 41.5 miles on I-45, exit at FM 1375, and turn left. Go 14 miles to FM 149. Turn right, go 4.3 miles to Forest Service 219, and turn left. The parking lot is on the left. (FS 219 is unsigned, but there is a sign telling you to turn here for hiking parking.)

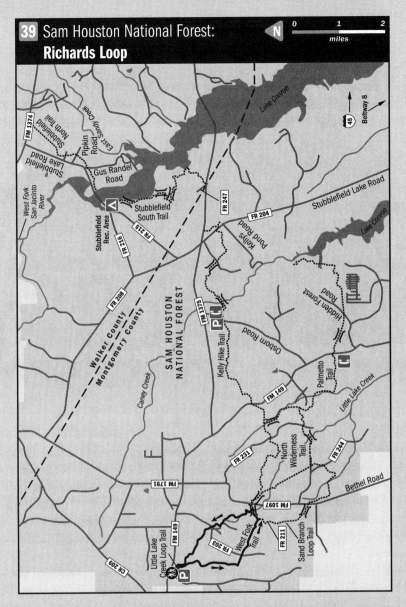

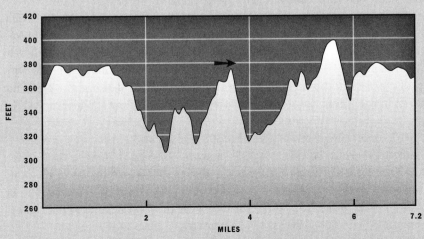

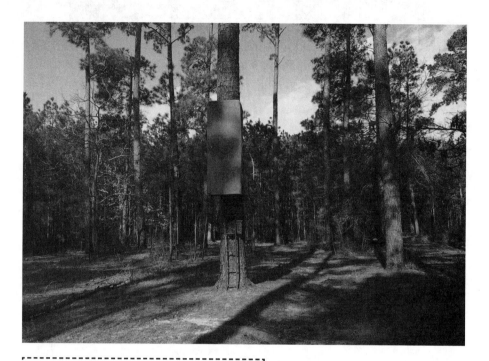

A ranger spotter ladder on the Richards Loop hike

markers on this part of the hike are white. Continue as the trail surface changes to grass and heads downhill through the trees. Most of the trees in the Sam Houston National Forest are loblolly pines; they are tall but allow sun to reach the forest floor. The vegetation is thick but only about 6 feet high in the densest areas. The trail is only about 2 feet wide, but there is another 3 feet of clearance on each side before the vegetation. There are some exposed tree roots, so watch your footing at all times.

Richards Loop is a winding trail but there are no major bends or turns. At the intersection and trail signs, go left and follow the sign for the Little Lake Creek Loop. The trail markers here are silver with an orange stripe. Cross a telephone easement, then go straight and slightly left to regain the trail. The trail winds through the trees and goes gradually downhill for several hundred feet. Watch for banana-spider webs across the trail from late spring to early fall. Continue as the trail surface gets grassier. It is still easy to follow, though, with the trail markers in the trees. Although the vegetation is dense, there are some openings in the forest floor due to controlled burns. Follow the markers as the trail heads uphill over exposed roots.

At the next intersection, cross FS 203 and go straight between two trees and look up ahead to see the next trail marker. Soon go slightly to the left and toward a small pond. Watch for snakes at all times. Hike to the left of the pond to find a trail marker just past the pond. The trail then heads left, away from the pond and uphill. When you come to a tree with an M on it, hike to the right of the tree and look ahead for an orange trail marker 5 in the distance. You may lose the trail here, so just stop and look ahead to find the next trail marker.

Go through a large open area and then head over some small humps in the trail that can make your footing a little precarious if you are not paying attention. Go through a bramble bush area where the vegetation is more than 5 feet high. Look to your right for a spotter ladder going up a tree. Forest rangers manage the forest, soil, timber, minerals, and wildlife, which include the endangered bald eagle and red-cockaded woodpecker. Continue past an old trail marker with the number 2 on it. This area has also been control burned: some of the markers in the trees may be difficult to see, since they have burned also. Follow the burned markers and step over several fallen trees. The trail bends left, with a creek on your right. Step to the right and go over some tree roots if there is water in the creek. Head downhill into the creek bed and up the other side. Go steeply uphill and to the right. The next part of the trail is not as heavily marked but is easy to follow. Keep looking up ahead for the next marker.

Continue through another motorized-vehicle barrier and cross FS 203 toward a hiker trail sign. The trail heads downhill with the trees canopying overhead, making for a shady part of the hike. At an intersection, go right. The trail narrows here but is still easy to hike. Follow the trail as it goes between two creeks. Hike downhill via steps into the creek bed. Go slightly left and up the other side. Look for pink blazes in the trees, as there are no trail markers in this section. As you come to an opening in the foliage, look for the familiar orange trail markers.

At the next intersection, go straight, passing by another ranger ladder in the trees on the right. The vegetation is more open on the forest floor, but there are still very tall pine trees growing on both sides of the trail. As the trail heads uphill steeply, the vegetation encroaches on the trail and gets tall and thick. Make sure you look for trail markers in this area. The trail jogs right, then quickly left, around a low, possibly wet area on the right. Look ahead for trail markers. At an intersection with the West Fork Trail, bear left. The trail markers for this trail are silver with a blue stripe in the middle. Descend to cross a small creek bed, then head up the other side. The creek is now on your left, with the forest on your right. Cross a small bridge and then angle right, putting the creek on your right.

Continue to the next intersection and a trail sign for the North and South Lone Star trails. Go left on the North Lone Star Trail to complete the loop. The trail markers are now white again as they were in the beginning of the hike. Head left and uphill, with the creek on your right. Go past a sign on the left warning that cars, ATVs, and bikes are not allowed on any part of the trail. Hike in and out of several small creek beds. Beyond these, at an intersection, head left and then right to get back on the trail. Once back in the trees, go left, heading uphill and past a creek on your left. Continue uphill and past a pond on your left. As the trail heads away from the pond it continues uphill and through another small creek bed. Go straight through the next intersection, passing another small creek on your left. The trail roller-coasters past another number 2 trail marker on the right. Cross FS 203 and head toward a hiker trail sign. At a tree with the double trail markers, go right. This is a very open part of the trail, with thick grass on the trail surface. Head downhill for several hundred yards and gradually return to shade. Cross another small creek bed and head uphill and left. At the next intersection, go right and follow a trail marker in a tree on the left. Hike by a number 1 trail marker on the left. Go through a gate and soon meet the telephone easement. Go left along the easement and then turn right to get back on the trail. At the intersection with the Little Lake Creek Loop, bear right. Go through the motorized-vehicle barrier and toward the parking lot to end the hike.

Note: The Richards Loop is part of the Lone Star Hiking Trail, a 128-mile trail that has gained National Recreation Trail recognition. The trail winds through the Sam Houston National Forest and consists of three major sections: a 40-mile Lake Conroe section, the Central section, and the Winters Bayou/Tarkington Creek section. The trails were developed and are now maintained by the Lone Star Hiking Trail Club.

NEARBY ACTIVITIES

Sam Houston Memorial and Park Complex (**samhouston.org**), the Texas Prison Museum (**txprisonmuseum.org**), H.E.A.R.T.S. Veterans Museum (**heartsmuseum .com**), Sam Houston National Forest, Lake Conroe.

SAM HOUSTON NATIONAL FOREST:
Sand Branch Loop

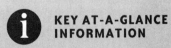

40

IN BRIEF

The Sam Houston National Forest is one of four national forests in Texas. It contains more than 163,000 acres and is located between Huntsville, Conroe, Cleveland, and Richards. The district ranger's office is located on FM 1375, 3 miles west of New Waverly. Archeological evidence that dates back 7,000 years has been found in a number of sites in the national forest. Any artifacts found must not be disturbed, as they are protected by federal and state regulations. Hiking, fishing, and hunting are allowed in most of the national forest. Check the website for the Sam Houston National Forest at **www.fs.fed.us** for more information.

DESCRIPTION

Start the Sand Branch Loop hike on FS 211, hiking past information signs to a hiker sign on the right side of the road. Go into the trees, following white trail markers. This is a 4-foot-wide dirt trail with tall loblolly pines and low forest-floor foliage. Continue as the trail heads downhill over exposed roots. Watch your footing at all times. There is a creek on your right and forest on your left. The middle of the trail has been washed out, so the ground is very uneven. As the trail goes uphill, the washed-out section ends, making for easier footing. The trail then heads downhill and right, into

---

Directions ⟶

From the intersection of Beltway 8 and I-45, head north 41.5 miles on I-45, exit at FM 1375, and turn left. Go 14 miles to FM 149. Turn right, go 1.3 miles to Forest Service 211/ Bethel Road, and turn left. Go 2 miles to the parking lot on the right.

ⓘ KEY AT-A-GLANCE INFORMATION

LENGTH: 6.1 miles

CONFIGURATION: Loop

DIFFICULTY: Moderate to difficult

SCENERY: Woodlands, creeks, ponds

EXPOSURE: Shady

TRAIL TRAFFIC: Light

TRAIL SURFACE: Dirt

HIKING TIME: 3.5 hours

DRIVING DISTANCE: 58 miles from the intersection of Beltway 8 and I-45

ACCESS: Free

MAPS: USGS Richards, Dacus, Montgomery, San Jacinto; trail map available at the Lone Star Hiking Trail Club website, lshtclub.com

WHEELCHAIR ACCESS: None

FACILITIES: Parking, trail markers

SPECIAL COMMENTS: There are no facilities on many of the trails in the Sam Houston National Forest except for parking, so make sure you bring sunscreen, bug repellent, water, and food. Pets must remain on a leash at all times. Motorized vehicles and bicycles are not allowed on the trails in the national forest. Wear appropriate footwear and long pants whenever hiking in the Sam Houston National Forest.

GPS TRAILHEAD COORDINATES

LATITUDE: N 30° 30.643'
LONGITUDE: W 95° 45.399'

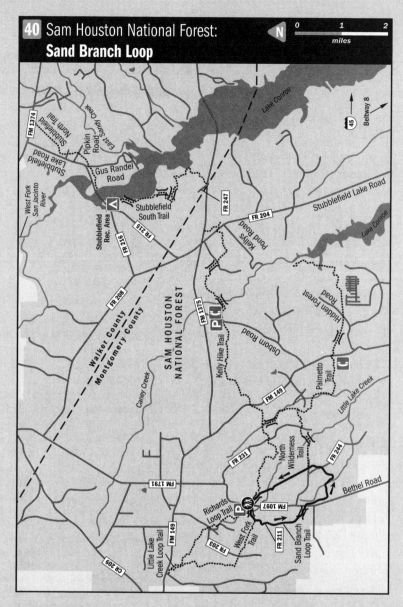

N

0   1   2
miles

Lake Conroe

45
Beltway 8

FM 1374
Stubblefield North Trail
Pipkin Road
East Sandy Creek
Gus Randel Road
Stubblefield Lake Road

West Fork San Jacinto River

Stubblefield Lake Road

Stubblefield South Trail

FR 247

FR 204

Stubblefield Rec. Area

FR 216

FR 215

Kellys Pond Road

Lake Conroe

Hidden Forest Road

FR 208

Walker County
Montgomery County

SAM HOUSTON NATIONAL FOREST

FM 1375

Kelly Hike Trail

Osborn Road

Caney Creek

FM 149

Palmetto Trail

Little Lake Creek

North Wilderness Trail

FR 231

FR 244

Bethel Road

FM 1791

FM 1097

Sand Branch Loop Trail

Richards Loop Trail

West Fork Trail

FR 203

FR 211

Little Lake Creek Loop Trail

FM 149

CR 209

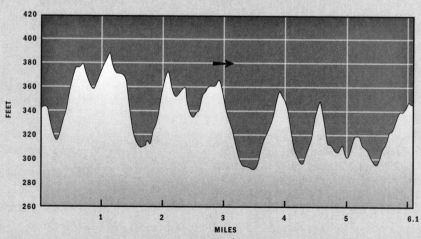

FEET

420
400
380
360
340
320
300
280
260

1   2   3   4   5   6.1

MILES

a deep creek bed. Hike up the other side using steps and follow the trail to the West Fork Trail sign. Take the left fork toward the blue-striped trail markers. The trail heads downhill into an area where it is not easy to tell which direction to go. Just follow the trail markers. If during any hike on the Lone Star Trail you have not seen a marker in a few minutes, stop and get your bearings. Look ahead and to both sides and you should be able to see a marker in the distance. There is a creek on your left.

Cross a bridge and head up the other side of the creek. The trail narrows to about 2 feet wide, with very thick, low-growing vegetation on both sides. Cross a small creek bed and head uphill. At the top of a hill, the trail bends left and then descends slightly. At a West Fork Trail sign, veer left, as it curves right past a brown-striped trail marker. Make sure you look for the trail markers as some of them in this area are difficult to see. FS 211 is now on your left, just past the trees. The trail heads downhill toward FS 211.

Cross FS 211, walking toward the orange trail markers on the other side of the road. Once back in the trees, the trail heads downhill and left. At a set of double trail markers in the trees, go left. You are heading uphill, with thick foliage on both sides of the trail. Some of the trail markers on this part of the hike are metal triangles rather than metal squares, but they still have an orange stripe in the middle of each marker. Because the trees are so tall and spread out and the forest floor vegetation is so low, there is considerable sunlight shining through the trees. Continue past a number 4 trail marker on the left as the trail goes downhill for several hundred yards.

Hike past an M trail marker in the trees on the right and some pink blazes in the trees ahead. At the pink blazes, go left and then take a quick right to climb down into a deep creek bed and up the other side. Now the trail goes uphill and left through a stand of young pines. Cross a dirt road and head toward orange trail markers on the other side. The trail again narrows, with bushes and weeds brushing up against your legs. The trail heads downhill over exposed roots and beneath a canopy of trees. Cross a creek bed and head up the other side. Hike over a small bridge and then cross another dirt road, passing a hiker trail sign. Go right, toward a tree with three trail markers. Pass a hiker trail sign and go through a motorized-vehicle barrier. The trail is not well marked past the barrier, so just stay on the trail and look for a trail marker ahead. Cross a creek bed via steps on both sides. Now the trail heads steeply uphill and then goes left, with vegetation encroaching from both sides.

At an intersection, go straight. Hike across a dirt road, go through a motorized-vehicle barrier, and then go left. Some of the trail markers here have been burned and are a bit difficult to see. Follow the trail and keep a sharp eye out for markers as you hike. Continue past a private residence and a road on the right: stay on the trail here. At an intersection, angle left, away from the private road. The trail heads gradually uphill and then downhill past thick foliage. After a short clearing, the trail heads downhill and back into the trees. There is a creek on your right with the forest floor opening up considerably. Cross a small creek bed and then head downhill past a creek on your right. After the trail goes uphill, cross a deep creek bed using steps. Now bear right, keeping the creek on your right.

Soon veer left, away from the creek, and head down steps into another creek bed and up the other side. Go past a number 6 trail marker on the right. After the trail goes to the left, look for a pond on your right and trailhead signs for the Sand Branch and Little Lake Creek Loop trails. Take the left fork to follow the Sand Branch Trail. The trail markers are now yellow. As the trail bends left and climbs away from the pond, it enters a more open, less overgrown realm. There is a small creek on your left, as you pass by a sign for a primitive campsite. Continue straight, following the trail. At FS 244, cross the road and head toward the hiker trail sign on the other side. The trail heads downhill and through another motorized-vehicle barrier. A creek is to the left of the sandy trail. Cross the creek bed and head up the other side to the yellow trail marker.

At the next two creek beds, use steps to descend and then ascend the other side. Follow the trail as it winds uphill. At a Lone Star Hiking Trail sign, go straight. The trail markers are again all white. Continue on another straight stretch that heads gradually uphill. There is an old logging road running parallel to the trail. Cross the next creek bed and head up a very steep bank on the other side. Once out of the creek bed, bear right at an intersection. The trail markers here are at least 10 feet high in the trees and may be difficult to see. Follow the trail and look for markers as the trail heads downhill and across another creek bed.

The trail levels before again heading downhill and into another creek bed. Head up the other side and follow the trail as it continues uphill. Cross two more small creek beds and then hike past a Lone Star Hiking Trail sign, continuing straight. Head downhill and cross one last creek bed before heading back uphill and through a motorized-vehicle barrier. Cross a large bridge and head up the steps on the other side toward another vehicle barrier and a hiker trail sign. Cross FS 211 and head toward your car in the parking lot across the road.

Note: The Sand Branch Loop is part of the Lone Star Hiking Trail, a 128-mile trail that has gained National Recreation Trail recognition. The trail winds through the Sam Houston National Forest and consists of three major sections: a 40-mile Lake Conroe section, the Central section, and the Winters Bayou/Tarkington Creek section. The trails were developed and are now maintained by the Lone Star Hiking Trail Club.

NEARBY ACTIVITIES

Sam Houston Memorial and Park Complex (**samhouston.org**), the Texas Prison Museum (**txprisonmuseum.org**), H.E.A.R.T.S. Veterans Museum (**heartsmuseum .com**), Sam Houston National Forest, Lake Conroe.

SAM HOUSTON NATIONAL FOREST:
North Wilderness Loop

41

IN BRIEF

The Sam Houston National Forest is one of four national forests in Texas. It contains more than 163,000 acres and is located between Huntsville, Conroe, Cleveland, and Richards. The district ranger's office is located on FM 1375, 3 miles west of New Waverly. Archeological evidence that dates back 7,000 years has been found in a number of sites in the national forest. Any artifacts found must not be disturbed, as they are protected by federal and state regulations. Hiking, fishing, and hunting are allowed in most of the national forest. Check the website for the Sam Houston National Forest at **www.fs.fed.us** for more information.

DESCRIPTION

To start the North Wilderness Loop hike, enter the woods at the hiker sign. Go past an information sign and through a motorized-vehicle barrier to reach the 1-foot-wide trail. The vegetation is thick on both sides, with FM 149 running on your left just past the trees. The markers on this trail are silver and are located about 6 feet high in the trees. If during any hike on the Lone Star Trail you have not seen a marker in a few minutes, stop and get your bearings. Look ahead and to both sides and you should be able to see a marker in the distance. Hike through a telephone easement and enter the forest on the other side. The trail

- -

Directions ⎯⎯⎯⎯⎯⎯⎯⎯⎯⎯⎯⟶

From the intersection of Beltway 8 and I-45, head north 41.5 miles on I-45, exit at FM 1375, and turn left. Go 14 miles to FM 149. Turn left and go 1.5 miles to the Lone Star Hiking Trail parking lot, on the right.

KEY AT-A-GLANCE INFORMATION

LENGTH: 7.9 miles

CONFIGURATION: Balloon

DIFFICULTY: Moderate to difficult

SCENERY: Woodlands, creeks, ponds

EXPOSURE: Shady

TRAIL TRAFFIC: Light

TRAIL SURFACE: Dirt

HIKING TIME: 3.5 hours

DRIVING DISTANCE: 60 miles from the intersection of Beltway 8 and I-45

ACCESS: Free

MAPS: USGS San Jacinto, Montgomery, Richards; trail map available at the Lone Star Hiking Trail Club website, lshtclub.com

WHEELCHAIR ACCESS: None

FACILITIES: Parking, trail markers

SPECIAL COMMENTS: There are no facilities on many of the trails in the Sam Houston National Forest, so make sure you bring sunscreen, bug repellent, water, and food. Pets must remain on a leash at all times. Motorized vehicles and bicycles are not allowed on the trails in the national forest. Wear appropriate footwear and long pants whenever hiking here.

GPS TRAILHEAD COORDINATES

LATITUDE: N 30° 30.604'
LONGITUDE: W 95° 43.059'

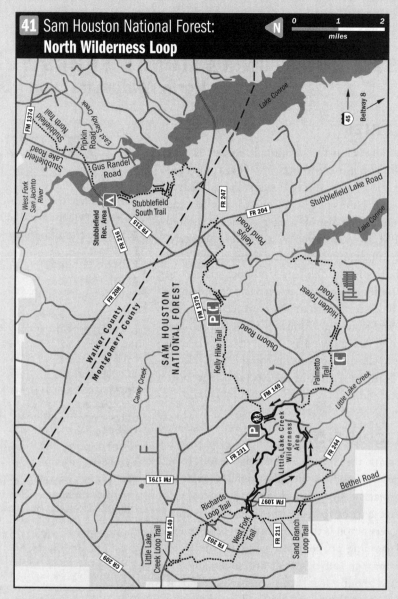

N

0 1 2
miles

45
Beltway 8

Lake Conroe

FM 1374

Stubblefield
North Trail

Pipkin
Road

East Saras Creek

Stubblefield
Lake Road

Gus Randel
Road

West Fork
San Jacinto River

Stubblefield
Rec. Area

Stubblefield
South Trail

FR 216

FR 215

FR 247

FR 204

Stubblefield Lake Road

Lake Conroe

Kellys
Pond Road

Hidden Forest
Road

SAM HOUSTON
NATIONAL FOREST

FR 208

Walker County
Montgomery County

Caney Creek

FM 1375

Kelly Hike Trail

Osborn Road

FM 149

Palmetto
Trail

Little Lake Creek

FR 231

Little Lake Creek
Wilderness
Area

FR 244

FM 1791

Bethel Road

Richards
Loop Trail

West Fork
Trail

FM 1097

FR 211

Sand Branch
Loop Trail

FM 149

Little Lake
Creek Loop Trail

FR 203

CR 209

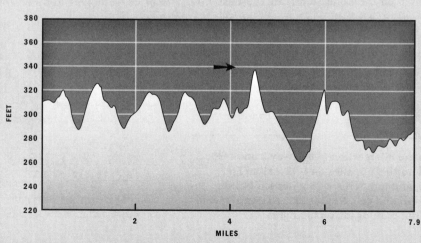

380
360
340
320
300
280
260
240
220

FEET

2   4   6   7.9

MILES

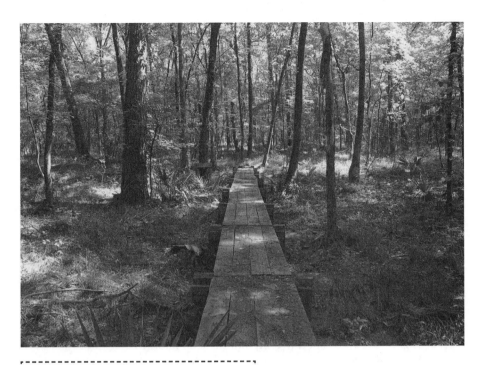

A makeshift bridge made of boards over a bog

widens to about 4 feet and moves away from the highway, which is now behind you. Go through a thick canopy of trees as the trail heads downhill. The vegetation opens up briefly, allowing you to see deeper into the forest. Once it heads back uphill, the trail starts to wind back and forth. Although there is considerable grass on the trail surface, it is still easy to follow.

The trail widens, becoming even more defined as it heads uphill. Climb over a fallen tree and continue on the straight path past a large stand of pine trees before the trail curves and goes downhill. Cross a creek bed and follow the markers to the next, deeper creek bed. Watch your footing both going down and back up out of the deep creek bed. The trail surface is sandier here and the footing is more difficult. At the intersection with the North Wilderness Trail, take the right fork. The markers on this part of the hike are pink on silver. The trail is wide with some exposed tree roots. There are thick weeds and grass growing on both sides of the trail, so stay on the trail at all times. Poisonous snakes do exist in the Sam Houston National Forest.

Hike across a dirt road and head back into the woods, following the trail markers in the trees. Watch out for spider webs from early spring to late fall. Although these spiders are not dangerous, the webs can be irritating. There is a creek on your right, past the trees and dense foliage. The trail, although very narrow here, is still easy to follow. Hike through a very deep creek bed, climbing (and I mean climbing) down one side and up the other. Once out of the creek bed, the trail curves right, with a trail marker in a tree on the right. There are considerable lichen and moss growing on the trail, indicating a damp environment. Watch your footing.

Continue along the trail, following a creek on your right. At the next creek, head to your right and climb down into the creek bed. Go to your left slightly where the creek turns, to see the trail up ahead and the trail marker in a tree on the right. The trail goes right and then heads uphill steeply. The creek is again on your right and the trail bends left. Beyond the creek, the vegetation opens up some but the trail is still very narrow. Look for trail markers in the trees to help you stay on the trail. After a long, straight, flat stretch the trail winds through cut logs and over fallen trees. When you come to a point where overgrown foliage has obscured the trail, head left and then go immediately to the right to get back on the trail. The trail opens some, with a creek on your right. There are not a lot of trail markers in this area, so just follow the trail. Head downhill into a creek bed and back up the other side to a flat section with a creek on your left. Follow the trail right and up a steep slope. There is a trail marker in a tree on the right as you exit the creek bed. The vegetation opens up as the trail heads downhill and toward another creek bed. It curves left just short of the creek and heads downhill into the creek bed. Hike to the other side and then follow the trail as it goes left and then downhill and through another creek bed. The trail bends right and uphill. After a long uphill climb, the trail curves right and the vegetation gets thicker. Go through a small campsite, continuing straight to the next trail marker. At the next intersection, take the left fork to get on the Lone Star Hiking Trail, indicated by silver markers.

Cross a creek over a small bridge. There is a service road on your right with a clearing just past the road. Head downhill through another creek bed and hike up the steps on the other side. Cross another creek bed using the steps on both sides. Pass by a sign for the National Wilderness Forest and a trail marker, both left. Continue hiking parallel to the dirt road on your right, as the trail narrows and heads uphill. This is a long, straight stretch of the trail that eventually heads downhill and through a creek bed. Out of the creek, the trail goes uphill through very thick vegetation. Cross a creek bed and climb the other side over exposed roots. Go through a low area that may be wet or muddy and then head gradually uphill. The road and clearing are still on your right, with the deep forest on your left.

As the trail widens, it follows a rolling course away from the service road. At an intersection, take the left fork to enter the Little Lake Creek Wilderness Area. The trail markers are still silver, since you are still on part of the Lone Star Hiking Trail. Hike through a small creek bed and into an area with much less dense vegetation. Cross a bridge, then head left to another bridge over a very low boggy area. To continue through the low area, use boards that have been laid end-to-end as a walkway. Beyond this area, head left to get back on the trail. At a trail sign on your right, go left. Pass through an intersection on the left and continue straight past a creek on your right. Take the left fork at the next intersection and follow the trail markers on the now-wider trail. Go past a house on the right and then through a creek bed.

Continue past an M marker and a number 7 marker in a tree on your right. Hike through some cut logs and head downhill into a creek bed. Go slightly to your right to head up the other side. A creek continues on your right for quite some distance. Cross a bridge and then hike past a number 8 marker on a post on the right. Cross another bridge and at the next intersection, take the right fork to head back to the parking lot. You have 0.7 miles from this intersection to the end of the hike.

Note: The North Wilderness Loop is part of the Lone Star Hiking Trail, a 128-mile trail that has gained National Recreation Trail recognition. The trail winds through the Sam Houston National Forest and consists of three major sections: a 40-mile Lake Conroe section, the Central section, and the Winters Bayou/Tarkington Creek section. The trails were developed and are now maintained by the Lone Star Hiking Trail Club.

NEARBY ACTIVITIES

Sam Houston Memorial and Park Complex (**samhouston.org**), the Texas Prison Museum (**txprisonmuseum.org**) H.E.A.R.T.S. Veterans Museum (**heartsmuseum .com**), Sam Houston National Forest, Lake Conroe.

42 SAM HOUSTON NATIONAL FOREST:
Huntsville Hike

GPS TRAILHEAD COORDINATES

LATITUDE: N 30° 38.995'
LONGITUDE: W 95° 30.632'

IN BRIEF

The Sam Houston National Forest is one of four national forests in Texas. It contains more than 163,000 acres and is located between Huntsville, Conroe, Cleveland, and Richards. The district ranger's office is located on FM 1375, 3 miles west of New Waverly. Archeological evidence that dates back 7,000 years has been found in a number of sites in the national forest. Any artifacts found must not be disturbed, as they are protected by federal and state regulations. Hiking, fishing, and hunting are allowed in most of the national forest. Check the website for the Sam Houston National Forest at **www.fs.fed.us** for more information.

DESCRIPTION

To start the Huntsville Hike, go into the woods at the hiker trail sign. Take a left and then a quick right to go toward another hiker trail sign. Pass by a number 35 trail marker on the right, opposite the sign. This is a dirt trail headed away from I-45 and into thick forest vegetation. The trail markers are silver and are located about 6 feet high in the trees along the trail. If during any hike on the Lone Star Trail you have not seen a marker in a few minutes, stop and get your bearings. Look ahead and to both sides and you should be able to see a marker in the distance. Watch for spider webs across the trail. While the webs are annoying,

----

Directions ⟶

From the intersection of Beltway 8 and I-45, head north 49 miles on I-45 and take the exit for Park Road 40. Cross under the freeway and go right on the two-way feeder road 0.7 miles to the trailhead on the left.

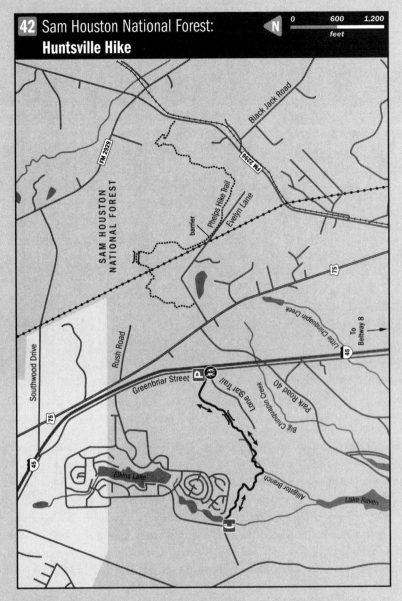

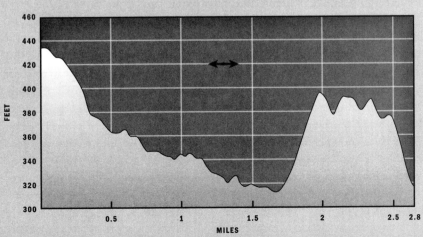

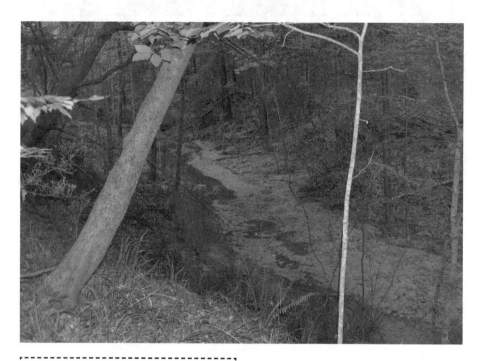

Alligator Branch that runs parallel to the trail

the spiders are not poisonous. Continue on the trail as it heads downhill gradually. Follow the trail uphill and left before it curves right. It then goes back downhill, winding through the trees. Step over some exposed roots, watching your footing at all times. At a trail marker on a tree on the right, go right. Step around a fallen pine tree and get back on the trail, looking for markers ahead. Once around the tree, the trail heads downhill. Follow the trail marker in a tree on the right and go left, away from a low sandy area on your right. Step through a cut fallen tree and go left, away from a small creek on the right. The trail narrows as it heads uphill and out of the low area.

There is a deep creek about 30 feet away on your right. Hike down into a small creek bed and head up the other side and to the right. Along with silver trail markers, there are also pink blazes in the trees to help guide you. The creek is still on your right, as you go under a canopy of old vines. Follow the trail downhill and across a bridge. Past the bridge, the trail goes right, past the creek that continues to run on your right. The banks of the creek are loose and sandy, so stay on the trail at all times. At a fork in the trail, bear left, toward a trail marker in a tree on the right.

Pass by a number 34 trail marker on the right and follow the trail as it winds uphill toward a creek. Go left around the large root ball of a fallen tree and then head right to get back on the trail. The trail heads uphill steeply over a bed of pine needles, making the trail surface a bit difficult to see. Look for the trail markers in the trees to guide you. Follow the trail to the right over exposed roots and down into a creek bed. Head up the other side and into an area with considerably more grass and fan palms on the forest floor. The trail narrows again and heads downhill into a more open area. Step through some cut fallen trees and into a sunnier area with small pine trees. Cross a small creek bed, following the trail markers on the other side. Parts of this trail have been washed out by heavy rains, so look for the markers in the trees. Hike through a low wet area, heading toward the creek. Go left past a pond on the right. The trail is not much higher than the creek bed that you have been hiking near: it can be muddy and at times very wet. Wear appropriate footwear and long pants whenever hiking in the Sam Houston National Forest. Continue on the sandy trail as it narrows to only a foot wide, with grass and weeds brushing up against your legs. Step over a fallen tree and back onto the trail, which is almost obscured here by grass and weeds. Look for trail markers and pink blazes to guide you through Alligator Creek. Go over another fallen tree, past a boggy area on your right and a small pond on your left. Turn right and look for the pink blazes. The trail surface is totally covered in low vegetation. At a trail marker in the trees, hike to the right over some debris. Go through some high weeds following the pink blazes. Hike toward two more pink blazes to get back on the trail. Cross a small stream heading toward the trail marker on the other side.

Beyond the creek bed, the trail heads steeply uphill. Go by trail marker number 33 on the right and an M trail marker in a tree on the left. Notice the lichen and moss growing on this part of the trail, indicating a damp environment. Now the trail roller-coasters along past a number 32 post and through a more open forest. As the trail heads downhill, you can see trail markers ahead. Cross another small creek bed and hike under a canopy of trees, heading downhill on the winding trail, which skirts the Elkins Lake subdivision. Cross a telephone easement, heading to the left and then quickly to the right up a small hill. At the end of the trail is the Elkins Lake subdivision and a lake. Turn around and retrace your route to the parking area.

Note: The Huntsville Hike is part of the Lone Star Hiking Trail, a 128-mile trail that has gained National Recreation Trail recognition. The trail winds through the Sam Houston National Forest and consists of three major sections: a 40-mile Lake Conroe section, the Central section, and the Winters Bayou/ Tarkington Creek section. The trails were developed and are now maintained by the Lone Star Hiking Trail Club.

NEARBY ACTIVITIES

Sam Houston Memorial and Park Complex (**samhouston.org**), the Texas Prison Museum (**txprisonmuseum.org**), H.E.A.R.T.S. Veterans Museum, (**heartsmuseum .com**), Sam Houston National Forest, Lake Conroe.

43 SAM HOUSTON NATIONAL FOREST:
Phelps Hike

KEY AT-A-GLANCE INFORMATION

LENGTH: 10.4 miles

CONFIGURATION: Out-and-back

DIFFICULTY: Difficult

SCENERY: Woodlands, creeks

EXPOSURE: Shady

TRAIL TRAFFIC: Light

TRAIL SURFACE: Dirt

HIKING TIME: 5.5 hours

DRIVING DISTANCE: 50 miles from the intersection of Beltway 8 and I-45

ACCESS: Free

MAPS: USGS Phelps; trail map available at the Lone Star Hiking Trail Club website, lshtclub.com

WHEELCHAIR ACCESS: None

FACILITIES: Trail markers

SPECIAL COMMENTS: There are no facilities on many of the trails in the Sam Houston National Forest except for parking, so make sure you bring sunscreen, bug repellent, water, and food. Pets must remain on a leash at all times. Motorized vehicles and bicycles are not allowed on the trails in the national forest. Wear appropriate footwear and long pants whenever hiking in the Sam Houston National Forest.

GPS TRAILHEAD COORDINATES

LATITUDE: N 30° 39.106'
LONGITUDE: W 95° 29.916'

IN BRIEF

The Sam Houston National Forest is one of four national forests in Texas. It contains more than 163,000 acres and is located between Huntsville, Conroe, Cleveland, and Richards. The district ranger's office is located on FM 1375, 3 miles west of New Waverly. Archeological evidence that dates back 7,000 years has been found in a number of sites in the national forest. Any artifacts found must not be disturbed, as they are protected by federal and state regulations. Hiking, fishing, and hunting are allowed in most of the national forest. Check the website for the Sam Houston National Forest at **www.fs.fed.us** for more information.

DESCRIPTION

To start the Phelps Hike, enter the woods at the hiker trail sign and head uphill. The trail is closed to horses, motor vehicles, and pack stock at all times. As you enter the woods, a fence and private road are left, and woods are right. Look for small white markers in the trees to guide you the length of the hike. If during any hike on the Lone Star Trail you have not seen a marker in a few minutes, stop and get your bearings. Look ahead and to both sides and you should be able to see a marker in the distance. The trail surface is dirt with pine

----

Directions ———————————➔

From the intersection of Beltway 8 and I-45, head north 49 miles on I-45 and take the exit for Park Road 40. Turn right, go 1 mile to US 75, and turn right. Turn left at the first street, Evelyn Lane, and go 0.3 miles to the trailhead, which is on the left side of the road just past a blue gate. Park on the grass next to the dirt road.

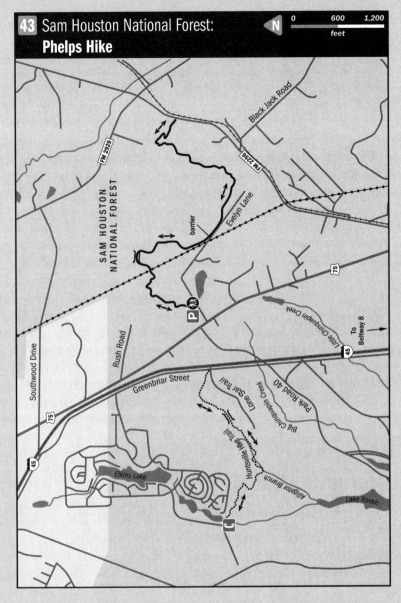

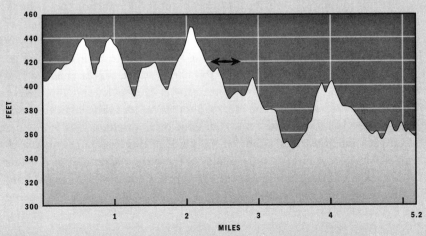

needles and heads uphill gradually, curving right, past white markers and pink blazes in the trees. The vegetation, which is thick on both sides of the trail, is made up of low-lying forest plants such as American holly and tall loblolly pines. Watch for spider webs across the trail. Most of the spiders are banana spiders and are harmless. Also remember that the Sam Houston National Forest is home to bears, alligators, and venomous snakes, so take precautions at all times.

Continue along the trail watching for trail markers, since parts of the trail are not easy to recognize without them. Go left of a fallen tree and then uphill. The middle of the trail has washed out, so watch your footing. Hike under a canopy of trees, following the trail as it curves left. As you head uphill, the trail winds past a more open area, on the right. It then swings right and downhill toward a creek. Cross the creek bed and follow the trail as it heads downhill. Eventually, the trail bends left and then heads back uphill. Go by marker 37 on the left side of the trail. Wander downhill and through a small creek bed, then climb uphill and right.

The next creek bed is fairly steep, so take it slowly. Use the step on the downhill side and then cross, heading uphill and straight, following markers in the trees. Go uphill and then to the right. The area on the left opens, letting in more sunlight and improving visibility into the woods. Cross an old road toward blazes and trail markers. Back in the trees, the trail heads uphill, losing some of the thick foliage. At the top of the climb, the trail heads downhill into thicker foliage. Hike by marker 38 on the right and then cross a telephone easement to the markers on the other side. The trail bends left and takes you into another creek bed. Go right and cross a small bridge, heading up the other side of the creek to the next trail marker.

Once out of the creek bed, the trail heads steeply downhill, taking you across another creek and up the other side. Cross a road toward the marker on the other side. Hike under a canopy of trees. Pass by another marker 38 on the left and head downhill. There is a creek on your right. Turn right to cross the creek bed and head up the other side and to the right. Now head away from the creek and uphill. Make sure you look for trail markers, since this part of the trail is more difficult to follow. Go by trail marker number 39 and continue straight. When you get to the top of the hill, the vegetation gets thicker. Cross another road and head left, toward the blazes in the trees. The telephone easement you crossed earlier is to your right. Head to your right at the trail marker and go back into the woods, heading downhill. You can now see the easement in the distance on your right. Pass through a motorized-vehicle barrier and onto Evelyn Lane. Hike down the left side of the dirt road for 0.3 miles to the hiker trail sign on the left. There is a lone house on Evelyn Lane on the right.

Head back into the trees. Many of the pines in this area are young, with slim trunks. The trail winds through an alley of these trees. Continue as it winds to a small stream and then uphill. Now the trail heads downhill for several hundred yards on a very straight stretch. At the next intersection, go straight passing marker 40. Hike under a fallen tree and follow the trail as it narrows considerably. Cross a creek bed and pass through very dense vegetation that makes finding the trail markers a bit of a challenge. Stop and take your time to find your bearings. At the next creek, hike across and then head to the right. Cross a bridge over a much deeper creek and continue straight. At a big marker on a tree to the left, go right, into another creek bed. Once across the creek, head left and then up the steep bank. The trail bends left and uphill. Head left and back down into the creek bed. You cross the creek again and go right. Look ahead to see a marker on a tree on the right.

The trail bends right to cross a creek bed and then goes left. If you do not see any metal markers in the trees, look for pink or orange blazes. Go by marker 41, then turn right at the double trail markers on a tree to the left. Pass by another number 41 trail marker on the right, with a small creek running on your left. The vegetation overhead opens up greatly here, letting in much more sunlight. At the next intersection, continue straight toward trail markers. The lower vegetation is thick enough in this area to hide some of the trail markers, so make sure you keep an eye out for blazes. As you continue along the trail, the vegetation opens up on the left, revealing a stand of newly planted pines. Go straight through an intersection, following orange blazes. This is a very shady part of the trail. Go under a canopy of trees and cross a small creek bed, looking for the blazes on the opposite side. The trail is heading uphill. Cross an easement, past a gate on the left, and head back into the trees. At the double markers on the trees, take a right and head downhill, toward a house in the distance on the left.

As you approach the house, the trail curves right. Go by a number 42 trail marker on the left. FM 2296 is now on your left, past the trees. At a fallen tree on the right, turn left, following blazes. Exit the trees at FM 2296, turn around, and retrace your route to the parking area.

Note: The Phelps Hike is part of the Lone Star Hiking Trail, a 128-mile trail that has gained National Recreation Trail recognition. The trail winds through the Sam Houston National Forest and consists of three major sections: a 40-mile Lake Conroe section, the Central section, and the Winters Bayou/Tarkington Creek section. The trails were developed and are now maintained by the Lone Star Hiking Trail Club.

NEARBY ACTIVITIES

Sam Houston Memorial and Park Complex (**samhouston.org**), the Texas Prison Museum (**txprisonmuseum.org**), H.E.A.R.T.S. Veterans Museum (**heartsmuseum .com**), Sam Houston National Forest, Lake Conroe.

44 SAM HOUSTON NATIONAL FOREST:
South Wilderness

KEY AT-A-GLANCE INFORMATION

LENGTH: 7 miles

CONFIGURATION: Out-and-back

DIFFICULTY: Difficult

SCENERY: Woodlands, creeks, ponds

EXPOSURE: Shady

TRAIL TRAFFIC: Light

TRAIL SURFACE: Dirt and grass

HIKING TIME: 3.5 hours

DRIVING DISTANCE: 62 miles from the intersection of Beltway 8 and I-45

ACCESS: Free

MAPS: USGS Montgomery; trail map available at the Lone Star Hiking Trail Club website, lshtclub.com

WHEELCHAIR ACCESS: None

FACILITIES: Parking, trail markers

SPECIAL COMMENTS: There are no facilities on many of the trails in the Sam Houston National Forest except for parking, so make sure you bring sunscreen, bug repellent, water, and food. Pets must remain on a leash at all times. Motorized vehicles and bicycles are not allowed on the trails in the national forest. Wear appropriate footwear and long pants whenever hiking in the Sam Houston National Forest.

GPS TRAILHEAD COORDINATES

LATITUDE: N 30° 28.959'
LONGITUDE: W 95° 41.838'

IN BRIEF

The Sam Houston National Forest is one of four national forests in Texas. It contains more than 163,000 acres and is located between Huntsville, Conroe, Cleveland, and Richards. The district ranger's office is located on FM 1375, 3 miles west of New Waverly. Archeological evidence that dates back 7,000 years has been found in a number of sites in the national forest. Any artifacts found must not be disturbed, as they are protected by federal and state regulations. Hiking, fishing, and hunting are allowed in most of the national forest. Check the website for the Sam Houston National Forest at **www.fs.fed.us** for more information.

DESCRIPTION

After parking, hike across FM 149 to the hiker trail sign. Watch for traffic, since this is a busy highway. Go into the trees to get on the narrow dirt trail. The trail markers are orange and are about six feet high in the trees. If during any hike on the Lone Star Trail you have not seen a marker in a few minutes, stop and get your bearings. Look ahead and to both sides and you should be able to see a marker in the distance. The trail heads downhill and curves left, past a creek on your left. Parts of this trail can be steep and may require some climbing in and out of creek beds, so make sure you wear proper footwear. Hike into a low area

Directions

From the intersection of Beltway 8 and I-45, head north 41.5 miles on I-45, exit at FM 1375, and turn left. Go 14 miles to FM 149. Turn left and go 3.5 miles to the first Lone Star Hiking Trail parking lot on the left.

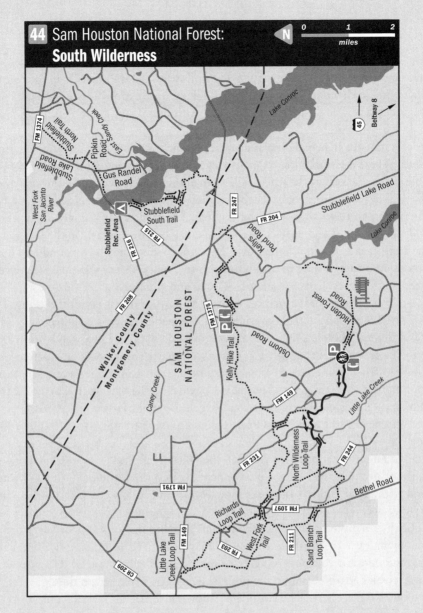

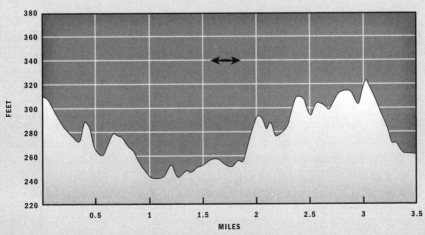

and up the other side. Take a quick left, following the trail marker in the tree on the right. Go downhill into a creek bed, hiking over exposed roots, and climb up the other side. This is a very rolling trail with many humps, or moguls. A creek is now on your right.

Notice the lichen and moss growing on the trail, indicating a damp environment. Where the trail narrows, it also levels and starts winding through the trees. Follow the markers as the trail bends right and into a creek bed. Out of the creek, the trail heads uphill steeply. The vegetation is thick and impenetrable, so stay on the trail at all times to prevent getting lost. The trail, which is only about a foot wide, curves right and heads down into a creek bed over steps. Up the other side, the trail zigzags uphill. Climb down into a deep creek bed, cross, and climb the other side. You may have to use your hands for balance, since these climbs are very steep and slippery. Cross another creek bed and climb the other side on steps.

Go by a number 12 marker and an M marker in a tree on the right. The trail, which gets shade from overhead foliage, widens and passes through a large stand of small pines. There are many exposed roots here, so watch your footing. The trail winds through a low area that may be wet or muddy: watch your footing. When you come to a black gumbo area that may be muddy, look for a trail marker. Go straight to see the trail, which is slightly right. There is a trail marker on a tree on the right, beyond which the trail heads uphill. Cross a creek bed and head right to a Pole Creek Trail sign, on the right. Go left and cross a deep creek bed, climbing the other side.

At an intersection, bear right on the Pole Creek Trail. The trail markers on this part of the hike are blue—you're heading into the Little Lake Creek Wilderness Area. Bear right at the next intersection and follow the blue markers into another deep creek bed. At a Pole Creek Trail sign, take the left fork, hiking past a boggy area on the right. The trail widens here but the foliage is still very dense, canopying over the trail. At times you may even need to duck under branches. Past the trees on your left is a creek running parallel to the trail. Go through a small creek bed and head up the other side, to a trail marker on the right. As the trail goes right, the vegetation opens, allowing some sunlight to come through the trees.

As the trail heads uphill onto drier ground, it narrows. The trail bends left and then goes straight for a long stretch. When you come to a point where the trail seems to swing right, stop: look for a marker in the large tree ahead and go straight. Head into another creek bed and hike toward the trail marker on the other side. Once out of the creek bed, the trail levels, with a creek on your right. Look through the trees to your right for a large horse farm and rolling fields. Just before you reach a fence on your right, the trail swings left and heads gradually uphill. Now it widens and becomes more defined before coming to a trail marker on the left. Here go straight, hiking through some cut fallen trees.

The trail curves right taking you past a national-forest wilderness sign on a tree to the left. Now curve left and cross a small creek. The trail is wide and shady here, with a predominance of pines. Hike through another small creek bed and then go steadily uphill. At an intersection, go across a dirt road, then hike through a cut log and past an open field on your right. At a Pole Creek Trail sign, take the left fork to get on the Lone Star Hiking Trail: the trail markers are now silver. Some of this area has recently been cleared, so there is more sunlight coming through, creating an open feel to the forest. Some of the trail can be difficult to see, so make sure you look for trail markers in the trees.

Now go through some motorized-vehicle barriers and cross a dirt road to the Little Lake Creek Wilderness Area sign. Go back into the woods; there is a deep creek on your left. At a trail sign, curve right and then go through a low, muddy area. Hike across some boards that have been laid end-to-end to create a makeshift walkway. Now cross a long bridge, go right, and then cross a short bridge heading left and out of the muddy area. Hike past marker 6 on the right. After crossing a small creek you reach a Little Lake Creek Wilderness Area sign. Here turn around and retrace your route to the parking area, remembering to follow the trail markers—silver, blue, and then orange.

Note: The South Wilderness hike is part of the Lone Star Hiking Trail, a 128-mile trail that has gained National Recreation Trail recognition. The trail winds through the Sam Houston National Forest and consists of three major sections: a 40-mile Lake Conroe section, the Central section, and the Winters Bayou/Tarkington Creek section. The trails were developed and are now maintained by the Lone Star Hiking Trail Club.

NEARBY ACTIVITIES

Sam Houston Memorial and Park Complex (**samhouston.org**), the Texas Prison Museum (**txprisonmuseum.org**), H.E.A.R.T.S. Veterans Museum (**heartsmuseum .com**), Sam Houston National Forest, Lake Conroe.

45 SAM HOUSTON NATIONAL FOREST:
Mercy Fire Tower Loop

KEY AT-A-GLANCE INFORMATION

LENGTH: 7.6 miles

CONFIGURATION: Loop

DIFFICULTY: Moderate

SCENERY: Woodlands, creeks, bayou, old logging road

EXPOSURE: Shady with some sun

TRAIL TRAFFIC: Light

TRAIL SURFACE: Dirt and grass

HIKING TIME: 4 hours

DRIVING DISTANCE: 37 miles from the intersection of Beltway 8 and I-59

ACCESS: Free

MAPS: USGS Westcott; trail map available at the Lone Star Hiking Trail Club website, lshtclub.com

WHEELCHAIR ACCESS: None

FACILITIES: Parking, trail markers

SPECIAL COMMENTS: There are no facilities on many of the trails in the Sam Houston National Forest except for parking, so make sure you bring sunscreen, bug repellent, water, and food. Pets must remain on a leash at all times. Motorized vehicles and bicycles are not allowed on the trails in the national forest. Wear appropriate footwear and long pants whenever hiking in the Sam Houston National Forest.

GPS TRAILHEAD COORDINATES

LATITUDE: N 30° 26.343'
LONGITUDE: W 95° 7.278'

IN BRIEF

The Sam Houston National Forest is one of four national forests in Texas. It contains more than 163,000 acres and is located between Huntsville, Conroe, Cleveland, and Richards. The district ranger's office is located on FM 1375, 3 miles west of New Waverly. Archeological evidence that dates back 7,000 years has been found in a number of sites in the national forest. Any artifacts found must not be disturbed, as they are protected by federal and state regulations. Hiking, fishing, and hunting are allowed in most of the national forest. Check the website for the Sam Houston National Forest at **www.fs.fed.us** for more information.

DESCRIPTION

The Mercy Fire Tower Loop starts in thick woodlands, goes through a riparian landscape, and finishes along an old logging road. To start the hike, head toward the hiker trail sign, going past an information sign and into the woods. Go through the motorized-vehicle barriers and get on a dirt trail. The trail markers are silver and are located about 6 feet high in the trees. If during any hike on the Lone Star Trail you have not seen a marker in a few minutes, stop and get your bearings. Look ahead and to both sides and you should be able to see a marker in the distance. The trail heads downhill winding right over exposed tree

----

Directions ———————————➤

From the intersection of Beltway 8 and I-59, head north 31 miles on I-59, exit at FM 2025, and turn left. Go 6.2 miles to the trailhead parking lot, on the right just past the lumber mill.

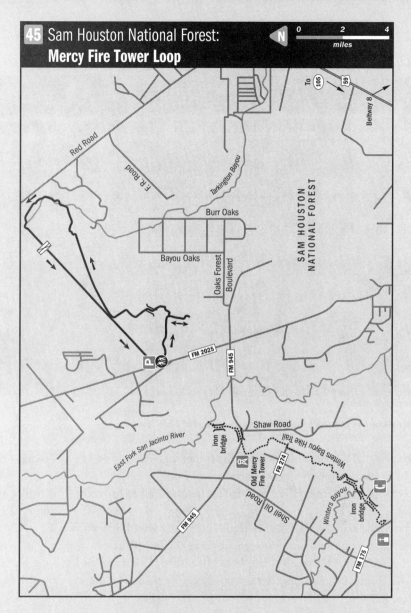

0   2   4
miles

N

To 105 59

Beltway 8

Red Road

F. R. Road

Tarkington Bayou

Burr Oaks

Bayou Oaks

Oaks Forest Boulevard

SAM HOUSTON NATIONAL FOREST

P

FM 2025

FM 945

Shaw Road

East Fork San Jacinto River

Iron bridge

Winters Bayou Hike Trail

Old Mercy Fire Tower

FR 274

Shell Oil Road

FM 945

Winters Bayou

Iron bridge

FM 1725

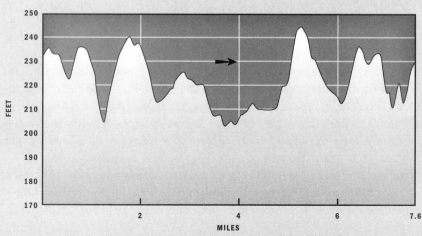

250
240
230
220
210
200
190
180
170

FEET

2   4   6   7.6

MILES

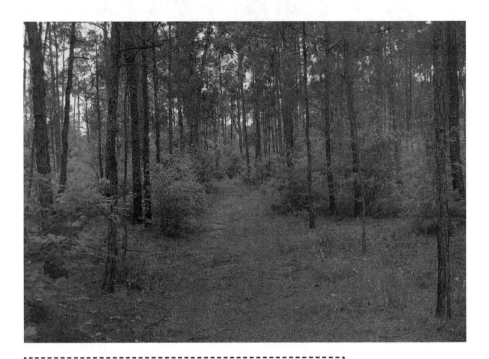

The Mercy Fire Loop trail meanders through a stand of loblolly pines.

roots. Watch your footing. Watch for spider webs across the trail. Although their webs are annoying, the spiders here are not poisonous.

Step over a large fallen tree, following the trail to the right. The trail, which now widens, goes downhill for several hundred yards. After a long straight stretch, the narrow trail curves right and heads uphill. It then widens to about 6 feet before coming to an intersection. Take the left fork, following a blue marker and a red flag in a tree on the left. Hike through an alley of foliage, ducking under some of the bushes that canopy over the trail. The markers are still in the trees, but some of them are obscured by tall bushes in front of them: look carefully to find them.

There is a gravel road on your left. When you come to a hiker trail sign, cross the gravel road and head into the trees, watching for a trail marker in a tree on the left. There are lichen and moss growing on the rocks and tree roots, indicating that this area stays damp. The trail winds through the trees before coming to a small bridge. Cross the bridge and head right, following trail markers in the trees. The trail goes uphill over roots on a long, straight course. There are not many tall trees in this part of the forest, allowing more sunlight to come in on the now-grassy trail. Pass by a Lone Star National Recreation Trail sign on the right. At an intersection, go right, entering a much more open area.

Now the trail heads uphill and goes under a canopy of trees. Hike by a second Lone Star National Recreation Trail sign with double trail markers indicating that the trail goes left. At an intersection, take the right fork, following a trail marker in a tree on the right. The trail widens and becomes more defined. At the next intersection, go straight. Continue on this straight section, heading downhill through an alleyway of pines. After curving left to cross a creek, the trail climbs, but there are some low spots on this part of the trail that may be wet after rain.

Cross a pipeline easement, then follow the trail through a low, possibly wet area. Some of the trail markers here are fire-charred, so follow pink blazes if you do not see a marker in a tree. At a trail marker on the left, go left, then curve right. The trail heads downhill through thick vegetation before coming into a clearing. Go straight, stepping through a large cut fallen tree. At a clearing, head toward a pink blaze and then go left. Hike toward a trail marker ahead in a tree on the right. The forest opens and transitions to a riparian landscape as the trail almost disappears under grass and weeds.

Tarkington Bayou is now on your right and will continue on your right for the next mile. Hike next to the bayou, looking ahead for some red markers in a tree on the left. Go toward a number 87 trail marker and letter M trail marker: the trail is obscured with grass and weeds, so make sure you look for trail markers. Cross a fallen tree and go slightly left. Cross a small creek bed to a trail marker on the other side. The trail comes to the edge of the bayou before heading left, toward a pink streamer. It then goes right and downhill, through another creek. Head toward a trail marker in a tree on the right, then go slightly right. Go through another creek bed, beyond which the trail becomes more defined and easier to follow. At a dirt road, go left to hike along the road and toward FM 2025.

The forest floor vegetation on both sides of the road is low, but there are tall pines overhead. Hike around several fallen trees as the trail heads uphill. Go through a gate, cross another road, and head back onto the trail, soon hiking through another gate. This is a very straight stretch—you can see for a mile or more. Continue across a pipeline easement, staying on the trail. At an intersection, go straight on the now-grassy trail. The trail heads downhill for a long stretch, allowing you to see FM 2025 up ahead. Hike through a small creek bed. Continue uphill to a gate and go left, up a small hill. At FM 2025, go left and hike along the edge of the road to the Lone Star Hiking Trail parking lot and the end of the hike.

NEARBY ACTIVITIES

Sam Houston Memorial and Park Complex (**samhouston.org**), the Texas Prison Museum (**txprisonmuseum.org**), H.E.A.R.T.S. Veterans Museum (**heartsmuseum .com**), Sam Houston National Forest, Lake Conroe.

46 SAM HOUSTON NATIONAL FOREST:
Kelly Hike

KEY AT-A-GLANCE INFORMATION

LENGTH: 13.4 miles

CONFIGURATION: Out-and-back

DIFFICULTY: Moderate to difficult

SCENERY: Woodlands, creeks, bogs

EXPOSURE: Shady

TRAIL TRAFFIC: Light

TRAIL SURFACE: Dirt and grass

HIKING TIME: 6.5 hours

DRIVING DISTANCE: 60 miles from the junction of Beltway 8 and 1-45

ACCESS: Free

MAPS: USGS San Jacinto; trail map available at the Lone Star Hiking Trail Club website, lshtclub.com

WHEELCHAIR ACCESS: None

FACILITIES: Parking, trail markers

SPECIAL COMMENTS: Be sure you bring sunscreen, bug repellent, water, and food. Pets must remain on a leash at all times. Motorized vehicles and bicycles are not allowed on the trails in the national forest. This area is very low and prone to flooding, so watch the weather and wait a few days before entering this area after a heavy rain. Wear appropriate footwear and long pants whenever hiking in the Sam Houston National Forest.

GPS TRAILHEAD COORDINATES

LATITUDE: N 30° 30.604'
LONGITUDE: W 95° 43.059'

IN BRIEF

The Sam Houston National Forest is one of four national forests in Texas. It contains more than 163,000 acres and is located between Huntsville, Conroe, Cleveland, and Richards. The district ranger's office is located on FM 1375, 3 miles west of New Waverly. Archeological evidence that dates back 7,000 years has been found in a number of sites in the national forest. Any artifacts found must not be disturbed, as they are protected by federal and state regulations. Hiking, fishing, and hunting are allowed in most of the national forest. Check the website for the Sam Houston National Forest at **www.fs.fed.us** for more information.

DESCRIPTION

To start the hike, go across FM 149 to the trailhead and enter the woods at the hiker sign. The trail markers on this hike are silver and are located about 6 feet high in the trees. If during any hike on the Lone Star Trail you have not seen a marker in a few minutes, stop and get your bearings. Look ahead and to both sides and you should be able to see a marker in the distance. The narrow dirt trail winds through thick woodlands vegetation. FM 149 is on your left as you hike over exposed roots. Watch your footing and wear proper footwear. The trail turns right and then goes

----

Directions ⟶

From the intersection of Beltway 8 and I-45, head north 41.5 miles on I-45, exit at FM 1375, and turn left. Go 14 miles to FM 149. Turn left and go 1.5 miles to the Lone Star Hiking Trail parking lot on the right. The trailhead is across FM 149 at the trailhead sign.

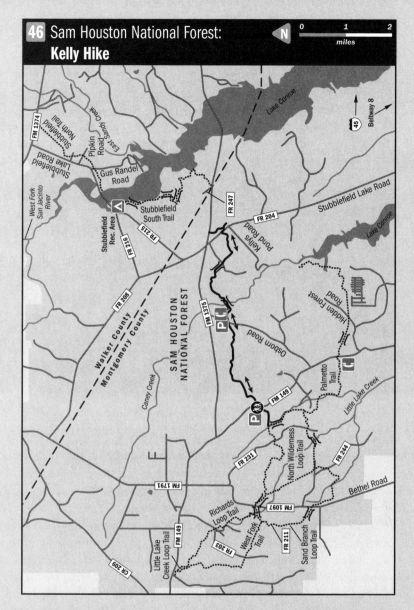

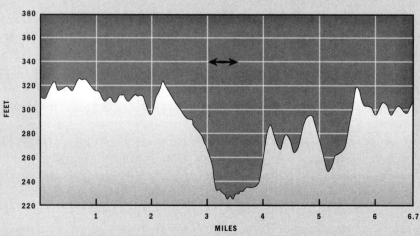

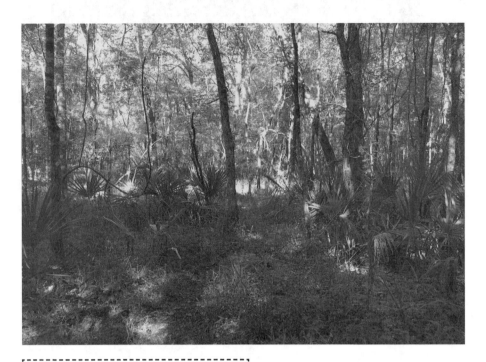

A tropical field of fan palms on the Kelly Hike

under a canopy of trees. Hike past a fence on the right and then take the right fork. Quickly turn left, following a tree marker in a tree up ahead. Watch for spider webs extending across the trail from early spring to late fall. While these spiders are not poisonous, their webs can be irritating.

The trail enters an area that has recently been cleared. At double markers in a tree on the right, take the right fork. At the next set of double markers, go left, entering a more open, sunlit area. The trail heads downhill, curves right, and then passes a number 9 trail marker on a metal post on the left. Hike past a tree on the left with steps going up it, reminiscent of a tree-house ladder. These ladders are used by the forest rangers to get high in the trees as spotters. At the next set of double markers on the left, go left. This is a grassy trail that is difficult to see at times, so follow the trail markers in the trees. Follow markers on the left to an intersection and take the right fork, stepping through a cut fallen tree. Go through a cleared area and follow the trail markers; it is easy to get off route here. The trail, which heads downhill and narrows, is more defined as it winds through the trees. Duck under a large fallen tree and look for a trail marker on a tree ahead. There is a small creek on your left as you hike over a rolling part of the trail.

At an intersection marked by double markers on the left, take the right fork, hiking over exposed roots. Once it goes right, the trail heads slightly uphill and back into thicker and taller vegetation. Hike between two trees with trail markers on each of them and then curve right. Go slightly uphill, passing a number 10 trail marker on a post on the right and an M trail marker on a tree on the left. At the top of the slope the trail heads downhill on a foot-wide trail. It then widens in a more open area and heads downhill. Follow the trail as it bends left and uphill. The grassy trail winds right and downhill. Step over a fallen tree and continue downhill through thick foliage. Go over two more fallen trees and follow the trail to the left. Continue as the trail goes uphill, downhill, and then through an alley of bushes. Hike past an old fence on the right. The trail heads downhill past a forest-service marker on the left. At a junction, take the right fork into a flat open area. Hike through some motorized-vehicle barriers and through a Lone Star Hiking Trail parking lot. Cross Osborn Road and head back into the trees at the hiker sign. Go through motorized-vehicle barriers and get on the wide dirt trail. The vegetation is thicker here and has a more East Texas woodlands feel. Continue across a telephone easement and back into the trees. The trail is very easy to follow in this section, as you come out of the trees and into a clearing that has recently been burned. The trail goes right and downhill over some humps. At the Little Lake Creek and Lone Star trail signs, go straight to stay on the Lone Star Trail. Go through a cut fallen tree and follow the trail as it curves left. There is a tropical feel in this low area, with fan palms, bogs, and mud. The trail narrows to about a foot wide and curves right at a marker on the right. Cross a small creek bed and go right on the other side. This is a very overgrown trail so make sure you watch for the trail markers in the trees.

Cross another creek bed and climb the other side, past a larger creek on your left. The trail narrows and bends left over exposed roots. Climb over a fallen tree, making sure that you look for trail markers in the trees. Hike over a bridge and follow the trail marker to the right over a fallen tree. Continue left of that tree and toward a trail marker ahead. Go past a number 12 trail marker on a post on the right and an M marker on a tree on the left, hiking past a bog on the left. At a trail marker on the right, head slightly left on the primitive, over-grown trail. When you come to foliage debris, go right and then left to get back on the trail. Go under a very large fallen tree, past a creek on your left. The trail swings right through a low, potentially wet and muddy area. Again, look for the trail markers here since the trail surface is not easy to see.

Cross a small creek bed and follow the trail to the right, putting the creek on your left. Go through another creek bed and then follow the trail left past another bog on your right. The trail bends right past the bog and enters a more open area with a large number of dead bushes. The trail is more defined here as you go uphill and onto drier ground. This is a long uphill climb that takes you through an open area. Some of the trail markers are fire-charred and difficult to see, so watch closely for them. Cross a dirt road and go slightly left to find the trail on the other side. Go through a creek bed, using tree roots on the other side to help you climb out. The trail swings right and then goes past a number 13 marker on a post on the left and an M marker on a tree on the right. Hike down-hill toward another creek. Cross the creek using a bridge that is very unstable and leaning greatly right. Once off the bridge, head left and uphill.

Hike through a large burned area with few trail markers. As you hike, turn around to see the trail markers going in the opposite direction to ensure that you are still on the trail. Cross a gas pipeline road to the hiker trail sign on the other side. Go through a gap in a fence and onto a dirt trail. Hike over a fallen tree and continue through the trees, with a creek on your left. At a trail marker, go left as indicated and then down into a creek bed. Beyond the creek, the trail goes right and then bends left, with the creek on your left. The vegetation is thicker here. Go through another creek bed and follow the double trail markers on a tree on the right. The creek is now on your right. Hike past a number 14 trail marker on a post on the right and an M marker on a tree on the left. The trail is very grassy and is heading gradually uphill.

At the next road, turn left. Follow the road until you reach Forest Service Road 204, then cross the road to the trail and stop sign on the other side. This is a wide dirt trail through thick forest vegetation. At an intersection go straight and head uphill on a very well-defined trail. At FM 1375, turn around and retrace the route to the parking area.

NEARBY ACTIVITIES

Sam Houston Memorial and Park Complex (**samhouston.org**), the Texas Prison Museum (**txprisonmuseum.org**), H.E.A.R.T.S. Veterans Museum (**heartsmuseum .com**), Sam Houston National Forest, Lake Conroe.

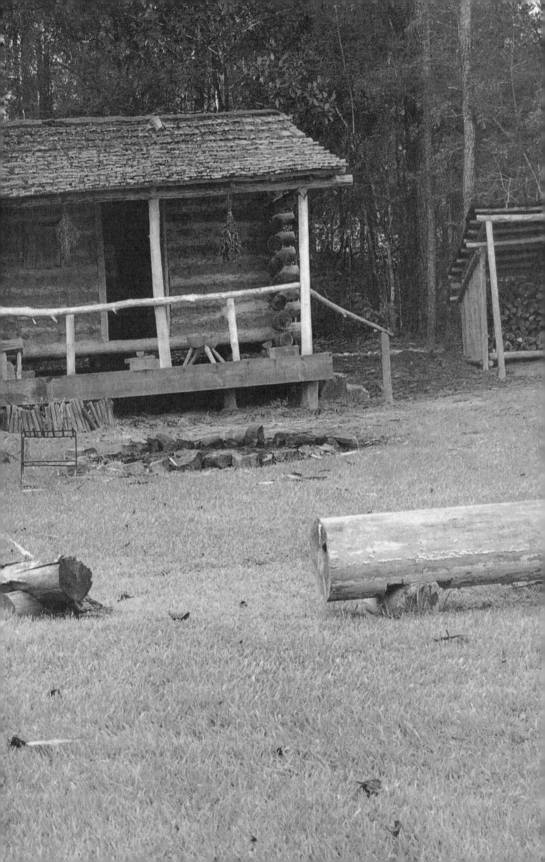

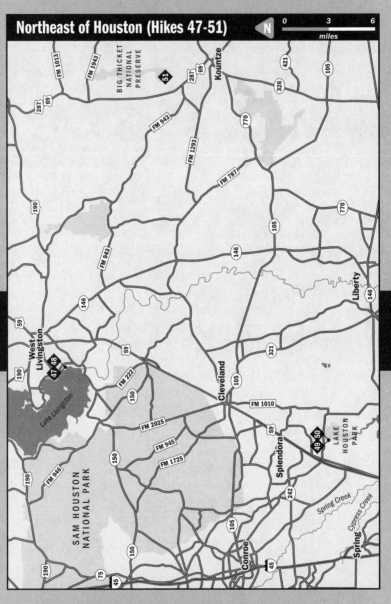

BIG THICKET NATIONAL PRESERVE

FM 1013

FM 1943

51

287

69

Kountze

421

105

287

69

326

FM 943

770

FM 1293

FM 787

190

770

105

FM 943

146

146

Liberty

146

59

West Livingston

59

321

105

Cleveland

Liberty

190

47 48

FM 222

150

Lake Livingston

Splendora

FM 1010

59

49 50

LAKE HOUSTON PARK

FM 2025

FM 945

FM 1725

190

FM 946

SAM HOUSTON NATIONAL PARK

150

242

Spring Creek

Cypress Creek

Spring

105

Conroe

45

190

75

45

150

NORTHEAST of HOUSTON

47 LAKE LIVINGSTON STATE PARK:
Pineywoods Nature and Briar Loop Trails

KEY AT-A-GLANCE INFORMATION

LENGTH: 3 miles

CONFIGURATION: Two loops

DIFFICULTY: Easy

SCENERY: Ponds, piney woods, butterfly garden, boardwalk

EXPOSURE: Shady with some sunny areas

TRAIL TRAFFIC: Light

TRAIL SURFACE: Boardwalk on Pineywoods Nature Trail, dirt and pine needles on Briar Loop

HIKING TIME: 1.25 hours

DRIVING DISTANCE: 55 miles from intersection of Beltway 8 and I-59

ACCESS: $3 per person age 13 and older, or buy a yearly Texas State Parks Pass; open 8 a.m.–10 p.m.

MAPS: USGS Blanchard; trail maps available at park headquarters

WHEELCHAIR ACCESS: Yes—the Pineywoods Nature Trail part of the hike is accessible

FACILITIES: Restrooms, camping, picnicking, swimming, boating, fishing, park store, showers, trail signs, horseback riding

SPECIAL COMMENTS: Pets must be leashed at all times.

GPS TRAILHEAD COORDINATES

LATITUDE: N 30° 39.885'
LONGITUDE: W 95° 0.317'

IN BRIEF

This hike combines the Pineywoods Nature Trail with the Briar Loop to create a nice hike for young children. It is flat and easy to follow. Along Lake Livingston, an 84,800-acre reservoir, are the 635.5 acres of Lake Livingston State Park. Along with easy, well-maintained hiking trails with a variety of views, the park offers camping, picnicking, swimming, mountain biking, horseback riding, fishing, and boating. A special attraction is a 30-foot observation tower, located near the park store and boat ramp, offering views of the park and the lake. Park vegetation includes loblolly pines and water oak in the pine-oak woodlands. Typical wildlife includes white-tailed deer, raccoons, mallard ducks, swamp rabbits, armadillos, and squirrels. The park is most crowded in the fall and spring on weekends, but summer weekends find very few campers here.

DESCRIPTION

Lake Livingston State Park is best known for its boating and fishing opportunities, but don't miss out on the great hikes in the park. The Pineywoods Nature and Briar Loop trails hike combines the 1-mile boardwalk Pineywoods Nature Trail with the 2-mile horseback Briar Loop Trail, which according to park rangers is open to hikers.

Directions ———————————————→

From Beltway 8 and I-59, head north on I-59 for 51 miles and turn left onto FM 1988. Drive 4 miles to FM 3126 and turn right. Drive 0.5 miles to Park Road 65 and turn left. From park headquarters, take Park Road 65 to the first intersection and turn right. The parking lot for the Pineywoods Nature Trail is on the right.

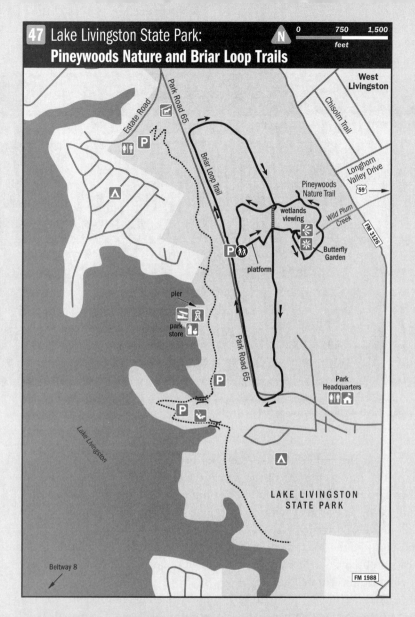

47 Lake Livingston State Park:
Pineywoods Nature and Briar Loop Trails

N

| 0 | 750 | 1,500 |

feet

West Livingston

Estate Road

Park Road 65

Chisolm Trail

Longhorn Valley Drive

59

Briar Loop Trail

Pineywoods Nature Trail

Wild Plum Creek

FM 3126

wetlands viewing

Butterfly Garden

platform

pier

park store

Park Road 65

Park Headquarters

Lake Livingston

LAKE LIVINGSTON STATE PARK

Beltway 8

FM 1988

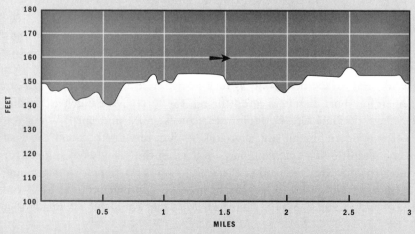

FEET						
180						
170						
160						
150						
140						
130						
120						
110						
100						

| | 0.5 | 1 | 1.5 | 2 | 2.5 | 3 |

MILES

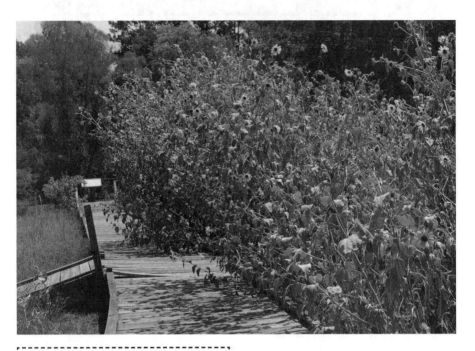

A boardwalk on the Pineywoods Nature Trail

From the trailhead, take the boardwalk trail located to the right of the sign. The trail to the left of the sign is the trail you will come out on after you have completed the Pineywoods Nature Trail. The boardwalk, which is wide and sturdy, is elevated, with a dense pine forest on both sides. Continue down the boardwalk until you reach an open platform with a nature sign describing the birds in the area, such as wood duck, pileated woodpecker, and brown-headed nuthatch. Other area birds include the osprey, bald eagle, scissor-tailed flycatcher, and painted bunting.

Continue along the boardwalk and past the horse trail, until you come to a butterfly garden with a bench and 7-foot-tall sunflowers. Go past the sunflowers to a viewing platform next to a duck pond. Although it's called a duck pond on the park map, it's more of a small lily pond. To continue the hike, retrace your route to the sunflowers, then turn left. There are numerous signs throughout the hike requesting that you stay on the boardwalk and not venture off of it.

While most of the boardwalk is very shady, there are some areas that are quite open for short distances, even though the forest is very dense. Beyond a bridge at Wild Plum Creek, the forest becomes grassy and open. When you spot a frog pond and picnic area sign, take a right to view the pond and visit the picnic platform. The picnic tables are deep in the piney woods, great for a secluded picnic. Go back along the trail and take a right. After crossing another horse trail while still on the boardwalk, continue straight until you come to benches and a nature sign describing the woodland mammals that are present in the park, including white-tailed deer, raccoons, armadillos, and swamp rabbits.

Continue on the boardwalk until you see a IS THIS WOODLANDS OR WETLANDS? sign. Lake Livingston State Park receives on average 48 inches of rain each year, and during the winter months, when most of this rain occurs, the area can look more like a wetland than a woodland. But despite the wetness, loblolly pines and water oaks thrive here—two trees that are considered woodland trees. Continue along the boardwalk and into the parking lot where you started the hike.

To begin the Briar Loop Trail, head out of the parking lot toward the park road. At the park road turn right at the trailhead. Again, the park rangers indicate that hikers are welcome on the trail; just watch out for horses and horse manure. This is a very well-maintained trail, with a dirt and pine needle surface for easy hiking. The trail is shady, wide, and straight, with the road on your left for the first 0.25 miles or so. At the end of the road are the horse stables. If you wish to ride, you must rent horses from the park, as you are not allowed to bring in horses.

Once past the stables, follow the trail right to reenter the woods. Be aware from spring to early fall that numerous spider webs often span the trail. Most of the webs are high enough to duck under. Cross the Pineywoods Nature Trail and continue along the winding trail. Cross the Pineywoods Nature Trail again and continue straight. The trail heads slightly left and becomes narrower as you approach the road. Once at the road, the park headquarters are visible on your left. Follow the trail to the right, along Park Road 65, and then right again as you continue next to the road where you parked. As you hike, listen for the numerous lizards and salamanders scurrying near your feet. Try not to step on them; they are harmless and are a benefit to any woodland area. Continue down the trail until you come to the parking lot and the end of the Briar Loop Trail. A park concession and boat ramp are located about 0.25 miles southwest of the parking lot.

Note: The Briar Loop section of this trail indicates that it is for horseback riding only, but park rangers indicate that hikers are welcome. The trail could be a bit messy if horses are on the trail, but I did not see any; manure on the trail is easily walked over. Although Lake Livingston State Park is a relatively small park, it is a very attractive park that runs along Lake Livingston, giving most campers lakeside views. Boat ramps and fishing piers provide easy access to the lake, where you can catch largemouth bass, white bass, striped bass, flathead catfish, channel catfish, and blue catfish. A fishing license is required for anyone under the age of 17; however, the Texas Parks and Wildlife Department often runs "Family Fishing Celebration" events, which offer free fishing in all state parks. Check the website **tpwd.state.tx.us** for details.

48 LAKE LIVINGSTON STATE PARK:
Lake Trail

KEY AT-A-GLANCE INFORMATION

LENGTH: 4 miles

CONFIGURATION: Out-and-back

DIFFICULTY: Easy

SCENERY: Lake Livingston, piney woods, campsites

EXPOSURE: Shady

TRAIL TRAFFIC: Light

TRAIL SURFACE: Dirt with some crushed granite

HIKING TIME: 2 hours

DRIVING DISTANCE: 55 miles from intersection of Beltway 8 and I-59

ACCESS: $3 per person age 13 and older, or buy a yearly Texas State Parks Pass; open 8 a.m.–10 p.m.

MAPS: USGS Blanchard; trail maps available at park headquarters

WHEELCHAIR ACCESS: None

FACILITIES: Restrooms, camping, picnicking, swimming, boating, fishing, park store, showers, trail signs, horseback riding

SPECIAL COMMENTS: Although the Lake Trail takes you through some campsites, you probably won't encounter many campers during the week. Pets must be leashed at all times.

GPS TRAILHEAD COORDINATES

LATITUDE: N 30° 40.196'
LONGITUDE: W 95° 0.477'

IN BRIEF

The Lake Trail is the only hike in Lake Livingston State Park that takes you along the shores of the lake. It winds through the campgrounds and past the fishing piers. Along Lake Livingston, an 84,800-acre reservoir, are the 635.5 acres of Lake Livingston State Park. Along with easy, well-maintained hiking trails with a variety of views, the park offers camping, picnicking, swimming, mountain biking, horseback riding, fishing, and boating. A special attraction is a 30-foot observation tower, located near the park store and boat ramp, featuring views of the park and the lake. Park vegetation includes loblolly pines and water oak in the pine-oak woodlands. Typical wildlife includes white-tailed deer, raccoons, mallard ducks, swamp rabbits, armadillos, and squirrels. The park is most crowded in the fall and spring on weekends, but summer weekends find very few campers here.

DESCRIPTION

Start the hike on the trailhead located left of the restrooms. Once on the trail, go straight passing by campsites on your right. The trail surface is dirt with leaves, pine needles, and some horse manure. Even though this is not designated as an equestrian trail, it is obviously used by horses: watch your step. After

----

Directions ⟶

From Beltway 8 and I-59, head north on I-59 for 51 miles and turn left onto FM 1988. Drive 4 miles to FM 3126 and turn right. Drive 0.5 miles to Park Road 65 and turn left. To get to the trailhead of the Lake Trail, take Park Road 65 to the first intersection and turn right. At the end of the road, turn left and park in the lot to the left of the restrooms.

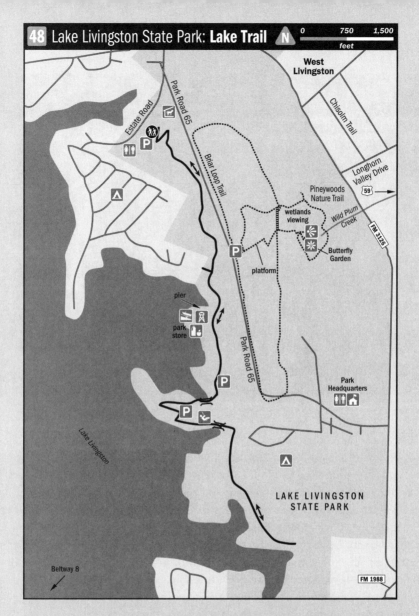

N

0   750   1,500
feet

West
Livingston

Chisolm Trail

Estate Road

Park Road 65

Longhorn
Valley Drive

59

Briar Loop Trail

Pineywoods
Nature Trail

wetlands
viewing

Wild Plum
Creek

Butterfly
Garden

FM 3126

platform

P

P

pier

park
store

Park
Headquarters

Park Road 65

P

P

Lake Livingston

LAKE LIVINGSTON
STATE PARK

Beltway 8

FM 1988

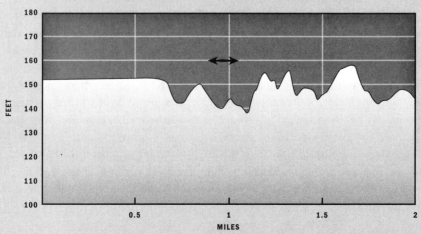

180

170

160

150

140

130

120

110

100

FEET

0.5   1   1.5   2

MILES

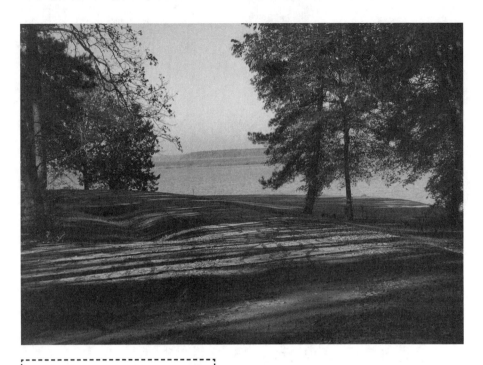

A view of Lake Livingston from the trail

heavy rains this part of the trail can have standing water, but there is room on both sides to go around it. Go left, away from the campsites and the parking lot. Now the trail becomes more defined and easier to follow.

The vegetation, which is not very dense, has numerous downed trees from recent storms. This allows you to see deeply into the trees and into the campsites just past them. Cross a paved road and soon come to an intersection. Go straight to stay on the tree-canopied and shady trail. You can now see glimpses of the lake to your right. After the trail bends left, you can clearly see the lake on the right, with picnic tables on a point jutting out into Lake Livingston. The ground slopes steeply downhill toward the lake, so make sure you stay on the trail.

Cross a road and pick up the trail on the other side. There are picnic sites on both sides of the trail now, with the lake in full view. If you hike during the week, most of the picnic tables and campsites will not be occupied, allowing for a quiet hike. Cross another road and go straight over culverts to get back on the trail. There is parking on your left, and fishing piers, an observation tower, and a park store with restrooms on your right. Veer slightly right toward the park store. Just left of the store, go left to get back on the trail. There are campsites on your left now, with picnic tables and the lake still on your right. Go through the next intersection and head straight. The trail surface is now crushed granite with some dirt and sand. There is a parking lot and boat launch down the hill at right. Continue straight across the boat-launch road; then head slightly left to stay on the trail.

Hike past more picnic tables and go straight toward a bridge on the right. The trail heads steeply downhill to the bridge, so watch your footing. Cross the bridge over a small inlet and go right to stay on the trail. Head left and uphill, past a swimming pool on the right. Continue across the swimming pool walkway and toward yellow motorized-vehicle barriers. Go through the barriers and toward two picnic tables out on a point in the lake. At the tables, turn around and bear left and back into the trees to get back on the trail. This part of the trail runs parallel to the trail you just used. It is about 10 feet wide and continues through another set of traffic barriers. At the barriers, go right to head toward the lake. There is a parking lot to your left. Before you get to the water, go left as you hike on an embankment above the water's edge.

Continue through the trees, with the lake on your immediate right and the road to your left. There is another small inlet right with a bridge that has been damaged and currently is not safe to cross. Continue straight, with a playground on your left and the trees to your right. At an intersection, turn right to get back on the trail. There are campsites on your left, and the lake is far to the right. The trail widens and goes left, past picnic tables on both sides of the trail. There are restrooms with showers on the right through the trees. Continue across a road and then left as the trail curves away from the lake. There are numerous paths that have been made by campers on both sides of the trail: do not take any of these. Stay on the trail and continue straight, past another set of restrooms on the left. As the trail swings left, the lake is no longer visible. Continue just past some benches and a nature trail sign on the right. The nature trail is 0.625 miles long but currently has a bridge out, so go straight to the other end of the nature trail and turn around. Now retrace your route to the parking area.

Note: This trail is not designated as an equestrian trail, but there is evidence of horse use: be careful where you step. Although Lake Livingston State Park is a relatively small park, it is a very attractive park that runs along Lake Livingston, giving most campers lakeside views. Boat ramps and fishing piers provide easy access to the lake, where you can catch largemouth bass, white bass, striped bass, flathead catfish, channel catfish, and blue catfish. A fishing license is required for anyone under the age of 17; however, the Texas Parks and Wildlife Department often runs "Family Fishing Celebration" events, which offer free fishing in all state parks. Check the website **tpwd.state.tx.us** for details.

NEARBY ACTIVITIES

The park is located near the ghost town of Swartwout, the meeting place of Polk County's first commissioner's court before Livingston was selected as the county seat. Swartwout was also a steamboat landing on the Trinity River in the 1830s and 1850s. The City of Livingston is only 10 miles from the park, providing all the amenities and conveniences of a small town. Hundreds of privately owned parks and marinas are in the area around Lake Livingston, providing access to the lake.

49 LAKE HOUSTON PARK:
Peach Creek Trail

**KEY AT-A-GLANCE
INFORMATION**

LENGTH: 4.7 miles

CONFIGURATION: Out-and-back

DIFFICULTY: Moderate

SCENERY: Woodlands, picnic areas, campsites, creeks, wetlands

EXPOSURE: Shady

TRAIL TRAFFIC: Light

TRAIL SURFACE: Dirt

HIKING TIME: 2 hours

DRIVING DISTANCE: 25.42 miles from the intersection of Beltway 8 and I-59

ACCESS: $3 per person age 13 and older; open 8 a.m.–10 p.m.

MAPS: USGS Moonshine Hill and Splendora; trail maps available

WHEELCHAIR ACCESS: None

FACILITIES: Restrooms, parking, picnic areas, campsites, bike trails, showers

SPECIAL COMMENTS: Lake Houston Park, previously known as Lake Houston State Park, was acquired by the City of Houston and Montgomery County in August 2006 from the State of Texas. Due to the acquisition, some of the signs directing you to the park may still say Lake Houston State Park.

GPS TRAILHEAD COORDINATES

LATITUDE: N 30° 8.307'
LONGITUDE: W 95° 10.404'

IN BRIEF

Peach Creek Trail is seldom used, creating an opportunity to hike in solitude most of the year. The trail leads to the park's primitive campsites and offers good views of Peach Creek and eventually Caney Creek, at the end of the hike. Lake Houston Park, which encompasses 4,919 acres, is located in New Caney, just north of Houston. The land was purchased from Champion Paper Company in 1981 by the State of Texas and opened for day use in 1992. Now part of the City of Houston Parks and Recreation Department, Lake Houston Park continues to offer facilities for campers, hikers, cyclists, and picnickers.

DESCRIPTION

All hikers must check in with park headquarters before beginning their hike to obtain a trail map and pay the daily fee. To reach Peach Creek Trail, start on the Forest Trail at the park headquarters by heading left out of the headquarters door. Once on the Forest Trail, head toward the sign that directs you to the restrooms. Head along the trail past the Lazy Creek Cottage and volleyball court, both on your left. The trail surface is dirt with some asphalt, showing remnants of an old road. Loblolly pines are the predominant tree in this part of the park, creating a high, thick canopy over the forest floor.

Directions ———————————————→

From the intersection of Beltway 8 and I-59, head north 21.78 miles on I-59 to FM 1485 and turn right. Go 0.22 miles and turn right onto Loop 494. Go 0.31 miles, turn left onto FM 1485, and go 1.55 miles to Baptist Encampment Road. Turn right and go 1.56 miles to the entrance of the park, on the left. Follow signs to park headquarters.

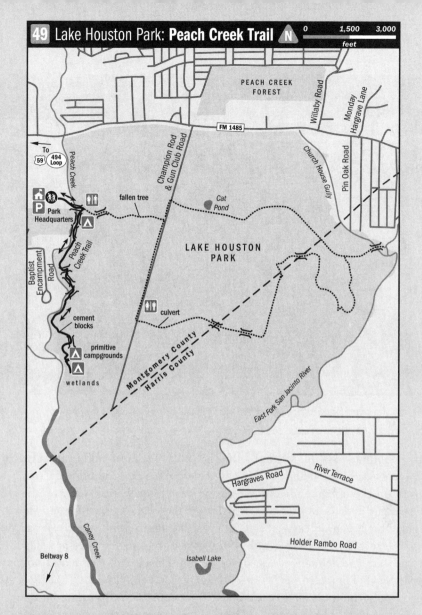

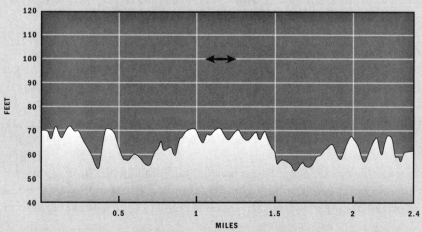

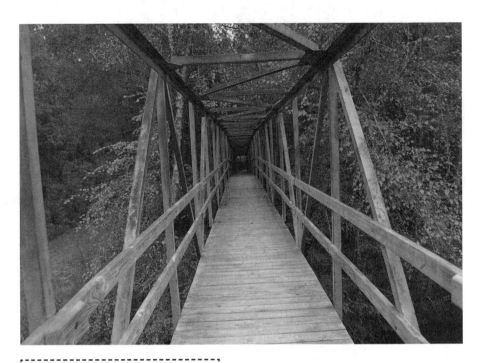

Continue past the Magnolia Interpretative Trail sign and trail on the right and cross a large metal bridge that resembles an old railroad bridge. Cross Peach Creek on the bridge and continue to the Peach Creek Trail sign, on the right. Restrooms and showers are located left of the trail, about 50 feet away. Bear right at the Peach Creek Trail sign. Go past the next Peach Creek Trail sign, with a bench to the right of the trail. Many of the trees in this area are magnolias, sycamores, and loblolly pines; other plants include elderberry and nonnative Japanese climbing fern.

Bear right at the next Peach Creek Trail sign. The trail surface here consists mainly of dirt and pine needles. Notice the blazes on trees—these assure you that you are still on the trail. This is a wooded trail with some elevation change, as you wind across creeks, bayous, and streambeds. Peach Creek is on your right, with numerous paths leading down to the creek. A group camping area is on your left. Continue over a bridge and onto a much sandier surface as you get closer to Peach Creek. This part of the trail is a little difficult to hike because of the loose sand, but this only continues for a short distance. Go past a bench on the right overlooking Peach Creek and continue as the trail curves left.

At the next intersection, bear right. As you hike, you may hear squirrels in the treetops. Cross the next bridge and at the next intersection go left, following blazes in the trees. Take the next fork left and head uphill. Once at the next Peach Creek Trail sign, take the right fork. Continue on the trail past a row of fence posts on the right side of the trail. There are no connecting fence rails or barbed wire, but the posts are obviously going to be part of a future fence. Go past another Peach Creek Trail sign, pointing straight ahead, until you reach the Peach Creek Loop Trail and Peach Creek Trail signs. Take the right fork to follow the Peach Creek Trail sign. The trail surface, which is now dirt mixed with considerable leaf litter, narrows to only about 3 feet wide. Be aware of spider webs along parts of the trail between trees. Most of the webs are from the banana spider, a harmless but rather large spider that is present from spring to late fall. Continue down the trail as it curves left, away from Peach Creek.

Cross a bridge and head right. There is a small creek to your right, creating more elevation changes in the trail as you hike in and out of small waterways. Cross another bridge and head right as the trail again gets more primitive, with underbrush pressing against you as you walk. Go down an embankment and up the other side. Peach Creek is still on your right as you cross another bridge. There are deer, raccoons, armadillos, and wild pigs in the area so stay alert as you get deeper into the park. Go downhill and then up an embankment, hiking away from the creek.

As the trail swings left, it goes uphill. Cross a new bridge that has sustained damage from a fallen tree. The trail curves right and over another bridge before going left and into an open area. Cross the next bridge and go past the first primitive campsite on your left. Caney Creek is now on your right, with paths leading to it. Stay on the trail until you reach the second primitive campsite on your left. Each campsite has a metal fire ring and a sign indicating a campsite number. Continue straight until you come to the end of the Peach Creek Trail. There is a large opening with power lines running down the middle of the easement and a sign for hikers coming the other way on the Peach Creek Trail. There is also a sign stating that you are entering a wetlands area. Because the grass is very long and provides good coverage for snakes, it is recommended that you not enter this area without adequate footwear and long pants. Turn around and retrace your route to the parking area.

Note: While hiking, be aware of wild pigs, especially during the spring, and poisonous snakes, which are very common along the creeks and rivers. There are more than 30 species of snakes in Lake Houston Park, but only four of them are poisonous. The three most common are copperhead, cottonmouth, and coral snake. The canebrake rattlesnake, although native to the area, is rarely seen. It's best to hike in boots and long pants if you plan to hike in the wetlands area or near the creeks.

NEARBY ACTIVITIES

Lake Houston, which includes fishing, boating, and picnicking facilities, is only a few miles south of Lake Houston Park. Jesse H. Jones Park and Nature Center are less than 10 miles away, and Kingwood Park is just a few miles south on I-59.

50 LAKE HOUSTON PARK:
Forest Trail

KEY AT-A-GLANCE INFORMATION

LENGTH: 8.8 miles

CONFIGURATION: Balloon

DIFFICULTY: Difficult

SCENERY: Woodlands, marsh, river, creek, picnic areas, campsites

EXPOSURE: Shady

TRAIL TRAFFIC: Light

TRAIL SURFACE: Dirt

HIKING TIME: 4.5 hours

DRIVING DISTANCE: 25.42 miles from the intersection of Beltway 8 and I-59

ACCESS: $3 per person age 13 and older; open 8 a.m.–10 p.m.

MAPS: USGS Moonshine Hill and Splendora; trail maps available

WHEELCHAIR ACCESS: None

FACILITIES: Restrooms, parking, picnic areas, campsites, bike trails, showers

SPECIAL COMMENTS: Lake Houston Park, previously known as Lake Houston State Park, was acquired by the City of Houston and Montgomery County in August 2006 from the State of Texas. Due to the acquisition, many of the signs directing you to the park may still say Lake Houston State Park.

GPS TRAILHEAD COORDINATES

LATITUDE: N 30° 8.307'
LONGITUDE: W 95° 10.404'

IN BRIEF

The Forest Trail, which does not feature much elevation change, is difficult due to its length. It starts at the parking lot and heads east toward the San Jacinto River before turning around and looping back. Lake Houston Park, which encompasses 4,919 acres, is located in New Caney, just north of Houston. The land was purchased from Champion Paper Company in 1981 by the State of Texas and opened for day use in 1992. Now part of the City of Houston Parks and Recreation Department, Lake Houston Park continues to offer facilities for campers, hikers, bikers, and picnickers.

DESCRIPTION

To start the Forest Trail, head left from the parking lot and go to park headquarters. All hikers must check in with park headquarters before beginning their hike to obtain a trail map and pay the daily fee. After doing so, head left out of headquarters and toward the sign that directs you to the restrooms. Head along the trail past the Lazy Creek Cottage and volleyball court, both on your left. The trail surface is dirt with some asphalt, showing remnants of an old road. Loblolly pines are the predominant tree in this part of the park, creating a high, thick canopy over the forest floor.

Directions ⟶

From the intersection of Beltway 8 and I-59, head north 21.78 miles on I-59 to FM 1485 and turn right. Go 0.22 miles and turn right onto Loop 494. Go 0.31 miles, turn left onto FM 1485, and go 1.55 miles to Baptist Encampment Road. Turn right and go 1.56 miles to the entrance of the park on the left. Follow signs to park headquarters.

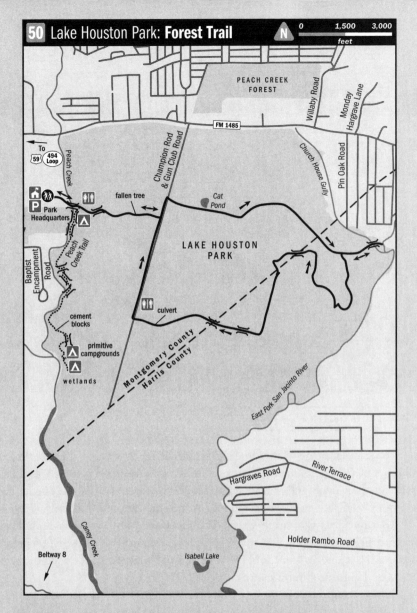

0   1,500   3,000
feet

N

PEACH CREEK
FOREST

Willaby Road

Monday
Hargrave Lane

FM 1485

To
59 494
     Loop

Peach Creek

Champion Road
& Gun Club Road

Church House Gully

Pin Oak Road

fallen tree

Cat
Pond

Park
Headquarters

P

LAKE HOUSTON
PARK

Baptist
Encampment
Road

Peach
Creek Trail

cement
blocks

primitive
campgrounds

culvert

wetlands

Montgomery County
Harris County

East Fork San Jacinto River

Hargraves Road

River Terrace

Beltway 8

Caney Creek

Isabell Lake

Holder Rambo Road

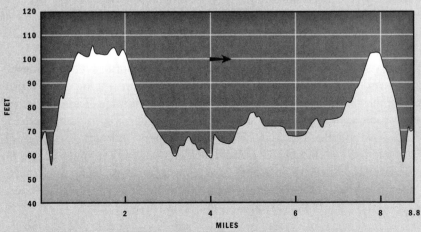

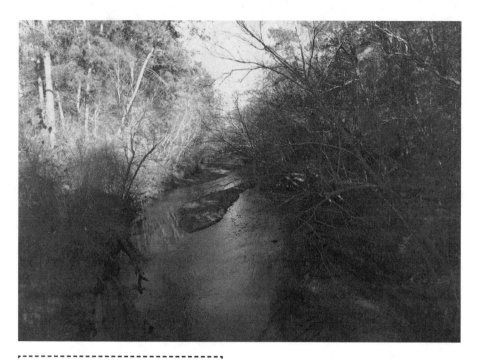

A view of Peach Creek after heavy rainfall

Continue past the Magnolia Interpretative Trail sign and trail on the right and cross a large metal bridge that resembles an old railroad bridge. Cross Peach Creek on the bridge and continue to the Peach Creek Trail sign, on the right. Restrooms and showers are located left of the trail, about 50 feet away.

Continue past the Peach Creek Trail and head left down an asphalt road to a trail sign instructing you to go straight. Many of the trees in this area are magnolias, sycamores, and loblolly pines; other plants include elderberry and nonnative Japanese climbing fern.

Hike through the campground to a trail sign on the left, directing you to go left between an old swimming pool and a building on the right. There are signs warning of poisonous snakes, so be aware of where you step at all times. Head into the trees away from the campsites and get on a dirt trail. Cross a bridge and then follow the trail as it curves right.

The trail goes uphill over roots and winds between borders of dense vegetation. Go past a bench on the left and then through an intersection where a trail joins from the right. Continue straight, following the trail sign. There are lichen and moss growing on the base of many of the trees, indicating a damp environment. Step over a fallen tree and then go left. Go past a horse-crossing sign on the right and then a trail sign. The trail winds to a small bridge and a bench, on the left. Cross the bridge to an asphalt road. Go left and hike along the road for 0.43 miles to a hiking trail sign on the right. While on the road, you are between forest, left, and a telephone easement, right.

Go right to get on the hiking trail and head back into the trees. Past a bench on the right, the trail angles left. Look left for a marsh beyond the trees. At a fork, bear left and hike past a bench, on the right. The mostly dirt trail now narrows, with tall loblolly pines lining both sides of the route. After passing trail marker 7, on the right, continue straight along the trail before curving left. A North River Trail and South River Trail sign is now on your left, with a bench and trail marker 6 sign on the right. Go straight to get on the North River Trail. After a long straight stretch, the trail bends left, heads slightly downhill, and takes you across a long bridge. Beyond the bridge, the trail narrows and curves right. Cross a small bridge and head uphill and left. As the trail traces a winding course, look for a tall structure up ahead. The trail heads uphill toward a covered bench on the left and the San Jacinto River straight ahead. At the covered bench, turn around and retrace your route to the previous intersection, at trail marker 6. Here turn left, keeping the bench on your right. After the trail bends right and widens, there is a large stand of fan palms on the right. After a long straight stretch, the trail goes right and heads steeply uphill. Continue past trail marker 5 and a South River Trail sign, on the left. At a fork, bear right, hiking past a bench on your left. This is a very shady and primitive part of the trail, narrowing to about 2 feet wide. Thick vegetation is on both sides as you pass trail marker 4. Take the trail to the left as it winds past a bench on the right. Cross a long boardwalk that is only a few inches off the forest floor. Once off the boardwalk, the trail becomes wider and more defined. Go over a small bridge and head slightly right. At trail marker 3, go left past a bench, which is on the right. The trail takes a big rightward bend and then goes straight and uphill. Pass trail marker 2 and a bench, both on the left. Go over a small bridge and then follow a boardwalk. After a third bridge, the trail goes downhill and then left. Step over a culvert and follow the trail as it swings right and widens. Pass trail marker 1 and go right to get back on the asphalt road you were on earlier. The telephone easement is again on your right with forest on your left. Go uphill past a trail rest stop with a bench and cover on the left, and through an intersection to reach the Peach Creek Camp Area. This part of the trail is very open and can be quite hot. At a bench on the left, go left, back into the trees to get back on the Forest Trail. Retrace your route past the pool and restrooms, and over the long metal bridge. Just past the sign about local birds is the parking lot.

Note: While hiking, be aware of wild pigs, especially during the spring, and poisonous snakes, which are very common along the creeks and rivers. There are more than 30 species of snakes in Lake Houston Park, but only four of them are poisonous. The three most common are copperhead, cottonmouth, and coral snake. The canebrake rattlesnake, although native to the area, is rarely seen. It's best to hike in boots and long pants if you plan to hike in the wetlands area or near the creeks.

51 BIG THICKET NATIONAL PRESERVE:
Kirby Nature Trail

KEY AT-A-GLANCE INFORMATION

LENGTH: 3.3 miles

CONFIGURATION: Balloon

DIFFICULTY: Easy

SCENERY: Big thicket, woodlands, cypress swamps, creeks, sloughs, boardwalks

EXPOSURE: Shady

TRAIL TRAFFIC: Light to moderate

TRAIL SURFACE: Dirt

HIKING TIME: 1.5 hours

DRIVING DISTANCE: 102 miles from the intersection of Beltway 8 and I-10 east

ACCESS: Free; visitor center open 9 a.m.–5 p.m.

MAPS: USGS Kountze North; trail maps available at trailhead

WHEELCHAIR ACCESS: None

FACILITIES: Restrooms, visitor center, parking, picnic tables, water fountains, fishing

SPECIAL COMMENTS: All hikers should register at the trailhead. Stay on the trail at all times. Bicycles and pets are not allowed on the trail. Because this is a national preserve, the removal of anything such as plants, rocks, or animals is prohibited. Use insect repellent and avoid disturbing bee, wasp, or fireant nests.

GPS TRAILHEAD COORDINATES

LATITUDE: N 30° 27.652'
LONGITUDE: W 94° 21.085'

IN BRIEF

Big Thicket was the first preserve in the U.S. national park system and encompasses more than 97,000 acres in nine land units. It was established in 1974 and was recognized in 2001 by the American Bird Conservancy as a Globally Important Bird Area. The preserve has many different ecosystems, including eastern hardwood forests, Gulf coastal plains, and Midwest prairies. There are nine trails in five of the land units, ranging from 0.5 to 18 miles in length.

DESCRIPTION

Start the hike at the Kirby Nature Trail parking lot and head east toward the trail sign at the east end of the lot. The trail surface is asphalt with landscaping timbers as edging. The trail curves right and then slightly left as you enter a picnic area. Continue through the picnic area on a wooden boardwalk toward the forest entrance. There are also water fountains, restrooms, and a small nature center in this area. Go past a sign on your left describing the nature trail and what you might expect to see. Head toward the trees and go through an intersection, passing restrooms on your right. Once in the forest, there is a sign about the important relationship between the air we breathe and the existence of large forests. At

----

Directions

From the intersection of Beltway 8 and I-10, head east 69 miles on I-10 to the Highway 69/96 North exit in Beaumont. Go 32 miles on Highway 69/96 to FM 420 and turn right. Follow signs to the visitor center, which is on the left. The trailhead for the Kirby Nature Trail is 2.5 miles east of the visitor center on FM 420.

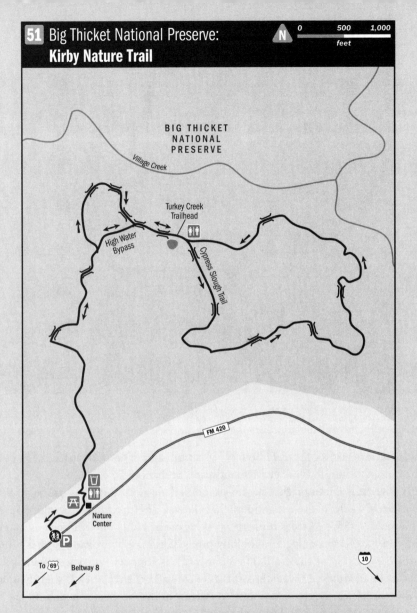

N

0   500   1,000

feet

BIG THICKET
NATIONAL
PRESERVE

Village Creek

Turkey Creek
Trailhead

High Water
Bypass

Cypress Slough Trail

FM 420

Nature
Center

P

To 69   Beltway 8

10

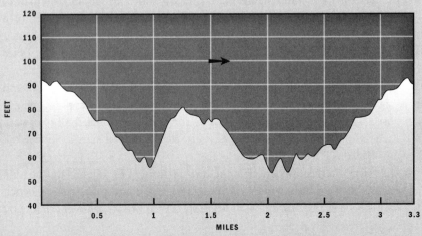

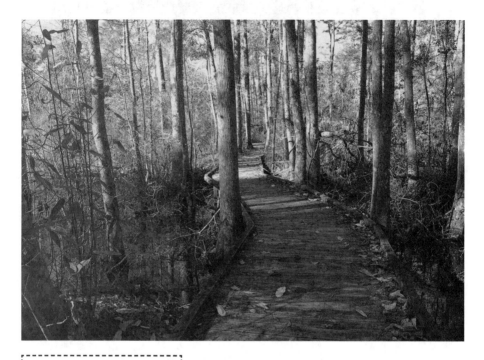

A boardwalk on the Kirby Trail

the next intersection, go left, following a trail sign. The trail surface changes to dirt but continues to be edged by landscape timbers.

The trail curves right, past a numbered marker and a nature sign about American beech. There is considerable evidence of Hurricane Rita in 2005, with a number of downed trees lining both sides of the trail. The trail passes magnolias, beeches, water oaks, and loblolly pines. Get on a boardwalk with a cypress bog on each side of the trail. The boardwalk is slippery when wet: watch your footing at all times. As you step off the boardwalk, the trail heads slightly uphill. Continue past a nature sign about American holly. Go past a bench on the left and then a nature sign about white oak. Cross a short bridge and then head left. The trail narrows to about 4 feet wide, just past nature signs about Eastern hornbeam and American hornbeam. Wind past a bench on the right. Cross a boardwalk and then head uphill as the trail surface changes to sand and takes a big bend left. After a straight stretch, the trail bends right and past a bench on the right. Continue to another boardwalk and past another trail marker and a nature sign for bald cypress. The boardwalk takes you over a cypress swamp with exposed cypress knees on both sides of the trail. Once off the boardwalk the trail heads uphill and right. Take the right fork at a trail sign to follow the High Water Bypass.

At the next intersection go straight on the Inner Loop Trail and cross a bridge over another cypress swamp. As you get off the boardwalk, go by a bench on the left, then head uphill and left. Passing trail marker 18 on the left, you go by a bench overlooking a large pond, on the left. At an intersection, turn right to stay on the Inner Loop Trail. Pass a nature sign about sweetgum trees and trail marker 19. Cross a bridge and then head uphill as the trail curves left. Continue past trail markers 20, 21, and a bench on the left. The trail bends right and then goes over a bridge, past a sign on the rattan-vine. Beyond the bridge, the trail swings right and uphill. Go past trail marker 23, a sign about the water oak on the right, and a bench on the left. At an intersection, take the left fork heading uphill. Cross a bridge and go past a bench on the left. The trail heads uphill and left, changing to dirt and grass. Continue past a bench on the right, cross a bridge, and go past another bench on the right as the trail heads uphill. After a sweeping rightward bend, go by a bench on the right as the trail heads uphill and left. There are lichen and moss growing on the trail here, indicating that this part of the Kirby Nature Trail is not used as much as other parts. The trail heads downhill and past two benches, one on the left and one on the right. Cross a bridge and follow the trail as it winds past a bridge on the left. Continue past a bench on the left and onto a short boardwalk over a cypress swamp. Once off the boardwalk, go by another bench as the trail heads uphill. The vegetation is very thick here, as you cross another bridge and hike past a bench on the right overlooking a pond on the right.

Go past a bench on the right as the trail winds right, past a trailhead sign for the Turkey Creek Trail. Continue straight to stay on the Kirby Nature Trail. At an intersection, head straight and then slightly right. Go past a bench on the right overlooking a pond on the right. Cross a boardwalk and then take the right fork to get on the Cypress Slough Trail. Cross a bridge and then continue past a bench on the left and trail marker 16. Cross another bridge and hike past a nature sign about water tupelo. The trail heads uphill, with a bench on the right and a bog on the left. Go past trail marker 15 and then cross a bridge. Once off the bridge, hike past a bench on the left. Continue along the trail to another bridge over a cypress swamp, and then head uphill to trail marker 14. At a fork, bear right and retrace your steps. As you exit the woods, the restrooms are on your left. Continue along the wooden boardwalk to the parking lot and the end of the hike.

Note: The weather during the summer months is hot and humid, so try to hike from late fall to late spring. There are poisonous snakes, feral hogs, and a recent reappearance of mountain lions. Use caution and stay on the trail at all times. Some of the snakes you may see include the coral snake (poisonous) and speckled king snake (nonpoisonous). Other animals in the preserve include bobcats, mountain lions, armadillos, white-tailed deer, skunks, raccoons, and coyotes. Birds you may see include the yellow-billed cuckoo, wood duck, road-runner, pileated woodpecker, brown-headed nuthatch, and Bachman's sparrow. Due to the dense tree canopy, migratory songbirds are difficult to spot but they do exist in great numbers at certain times of the year and you may be able to identify their songs.

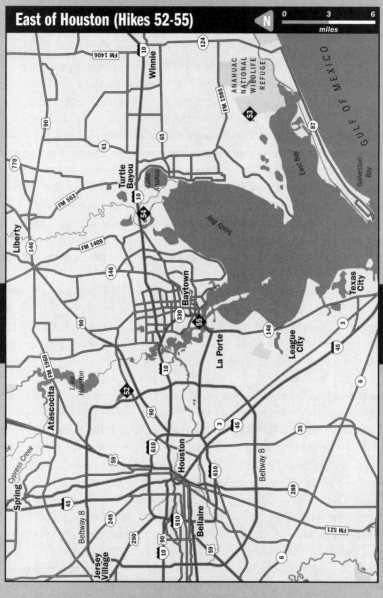

East of Houston (Hikes 52-55)

N

0   3   6
miles

GULF OF MEXICO

ANAHUAC NATIONAL WILDLIFE REFUGE

Galveston Bay

East Bay

Trinity Bay

Lake Anahuac

Turtle Bayou

Winnie

Liberty

Baytown

La Porte

League City

Texas City

Houston

Bellaire

Jersey Village

Atascocita

Lake Houston

Spring

Cypress Creek

FM 1406

FM 1985

FM 563

FM 1409

FM 1960

FM 521

EAST of HOUSTON
(INCLUDING BEAUMONT)

52

SHELDON LAKE STATE PARK:
Nature Trail

KEY AT-A-GLANCE INFORMATION

LENGTH: 1.1 miles

CONFIGURATION: Loops

DIFFICULTY: Easy

SCENERY: Ponds, rookeries, native vegetation, forestland, wildscape garden

EXPOSURE: Shady

TRAIL TRAFFIC: Light

HIKING TIME: 30 minutes

DRIVING DISTANCE: 2 miles from Beltway 8 and Hwy. 90

ACCESS: Free

MAPS: USGS San Jacinto, trail map

WHEELCHAIR ACCESS: Yes

FACILITIES: Restrooms, picnic tables, Learning Center, water fountain, fishing, boat ramp, nature-hike tours

SPECIAL COMMENTS: Sheldon Lake State Park is one of the newer parks in the Texas Parks & Wildlife family and one of the only free parks. It's a good choice for those who may not have the opportunity to visit many of the other parks. There are poisonous snakes, so use caution with young children and dogs. The park is open to school groups, Scout groups, and anyone who wants to feel a part of nature just minutes from downtown Houston.

GPS TRAILHEAD COORDINATES

LATITUDE: N 29° 51.500'
LONGITUDE: W 95° 9.650'

IN BRIEF

This 2,800-acre urban state park was originally established as Sheldon Reservoir in 1941 by the federal government. At that time Carpenter's Bayou was dammed to impound water for war-critical industries in the area. After the war ended, the land was purchased by the state of Texas as one of the first wildlife-management areas in the state. In 1954, half of the area of the reservoir was drained to open a fish hatchery with 28 ponds. The fish hatchery closed in 1975 and was made a state park in 1984. In 2005, the park was renovated using "green building" and "alternative energy" for all of its buildings and structures. Geothermal heating and cooling, wind turbines, and solar panels are used to power the park. Most materials used in the buildings are from torn-down buildings in Houston or surplus oilfield pipe.

DESCRIPTION

Park in the lot next to the Pond Center and head across the park road to start the hike. The trail surface is concrete initially but quickly changes to crushed granite. There are native Texas plants on each side with labels helping you identify the names of each plant. Hike past a park-rules sign on the left as you head toward a pavilion straight ahead. There are restrooms here, as well as a water fountain.

Directions ———————————————➤

From the intersection of Beltway 8 and Highway 90 (Beaumont Highway), head east 2 miles to Park Road 138. Look for the brown park signs and turn left over the railroad tracks, following the road to the Pond Center parking lot.

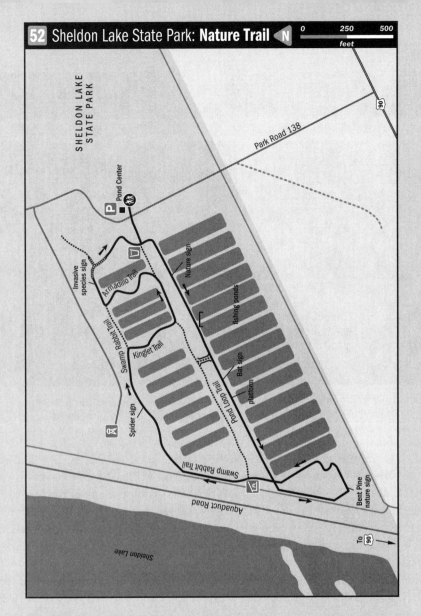

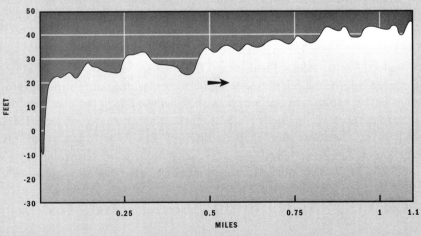

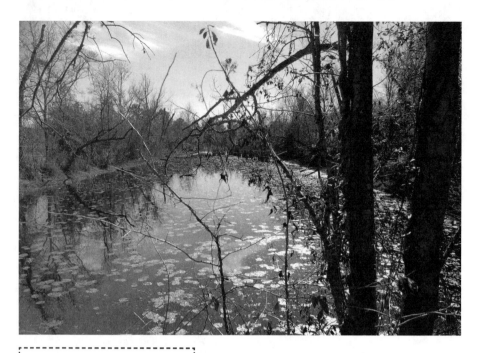

This old fish pond is now a rookery.

Get on the crushed granite trail headed away from the pavilion and past some benches on the left. Once on the trail, you will pass by 14 ponds on your left. Called Pond Loop Trail, this was the access trail to many of the fish hatchery ponds. Most of the ponds are now rookeries for the many wintering birds that make Texas home. As you continue, pass the first two ponds, which are still maintained as catch-and-release fishing ponds for children to try their hand at fishing. Poles are supplied.

As you pass the ponds on your left, most of them have trails that flank both sides of the pond. There are bridges across some of the ponds, as well as observation decks to give you access to the wildlife in the area. If you head down any of these trails, just return the way you came and go left to get back on this hike. The third pond is an aquatic study lab.

Pass another bench on your left and hike past a bridge on your right that takes you to the other side of Pond Loop Trail. Stop at the bridge to read a sign about the repurposed materials used to build the bridge, including oilfield pipes. Continue past a nature sign on local bats and past the last of the ponds on the left. At the next trail intersection, head slightly left to get on Bent Pine Trail, a .2-mile loop. There is a small trail pavilion on your right as you get on the small balloon loop trail and head toward the edge of the park. The trail narrows slightly and becomes a bit more winding as it travels past a trail sign and slightly downhill.

Hike past a Bent Pine nature sign on the right as the trail winds left and past another nature sign on poison ivy. Use caution, as there is poison ivy on almost any trail in southeast Texas; stay away from the vines climbing up trees and on the ground. As you exit Bent Pine Trail, head left past a large sign on your right and the trail pavilion on your left. Continue straight past the intersection to the other side of Pond Loop Trail and onto Swamp Rabbit Trail.

Hike on a long boardwalk over a low marshy area and then back onto the crushed granite trail. Just before the trail winds slightly right is a new observation tower on your left. If you wish, check out the tower and then return to the trail and go left off the tower trail. Pass a nature sign on spiders toward a small cement trail marker with a kinglet on it. The spiders here are not dangerous, but they do like to make their webs across the trail during the warmer months.

Take a right at the trail marker to get on the Kinglet Trail and head downhill. There are two nature signs on your left with information on the flora and fauna of the area. Continue on the trail until you come to an intersection, which is the other side of Pond Loop Trail. Turn left and pass a bench and another nature sign on spiders. At the next intersection, turn left onto the Armadillo Trail.

At the next intersection, turn right to get back on Swamp Rabbit Trail. Hike past a nature sign on invasive species and onto a boardwalk. There is a large picnic shelter to your left with the restrooms coming up on your right. Hike past the restrooms and water fountain on your right and back onto the concrete trail that leads to the parking lot and the end of the trail.

NEARBY ACTIVITIES

City Hall is only 16 miles west of Sheldon Lake. Other area attractions include the San Jacinto Monument, San Jacinto Battleground State Historic Site, Battleship Texas State Historic Site, and Lake Houston Park. Farther south is NASA Space Center and Mercer Arboretum.

53 ANAHUAC NATIONAL WILDLIFE REFUGE: Shoveler Pond Trail

KEY AT-A-GLANCE INFORMATION

LENGTH: 4.1 miles

CONFIGURATION: Loop

DIFFICULTY: Easy

SCENERY: Bayou, wetlands, ponds, willow stands, woodlot, butterfly and hummingbird habitat, coastal marsh, coastal prairie

EXPOSURE: Sunny

TRAIL TRAFFIC: Light

TRAIL SURFACE: Dirt and gravel, some paved and grass

HIKING TIME: 2 hours

DRIVING DISTANCE: 47.5 miles from the intersection of Beltway 8 and I-10 east

ACCESS: Free; main gate open 24 hours a day, seven days a week; public-use areas open one hour before sunrise to one hour after sunset

MAPS: USGS Frozen Point

WHEELCHAIR ACCESS: Yes

FACILITIES: Visitor information station, restrooms, gift shop, fishing, boating, canoe and kayak launch, parking, wildlife viewing areas

SPECIAL COMMENTS: This is a very open trail with no shade, so make sure you wear sunscreen, bring plenty of water, and plan to hike the refuge from late fall to early spring.

GPS TRAILHEAD COORDINATES

LATITUDE: N 29° 36.783'
LONGITUDE: W 94° 32.016'

IN BRIEF

Shoveler Pond Trail includes the Butterfly and Hummingbird Habitat, the Willows Trail, and the Shoveler Pond Loop, which encircles a 220-acre freshwater impoundment with opportunities to view alligators, birds, and other marsh wildlife. The refuge encompasses more than 34,000 acres bordering Galveston Bay. It contains bayous that meander through floodplains, creating an extensive coastal marsh-and-prairie landscape. Southerly breezes from the Gulf of Mexico result in high humidity and an average rainfall of more than 51 inches. Anahuac National Wildlife Refuge is a recognized stop on the Great Texas Coastal Birding Trail.

DESCRIPTION

Start the Shoveler Pond Trail at the Butterfly and Hummingbird Habitat behind the visitor information station, where restrooms are available. Head toward the flagpole to get on a paved surface that meanders through a garden built to attract hummingbirds and butterflies. At an intersection, go left. There is a pond on your left, with a bench and the garden on your right. Cross a small bridge and then follow the trail to the right. Look left to see a large expanse of water in the distance. The prairie stretches for miles on your right. Take the next fork left, as the trail goes between tall grasses and bushes.

Directions ──────────────────➤

From Beltway 8 and I-10 head east 31 miles on I-10 to exit 812 (TX 61). Go south on TX 61 for 4 miles to a stop sign. Continue through the stop sign as TX 61 becomes TX 562. Go another 8.5 miles to a fork. Bear left on FM 1985 and go 4 miles to the entrance of the refuge, on the right. The visitor information station is 3 miles ahead.

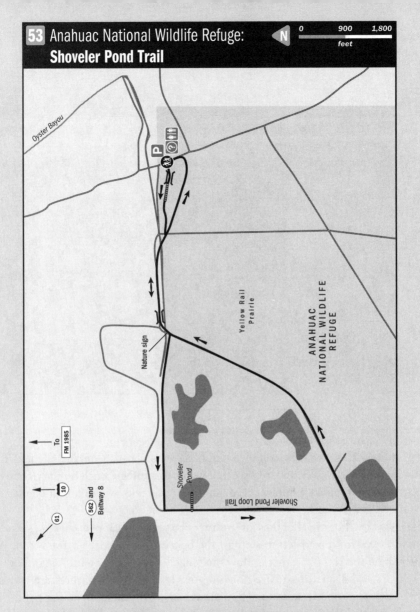

Oyster Bayou

P

Yellow Rail Prairie

ANAHUAC NATIONAL WILDLIFE REFUGE

Nature sign

To FM 1985

10

562 and Beltway 8

61

Shoveler Pond

Shoveler Pond Loop Trail

N

0   900   1,800
feet

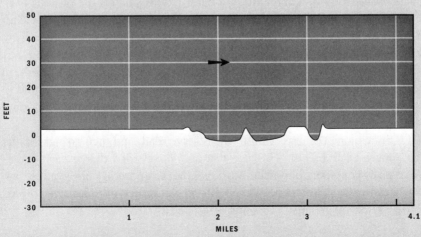

FEET

50
40
30
20
10
0
-10
-20
-30

1   2   3   4.1

MILES

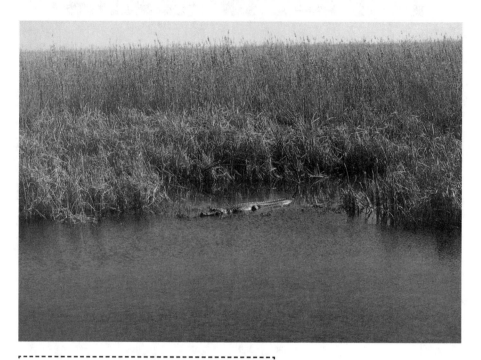

An alligator sunning itself off the Shoveler Pond Trail

Step onto a boardwalk to continue the hike. Pass a bench on the left and then another on the right. The boardwalk trail winds to another bench on the right overlooking a small pond. Continue through an intersection, where a trail departs left to an observation deck.

Now the boardwalk takes a right turn past a handicapped-parking space on the left. At a fork, bear left to step off the boardwalk and onto a grass trail. Pass a bench on the right and then follow the fence line on your right. A stand of willow trees and a small pond are now on your left. Stop at a nature sign to learn about the neotropical migratory birds that visit the refuge, including palm warbler, scissortail flycatcher, and eastern kingbird. This small stand of trees is an important habitat for the birds that make the 600-mile journey across the Gulf of Mexico. You may see more songbirds in the wooded areas and shorebirds on the mudflats and in the shallow water. As many as 27 species of ducks stop over between October and March, including green-winged teal, gadwall, northern shoveler, and northern pintail. Flocks of geese in excess of 80,000 are found in the marshes, rice fields, and mudflats. Roseate spoonbills, white-faced ibis, and great and snowy egrets are also plentiful.

Continue along the grass trail to the reserve road, and then go right to get on the Shoveler Pond Trail. This is a dirt-and-gravel road that is easy underfoot and gives you many opportunities to see ducks and other birds, alligators, snakes, and turtles. The nocturnal wildlife in the refuge includes river otters, raccoons, skunks, muskrats, opossums, and bobcats.

Continue along the road past a water channel on your left. Biking and driving are permitted on this road, so be aware of cyclists and cars coming from behind. Cross a bridge and continue past a gate on the right. The road bends left to the start of the Shoveler Pond Loop. Go right to get on the 2.5-mile trail. There is water on both sides of the trail here, with an amazing number of birds and turtles. Shoveler Pond is home to many alligators, so be wary at all times: there are no fences between you and them.

Continue toward an observation platform that overlooks Shoveler Pond, providing an excellent view of the area. Once off the platform, go left along a lengthy stretch of straight road. The terrain to your right is so flat that you can see for miles across marshes and mudflats to the East Bay of Galveston Bay. Soon you reach the Shoveler Pond boardwalk, left. There is a handicapped-parking space at the head of the boardwalk to accommodate wheelchairs. The boardwalk takes you into the middle of Shoveler Pond, offering views you can't see from the trail.

Once off the boardwalk, head left. Follow the trail as it bends left and past a gate on the right. There is water on both sides of the trail again as you head back in the direction of the visitor information station. At an intersection, continue straight over some culverts and a small channel of water. Look to your left for the Shoveler Pond Boardwalk jutting out into the pond. After another long straight stretch, the trail bends left, putting the visitor information station and the Yellow Rail Prairie on your right. The yellow rail is one of the most difficult birds to actually see in North America due to its preference for wet prairies and shallow marshes where bird-watchers rarely go. Yellow rail is listed on the National Audubon Society "Yellow" Watch List as those species that are also declining but at a slower rate than those in the red category. At an intersection, go straight and then follow the trail as it curves right and reverses direction. Walk past a stand of willows and a small pond.

Continue on the trail toward the visitor information station and past a sign describing a woodlot that was created to shelter and feed migratory birds. The visitor information station is now on your left as you approach the entrance road. At the entrance road, turn left to head back to your car. Turning right will take you to a boat launch and East Bay, but the distance makes it best to drive.

Note: Pets must be on leash at all times. Bicycles are permitted on gravel roads only; all-terrain vehicles, airboats, and personal watercraft are prohibited. There is no drinking water available anywhere in the refuge, so come prepared with water. Be aware at all times of snakes, alligators, fire ants, and mosquitoes.

NEARBY ACTIVITIES

Five miles west of I-10 and TX 61 is the J. J. Mayes Wildlife Trace. Other activities include Goose Creek Stream Greenbelt in Baytown, Baytown Nature Center, Eddie V. Gray Wetlands Center, San Jacinto Point Recreation Area, San Jacinto State Park, George and Freda Chandler Arboretum, and the Houston Raceway Park. East Bay and a boat launch are located just minutes south of the preserve entrance.

54 J. J. MAYES WILDLIFE TRACE:
Trinity River Trail

KEY AT-A-GLANCE INFORMATION

LENGTH: 4.8 miles

CONFIGURATION: Out-and-back

DIFFICULTY: Easy

SCENERY: Trinity River, cypress bogs, wetlands, marshes, prairies

EXPOSURE: Sunny

TRAIL TRAFFIC: Light

TRAIL SURFACE: Grass and asphalt

HIKING TIME: 2 hours

DRIVING DISTANCE: 24 miles from the intersection of Beltway 8 and I-10

ACCESS: Free

MAPS: USGS Cove and Anahuac; trail maps available

WHEELCHAIR ACCESS: None

FACILITIES: Restrooms, picnic pavilions and tables, boardwalks, Wallisville Lake Visitor Center, wildlife viewing areas, observation decks and towers

SPECIAL COMMENTS: This is an exposed trail, so take plenty of sunscreen and water. To get to the Wallisville Lake Visitor Center, exit the trace, get back on I-10 headed east, and take the first exit. Turn right at the first street and drive to the end of the road. The center is on your left, after the road winds to the right.

GPS TRAILHEAD COORDINATES

LATITUDE: N 29° 49.744'
LONGITUDE: W 94° 45.654'

IN BRIEF

This 2.4-mile (one-way) trail follows an old road along the banks of the Trinity River. It has an 0.8-mile paved section in the middle, with wheelchair access via boardwalks from parking lots located along the levee. The trace is named after Joshua Jackson Mayes, who owned one of the largest cattle ranches in the county. He fought in the Mexican-American War of 1846–1848 and served as a Texan Mounted Volunteer until 1847, when he left the military to start cattle ranching. The U.S. Army Corps of Engineers opened the J. J. Mayes Wildlife Trace in May of 2003.

DESCRIPTION

To start the Trinity River hike, park in the second parking lot on the left after you enter the trace. Go east through a gate and toward the gravel trail. The Trinity River, which is directly on your left, can run high and fast at times, so watch the weather before hiking and during your hike. This is a 20-foot-wide trail that follows the route, or trace, of the old road that ran through the Mayes cattle ranch parallel to the Trinity River. There is marshland on the right and the bank of the river on your left. Stay away from the bank of the river, as the soil is loose and sandy. Look right for the 4-mile nature auto-tour located atop the levee. Just before the trail bends slightly left, the trail surface changes to grass. There

----

Directions

From Beltway 8 and I-10 head east 24 miles on I-10 and exit just before you reach the bridge over the Trinity River. The entrance to the trace is on your right. Park in the second parking lot on the left after you enter the trace.

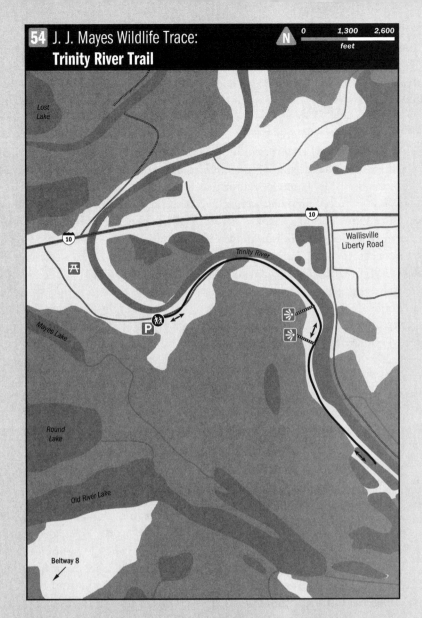

N

0   1,300   2,600
feet

Lost
Lake

10

Wallisville
Liberty Road

Trinity River

10

Mayes Lake

P

Round
Lake

Old River Lake

Beltway 8

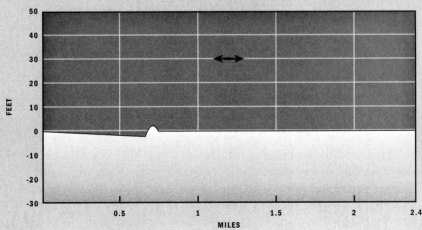

may be a considerable amount of animal scat on the trail, so watch your step. After a good rain you may see a number of tracks on the dirt parts of the trail, from animals such as deer, feral pigs, bobcats, river otters, raccoons, opossums, and coyotes. Besides a large variety of snakes (some poisonous) and turtles, the trace also is home to the American alligator. The bird life, which changes with each season, includes migrating songbirds, ducks, geese, waders, white and brown pelicans, and a large variety of raptors, such as ospreys and bald eagles.

While hiking, I did come across two feral pigs walking up the trail toward me. Once they spotted me, they left the trail quickly. Don't be afraid to be a little noisy, to let the wildlife know you are there. There is now some vegetation between the trail and the river, but it is still a low-lying area that could be inhabited by snakes. And there is now a marsh on your right.

As you go past the marsh, the vegetation on the right gets thicker and the water is less noticeable. With the marsh again on the right, there are a number of cypress trees and cypress knees sticking up out of the water, indicating a cypress bog. After a long straight stretch, the trail nears the river, and the bog on the right gives way to marshland. The area on the right now opens to a prairie marsh, with no trees and very low-lying grasses and reeds. After another long straight stretch, the trail bends right, bringing you to the 0.8-mile paved part of the trail. This is part of a wheelchair-accessible loop that contains more than 1,000 feet of boardwalk. Observation decks with benches are accessible from this part of the trail. When you get to the paved section, there is an observation deck on the left and a boardwalk on the right. At the end of the paved section, you come to another observation deck on the left and another boardwalk on the right, leading to a parking lot just below the levee. Once past the observation deck and boardwalk, the trail changes back to grass and remains this way until the turn-around point. There is a channel of water on the right, between the trail and bordering vegetation. Look right for a bridge and observation tower in the distance. The observation tower is for observing the trace from high above the marshes, prairies, and wildlife. Watch your footing as the trail dips down into a low area: this spot could be under water even though the rest of the trail is dry. Beyond the dip, the trail ends in a small field similar to a neighborhood cul-de-sac. Now turn around and retrace your route to the parking lot.

Note: Pets must be on leash at all times. Be aware of snakes, feral pigs, alligators, fire ants, and mosquitoes. This is a mowed grass trail that may be muddy after a good rain, so wear appropriate footwear.

NEARBY ACTIVITIES

Five miles east of I-10 and TX 61 is the exit for the Anahuac National Wildlife Refuge. Other activities in the area include the Goose Creek Stream Greenbelt in Baytown, the Baytown Nature Center, Eddie V. Gray Wetlands Center, San Jacinto Point Recreation Area, San Jacinto State Park, George and Freda Chandler Arboretum, and the Houston Raceway Park.

GOOSE CREEK STREAM GREENBELT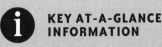

IN BRIEF

This 2.4-mile (one-way) trail follows the shores of Goose Creek from Tabbs Bay. It winds through two parks before exiting onto a hiking and biking trail that follows TX 255 and Goose Creek. The Greenbelt is an ongoing project, begun in 1990, that will eventually extend from downtown Baytown to Bayland Park Marina. Baytown boomed after the Civil War as a trading post along the Texas Gulf Coast and then again with the discovery of oil in 1916.

DESCRIPTION

The start of the Goose Creek Stream Greenbelt hike is in the Bayland Park Marina parking lot, just east of the Baytown Bridge. From the parking lot, head toward the no-fishing sign on the marina side of the park and then turn right to get on a concrete trail. There is a yellow stripe down the middle, indicating that this is a hiking and biking trail. Stay right of the yellow line at all times and give plenty of clearance to cyclists. The trail winds to a bridge. Once across, go left, hiking parallel to the marina road. Pass a small marsh on the left with a sign indicating that this is a Texas Parks and Wildlife Department Conservation Easement Project Area. At the sign, go right to cross the marina road and then get back on the trail. The trail curves left and downhill through a stand of trees. Continue through an intersection, where a trail joins from the right,

----

Directions ———————————➤

From Beltway 8 and TX 255, head east 10 miles on TX 255 over the Baytown Bridge. At the first stoplight past the bridge, turn right into the Bayland Park Marina parking lot.

KEY AT-A-GLANCE INFORMATION

LENGTH: 4.8 miles
CONFIGURATION: Out-and-back
DIFFICULTY: Easy
SCENERY: Tabbs Bay, woodlands, marsh, marina, Goose Creek
EXPOSURE: Sunny
TRAIL TRAFFIC: Light
TRAIL SURFACE: Concrete
HIKING TIME: 2 hours
DRIVING DISTANCE: 10 miles from the intersection of Beltway 8 and TX 255
ACCESS: Free
MAPS: USGS Morgans Point
WHEELCHAIR ACCESS: Yes
FACILITIES: Restrooms, picnic tables, playground, fishing piers, boat launch
SPECIAL COMMENTS: Pets on leash at all times. This is also a biking trail, so be aware of cyclists: stay right and give them plenty of room. There is no shade on the hike, so be sure to wear plenty of sunscreen and bring water. Some of the trail along the shore is secluded, so be sure to hike with a buddy. The only restrooms available along the hike are in portable toilets at Bayland Park Marina and W. C. Britton Park, but they are generally clean.

GPS TRAILHEAD COORDINATES

LATITUDE: N 29° 42.623'
LONGITUDE: W 94° 59.750'

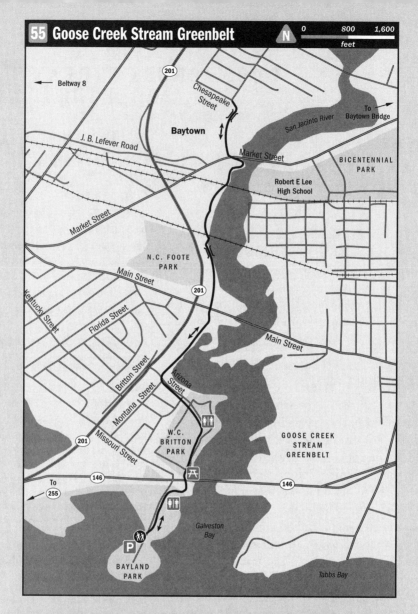

N

0   800   1,600
feet

Beltway 8

201

Chesapeake
Street

Baytown

J. B. Lefever Road

San Jacinto River

To
Baytown Bridge

Market Street

BICENTENNIAL
PARK

Robert E Lee
High School

Market Street

N.C. FOOTE
PARK

Main Street

201

Main Street

Kentucky Street

Florida Street

Britton Street

Montana Street

Arizona
Street

W.C.
BRITTON
PARK

GOOSE CREEK
STREAM
GREENBELT

201

Missouri Street

146

146

To
255

Galveston
Bay

BAYLAND
PARK

Tabbs Bay

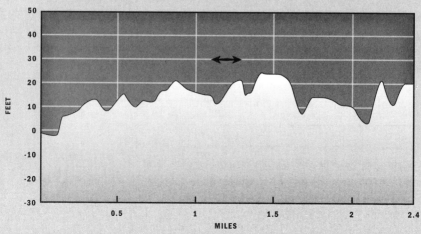

50
40
30
20
10
0
-10
-20
-30

FEET

0.5   1   1.5   2   2.4

MILES

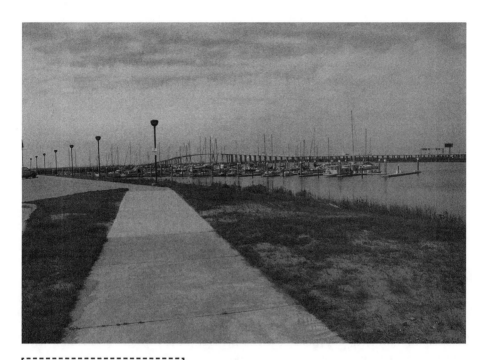

A view of Bayland Park Marina

and follow the trail as it runs parallel to the marina road. The trail heads uphill and right, passing through another parking lot. This is a boat-launch area, so the parking here may be limited on weekends.

You are now headed toward TX 146, with the marina road on your left and a parking lot on your right. Cross the road into the parking lot and continue straight to stay on the trail, which curves right, putting TX 146 on your left. The trail winds downhill toward a boat launch on the right. Tabbs Bay is to your right and also straight ahead. Go through the next intersection, continuing straight past the boat launch. Follow the trail as it swings left toward TX 146. Pass a small fishing pier on the right before the trail heads under TX 146. After crossing under the highway, the trail climbs away from the water and soon brings you into W. C. Britton Park. Look across the bay for working oil derricks on the opposite shore.

The trail curves left and downhill toward some fishing piers. Go by a picnic table and a water fountain on the right and through an intersection, where a trail joins on the left. Pass more picnic tables and basketball courts on the left, and continue through two more intersections, where paths go right, to fishing piers. Soon there is a playground on the left and a football field on the right. Just past the playground is a portable toilet on the left. You are heading away from the water and toward a parking lot on the right, with a neighborhood straight ahead. At a stop sign, continue straight to stay on the hiking and biking trail. This trail runs along the right side of Arizona Street where there are signs indicating that bikes must stay on the right side of the road. Cross Arizona Street and bear left walking up the right side of the road.

At the next stop sign, go right and follow signs to get on the protected hiking and biking trail that runs parallel to TX 146. There is a concrete barrier between the trail and traffic on the left to protect hikers and cyclists. Cross a bridge and now the highway is on your left and the water is back on your right. Because of the proximity of the highway, this part of the hike is very noisy. The water tower for Lee College is to your left and the bay is to your right. The trail bends right and then left just before you get to a street intersection. Cross a one-lane street and then wait for the light to change to cross the rest of the lanes. Continue straight toward the hike and bike sign and the Goose Creek Trail sign. There is water from an inlet into Tabbs Bay ahead and also right. As the trail heads left, it goes downhill past a high embankment on your left that muffles some of the traffic noise. Head downhill and right to cross a bridge. The trail curves right before heading back left and under a railroad trestle. Beyond the trestle, the trail heads uphill and right, past a bike trail sign on the right. Continue as the trail heads uphill and left, past an industrial complex on the left. The trail then goes left and under another railroad trestle before going back uphill and left. As it heads back to the right, the trail goes downhill, with Market Street now on your left. Hike under Market Street using the underpass and then go left, away from the water. The trail heads uphill past a marsh on the right. At the top of the hill, the trail goes right and into a stand of tall trees, then across a small bridge. Cross another small bridge and, at the end of the concrete trail, turn around and retrace your route to the parking lot. As you head out of the stand of tall trees and toward the Market Street underpass, look across the water for a small cemetery.

NEARBY ACTIVITIES

East of Baytown and the Goose Creek Stream Greenbelt are the Anahuac National Wildlife Refuge and the J. J. Mayes Wildlife Trace. Other activities in the area include the Baytown Nature Center, Eddie V. Gray Wetlands Center, San Jacinto Point Recreation Area, San Jacinto State Park, George and Freda Chandler Arboretum, and the Houston Raceway Park.

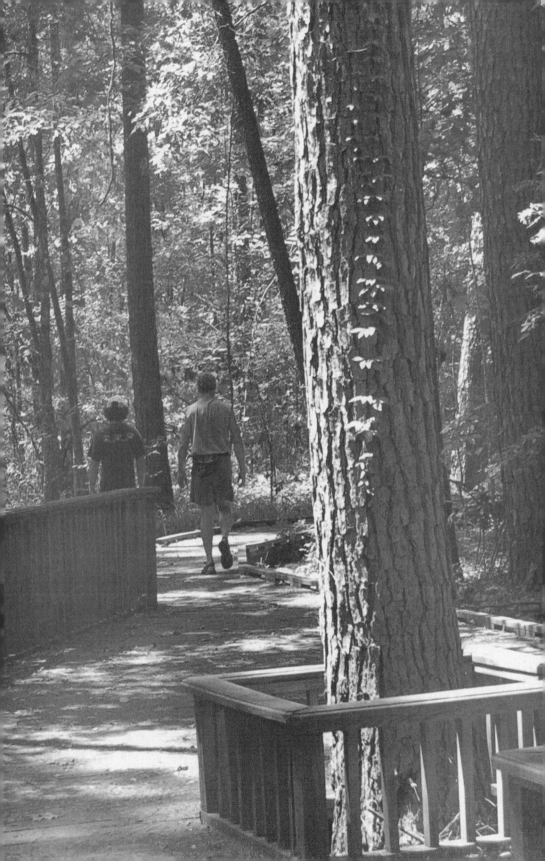

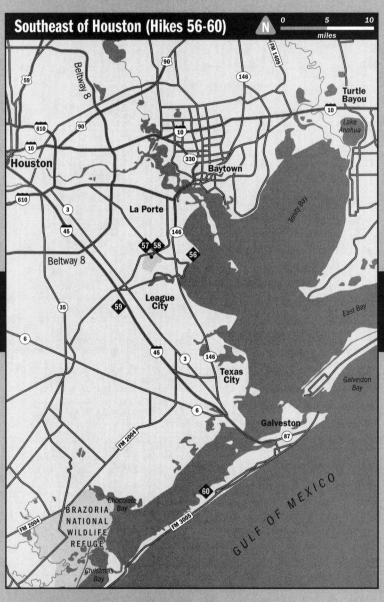

Southeast of Houston (Hikes 56-60)

N

| 0 | 5 | 10 |
| miles |

Houston

Baytown

La Porte

League City

Texas City

Galveston

Turtle Bayou

Lake Anahua

Trinity Bay

East Bay

Galveston Bay

GULF OF MEXICO

Chocolate Bay

BRAZORIA NATIONAL WILDLIFE REFUGE

Christmas Bay

SOUTHEAST of HOUSTON
(INCLUDING GALVESTON)

56 SEABROOK HIKE AND BIKE TRAIL

KEY AT-A-GLANCE INFORMATION

LENGTH: 6.8 miles

CONFIGURATION: Out-and-back

DIFFICULTY: Moderate

SCENERY: Marshes, bay, wilderness parks, urban parks

EXPOSURE: Sunny with some shade

TRAIL TRAFFIC: Moderate on weekends

HIKING TIME: 3 hours with lunch

DRIVING DISTANCE: 16 miles

ACCESS: Free

MAPS: USGS League City

WHEELCHAIR ACCESS: Yes

FACILITIES: Restrooms, picnic tables, ball fields, water fountains

SPECIAL COMMENTS: Be cautious while hiking in Seabrook Wilderness Park and Pine Gully Park; both are snake and alligator habitats. Stay on the trail at all times to avoid encounters with wildlife. If you park in Pine Gully Park, there is a $20 fee for nonresidents.

GPS TRAILHEAD COORDINATES

LATITUDE: N 29° 33.890'
LONGITUDE: W 95° 1.394'

IN BRIEF

This hike is a mixture of small-town neighborhood hiking and wilderness, solitary hiking in some of the best birding areas along the Texas Gulf Coast. Seabrook, which was founded in 1832 by Ritson Morris, received a league of land from the Mexican government. Parts of this league were sold to Seabrook W. Sydnor in 1895, giving the town its current name. Known for the bay and its accompanying wildlife, Seabrook has over 300 species of birds listed on the Great Texas Coastal Birding Trail. Look for pelicans, ospreys, warblers, egrets, sandpipers, buntings, and numerous migrant songbirds. Other wildlife includes white-tailed deer, alligators, bottlenose dolphins, armadillos, blue crabs, shrimp, and catfish.

DESCRIPTION

This 6.8-mile out-and-back hike can be shortened by parking at any of the other parking lots along the route. This hike, which is also popular with cyclists, takes you from the small town of Seabrook proper to Pine Gully Park on Galveston Bay. Park at either the Seabrook Community Center or City Hall and head right toward 2nd Street. You are walking on the side of the street so use caution. Turn left on 2nd Street and left again on N. Meyer and onto a sidewalk and the start of the trail.

Directions ———————→

From the intersection of Beltway 8 and I-45, drive south 7.6 miles and exit the Nasa Road 1 flyover into Clear Lake. Travel 8 miles to Highway 146/Bayport Blvd. and turn right. Quickly turn left onto Cook Street and drive one block to the Seabrook Community Center parking lot.

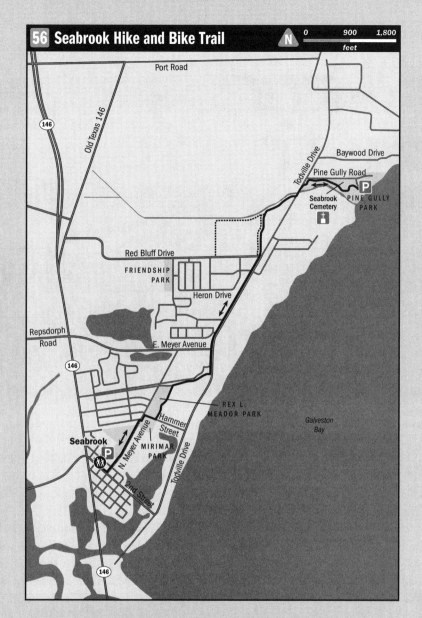

56 Seabrook Hike and Bike Trail

N

0   900   1,800
feet

Port Road

146

Old Texas 146

Baywood Drive

Todville Drive

Pine Gully Road

Seabrook Cemetery

PINE GULLY PARK

P

Red Bluff Drive

FRIENDSHIP PARK

Heron Drive

Repsdorph Road

E. Meyer Avenue

146

REX L MEADOR PARK

Galveston Bay

Seabrook

P

N. Meyer Avenue

Hammer Street

MIRIMAR PARK

Todville Drive

2nd Street

146

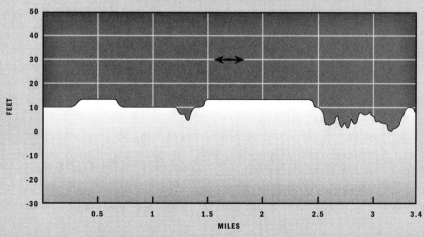

FEET

50
40
30
20
10
0
-10
-20
-30

0.5   1   1.5   2   2.5   3   3.4

MILES

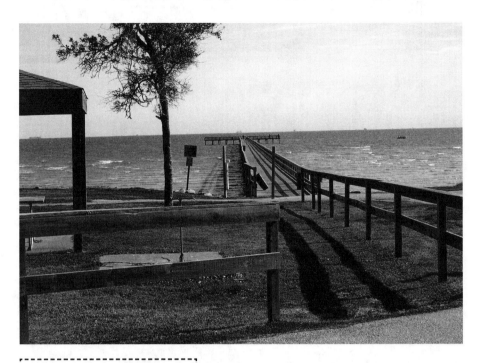

Galveston Bay at the end of the trail

The town of Seabrook is on the opposite side of the Kemah Bridge from the Kemah Boardwalk, a well-known tourist destination near Houston. With 18 parks, this small community is a favorite outdoor destination for hiking, cycling, kayaking, and fishing.

As you press on, you'll pass by beach cottages, small shops, and many parks. Continue down the concrete trail past an open field on the left until you come to Seabrook Sports Complex with numerous ball fields. Once past the complex, head toward Aspen and cross N. Meyer diagonally to get on the crushed granite trail in Miramar Park. Take the fork to the right at Hammer Street and head toward the swimming pool on your left. Hike past the pool, through a small parking lot, and take a left to follow the trail across Hammer Street. You will see a sign for a disc golf course to your left.

Continue down the crushed granite trail past a restroom on the right and a skate park on the left. As you hike, N. Meyer is far to your left, along with the other side of the loop for this trail. Continue straight past a small bridge on your right that goes to a private residence. Once you pass the intersection for the loop, the trail leaves the park and enters a more isolated area.

Hike past two benches on the left before coming to an intersection for another loop. Head right as you hike along the gully on your left and thick vegetation on your right. Again, you can easily see the other side of the loop to your left past the gully. Hike past a bridge on your left that takes you to the other side of the loop and continue straight through a large stand of bamboo trees on your left. While most of the trail is quite sunny, this section does offer some shade.

As you approach Todville Road, you get your first glimpse of Galveston Bay up ahead. At Todville, follow the trail to the left on a small bridge over Pine Gully. Continue past the parking lot to Hester Garden Park. Originally a nursery from 1925 to 1993, Hester Park was commissioned by the city in 1993. Many of the plants and trees for sale were simply left where they were set out and developed into a wooded area.

Continue past several subdivisions and cross E. Meyer Avenue, staying on the trail. The bay is on your right with houses on your left as you hike past crepe myrtles and oleanders toward Baybrook Park. Hike past tennis courts on your left and cross W. Flamingo Drive and then Red Bluff, entering the Seabrook Wildlife Park and the Galveston Bay Marsh. Turn right and pass a bench, water fountain, and trail signs. Expect to see numerous birds and other wildlife on this remote part of the hike. This section is also a loop, but you will only hike one side of it.

Continue straight past benches and a swing and large bridge on the left that not only takes you to the other side of the loop but also to additional trails heading north. Beware of snakes in this area, especially during the warmer months. Hike past a trail-marker sign as the trail winds to the right back toward Todville. Cross Todville to the bridge on the other side and head left. This is a very busy road; use caution when crossing.

Hike over Pine Gully and continue on the trail with the gully now to your right. At a small intersection go slightly left toward a fence. Enter Pine Gully Park, following the trail through the marsh. Pine Gully Road is now on your left and the bay on your right. Some of the trail is slightly elevated to accommodate high tide. Stay on the trail at all times because this is a snake and alligator habitat. Cross a long bridge over the marsh and pass a cemetery on the left. At a fork in the trail, head left past a bench on the right. At the next intersection, take the right fork into the Pine Gully Park parking lot. There you'll find a long fishing pier, picnic tables, and restrooms if you wish to take a break before heading back the same way you came.

NEARBY ACTIVITIES

Within a few minutes of Seabrook are the Carothers Coastal Garden ([281] 291-5713), 18 Seabrook parks, Armand Bayou Nature Center, NASA Space Center, Clear Lake, Kemah Boardwalk, University of Houston Clear Lake, Lunar Planetary Institute, and Challenger Seven Memorial Park. Galveston is 30 minutes south on I-45.

57 ARMAND BAYOU NATURE CENTER:
Martyn and Karankawa Trails

KEY AT-A-GLANCE INFORMATION

LENGTH: 2.9 miles

CONFIGURATION: Two loops

DIFFICULTY: Easy

SCENERY: Creek beds, woodlands, bayou, wetlands, boardwalk

EXPOSURE: Shady

TRAIL TRAFFIC: Light

TRAIL SURFACE: Dirt

HIKING TIME: 2 hours

DRIVING DISTANCE: 12 miles from the junction of Beltway 8 and I-45

ACCESS: $3 per person age 18 and older; $1 children ages 5–17 and seniors 60 and older; open Tuesday–Saturday, 9 a.m.–5 p.m., Sunday, noon–5 p.m.

MAPS: USGS League City; trail maps available

WHEELCHAIR ACCESS: None

FACILITIES: Restrooms, picnic tables, nature center, interpretative center, tours, trail signs

SPECIAL COMMENTS: Armand Bayou Nature Center also features a raptor house; the 1895 Hanson Farm House with a garden, barn, windmill, and pond; pontoon-boat rides; and canoe rides by reservation. Bikes and pets are not allowed on the hiking trails at any time. Bring plenty of insect repellent year-round.

GPS TRAILHEAD COORDINATES

LATITUDE: N 29° 35.657'
LONGITUDE: W 95° 4.344'

IN BRIEF

The Martyn and Karankawa trails are two trails combined into one hike. Although they run parallel to each other, they are very different trails. The Martyn Trail is narrower and goes into deeper woods, whereas the Karankawa Trail runs along the edge of a bayou. Combined, they make a fine hike of almost 3 miles, with helpful signage and rest benches along the way. The Armand Bayou Nature Center has been designated as one of only four Texas Coastal Preserves and is one of the largest bayous in the Houston area that is not channeled. It includes three different ecosystems: bayou, forest, and tall-grass prairie.

DESCRIPTION

To start the Martyn/Karankawa Trail, park in the first parking lot on the left as you enter the nature center. Go to the information center, which is just across the parking lot, to pay the entry fee and pick up a trail map. To start the hike, go left out of the building, past the raptor cage, and down the boardwalk. There are signs warning that the boardwalk is slippery when wet, so use caution. Continue past benches and nature signs along the extensive boardwalk, which is over wetlands. More than 370 species of birds, mammals, amphibians, and reptiles can be found in this 2,500-acre wildlife and nature preserve, including white-tailed deer, armadillos, bobcats, coyotes,

----

Directions

From Beltway 8 and I-45, head south 6 miles on I-45 and exit at Bay Area Boulevard. Turn left and go 6 miles to the entrance of the Armand Bayou Nature Center, on the right. Park in the first parking lot on the left.

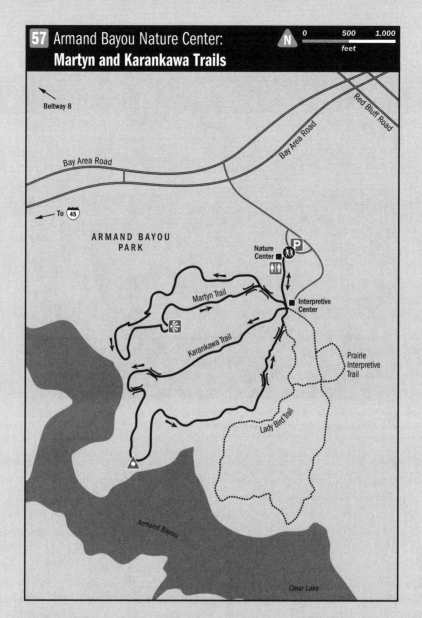

N

0   500   1,000
feet

Beltway 8

Red Bluff Road

Bay Area Road

Bay Area Road

To 45

ARMAND BAYOU
PARK

Nature
Center

P

Interpretive
Center

Martyn Trail

Karankawa Trail

Prairie
Interpretive
Trail

Lady Bird Trail

Armand Bayou

Clear Lake

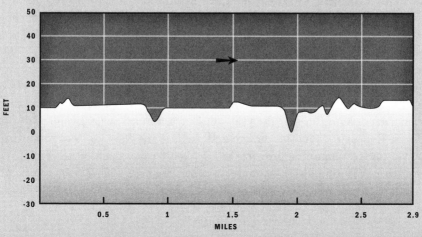

FEET

50
40
30
20
10
0
-10
-20
-30

0.5   1   1.5   2   2.5   2.9

MILES

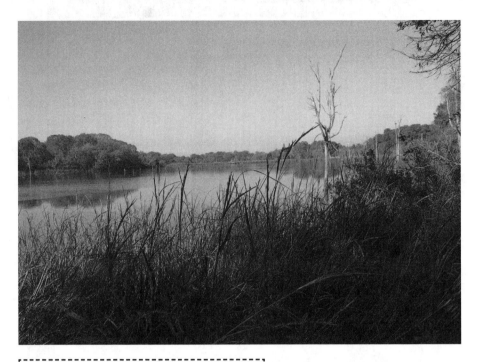

A view of Armand Bayou from the Karankawa Trail

swamp rabbits, turtles, alligators, and snakes (both poisonous and nonpoisonous). The bird population is extensive, with more than 220 species, including warblers, flycatchers, orioles, painted buntings, ospreys, owls, kites, and hawks.

Just before the boardwalk ends, there is a sign warning about poison ivy. Some of the other plants found in the preserve are yaupon, Spanish moss, white oak, black gum, ironwood, American beautyberry, and wax myrtle. Once off the boardwalk, go to the interpretative center, which is straight ahead. A trail sign and trail map are just past the center. The trailhead is just past an observation blind, on the right. The trail surface is dirt with some shale; the trail is about 9 feet wide here. Continue along the trail until you come to the first set of trail markers. Here turn right to get on the Martyn Trail. Cross a bridge and curve right as the trail narrows to about 6 feet wide. Notice the predominance of lichen on the trail, indicating that the preserve stays fairly wet and the trails are not heavily used.

Follow a curvy course past a bench on the right. A high tree canopy over a mostly level trail creates a shady environment. Due to the presence of standing water during certain times of the year, there is not much vegetative growth on the forest floor. Cross another bridge and then, at the Martyn Trail sign, turn right. Go under a naturally growing arbor, then past a bench on the right. As the trail goes slightly right, hike under another low arbor. Now holly trees and white oaks line the route. Go past another Martyn Trail sign on the left. Look right for Armand Bayou through the trees.

Hike past another Martyn Trail sign and then bear right at a fork to follow a spur trail to a bayou overlook. At the end of the spur are benches and a nature sign describing the Galveston Bay Marsh (one of the most diverse habitats in the Houston area). Galveston Bay Marsh is an estuary, one of Earth's most productive and important ecosystems. Estuaries are "nature's nurseries" where they nurture juvenile shrimp, oysters, crabs, and fin fish. Without a well-functioning estuary, there would be little local seafood in our restaurants, and overall populations would decline dramatically. After enjoying the view, retrace to the Martyn Trail sign and turn right. The trail heads slightly uphill and then winds through trees. Go straight through the next intersection, where a trail joins on the right. At the next trail marker, take the Martyn Trail to the left. The vegetation under the trees contains more tall grasses and low bushes, indicating that this area is not periodically covered in water, as in the previous section of the trail. Continue past the next trail marker and then go right to stay on the Martyn Trail. Turn right at the intersection to take a short spur to visit a wildlife observation platform. After visiting the platform, retrace to the previous intersection and then bear right. Go right, past numerous oak trees that regularly drop acorns on the trail, creating a bit of an uneven surface. Continue straight past a hiking sign and then follow the trail to the right, under a tree that is leaning over the trail.

Just past a bench on the left, the trail surface again gets grassy, making it a little more difficult to see. Once the trail goes left and then past a bench, it widens and is much more visible. The trail winds to a bridge, which you cross. At the next intersection, go right, following a sign that reads TO RETURN. Go back over the bridge you crossed at the beginning of the hike and then, at an intersection, turn right to get on the Karankawa Trail. The wide dirt trail goes by an area without much vegetation on the forest floor, indicating periodic flooding. Hike past a barbed-wire fence on your left continuing through the trees and past a bench on the left. Cross a bridge and then go past a clearing on the left with a picnic table; there is a trail marker on the right. Go straight to reach a small pier that juts into the bayou. There is a small fishing shack and some benches on the pier. Turn around and retrace to the previous intersection, then bear right to get back on the Karankawa Trail. Cross a wide bridge over a deep creek and then follow the twisty trail past a bench on the right. At a bayou overlook sign, turn right on a spur trail to visit the overlook, where there are benches for wildlife viewing. Now retrace along the spur to the previous intersection and turn right to regain the Karankawa Trail. Go past a bench on the left and then a trail marker on the right. Pass several benches and then cross a small bridge. At the next trail marker, go left and then over another small bridge. Cross a third bridge before reaching the interpretative center. Go around the interpretative center to get back on the boardwalk. Follow the boardwalk back to the parking lot and the end of the hike.

58 ARMAND BAYOU NATURE CENTER:
Lady Bird Trail

KEY AT-A-GLANCE INFORMATION

LENGTH: 1.6 miles

CONFIGURATION: Loop

DIFFICULTY: Easy

SCENERY: Creek beds, woodlands, bayou, wetlands, boardwalk, prairie, marsh

EXPOSURE: Shady with some sun

TRAIL TRAFFIC: Light

TRAIL SURFACE: Dirt

HIKING TIME: 1 hour

DRIVING DISTANCE: 12 miles from the junction of Beltway 8 and I-45

ACCESS: $3 per person age 18 and older; $1 children ages 5–17 and seniors 60 and older; open Tuesday–Saturday, 9 a.m.–5 p.m., Sunday, noon–5 p.m.

MAPS: USGS League City; trail maps available

WHEELCHAIR ACCESS: None

FACILITIES: Restrooms, picnic tables, nature center, interpretative center, tours, trail signs

SPECIAL COMMENTS: Armand Bayou Nature Center features a raptor house, the 1895 Hanson Farm House, pontoon-boat rides, and canoe rides by reservation. Bikes and pets are not allowed on the hiking trails at any time. Bring plenty of insect repellent year-round.

GPS TRAILHEAD COORDINATES

LATITUDE: N 29° 35.657'
LONGITUDE: W 95° 4.344'

IN BRIEF

The Lady Bird Trail takes you through each of the three ecosystems present at Armand Bayou Nature Center: bayou, forest, and prairie. The nature center has been designated as one of only four Texas Coastal Preserves and is one of the largest bayous in the Houston area that is not channeled. Although it is a short hike, you see many different and diverse habitats that border Armand Bayou, including woodlands, wetlands prairie, and marsh. This hike takes you by the Martyn Farm, an 1895 Texas farm; Armand Bayou; the prairie viewing platform; a Texas prairie marsh; and the interpretive center.

DESCRIPTION

Start the Lady Bird Trail at the interpretive center. To get there, park at the information center to pay your entry fee and then go left out of the information center and onto a boardwalk. The interpretative center is the building straight ahead. There are signs warning that the boardwalk is slippery when wet, so use caution. Continue past benches and nature signs along the extensive boardwalk, which is over wetlands. More than 370 species of birds, mammals, amphibians, and reptiles can be found in this 2,500-acre wildlife and nature preserve, including white-tailed deer, armadillos, bobcats, coyotes, swamp rabbits, turtles,

----

Directions ─────────────────────→

From Beltway 8 and I-45, head south 6 miles on I-45 and exit at Bay Area Boulevard. Turn left and go 6 miles to the entrance of the Armand Bayou Nature Center, on the right. Park in the first parking lot on the left.

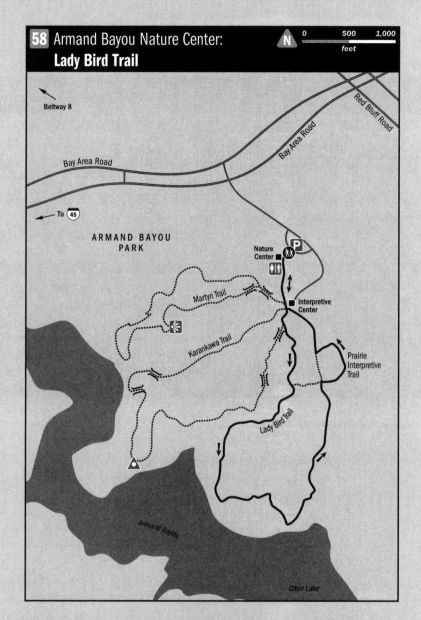

N

0   500   1,000
feet

Beltway 8

Red Bluff Road

Bay Area Road

Bay Area Road

To 45

ARMAND BAYOU
PARK

Nature
Center

P

Interpretive
Center

Martyn Trail

Karankawa Trail

Prairie
Interpretive
Trail

Lady Bird Trail

Armand Bayou

Clear Lake

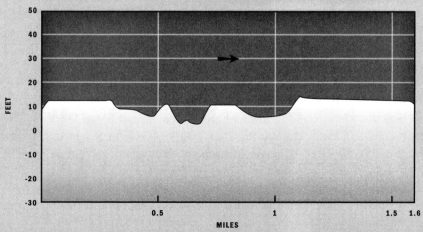

FEET

50
40
30
20
10
0
-10
-20
-30

0.5   1   1.5   1.6

MILES

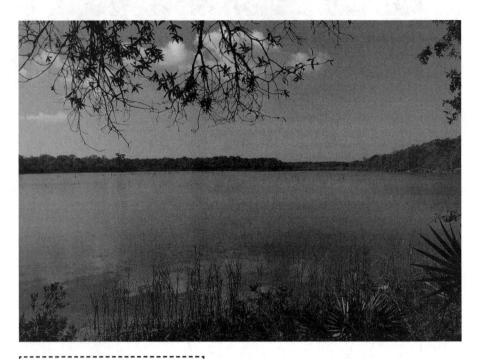

A view of Armand Bayou from the trail

alligators, and snakes (both poisonous and nonpoisonous). The bird population is extensive, with more than 220 species, including warblers, flycatchers, orioles, painted buntings, ospreys, owls, kites, and hawks.

Just before the boardwalk ends, there is a sign warning about poison ivy. Some of the other plants found in the preserve are yaupon, Spanish moss, white oak, black gum, ironwood, American beautyberry, and wax myrtle. Once off the boardwalk, go to the interpretative center, which is straight ahead. A trail sign and trail map are just past the center. The trailhead is just past an observation blind, on the right. The trail surface is dirt with some shale; the trail is about 9 feet wide here. Continue along the trail until you come to the first set of trail markers. Here go straight to get on the Lady Bird Trail. Go straight through the next intersection and cross a bridge. At the next Lady Bird Trail sign, go straight to stay on the trail. The vegetation on both sides of the trail is thick and impenetrable.

Hike past a nature sign, left, describing the sugarberry and hackberry tree. Continue past nature signs about willow oak, water oak, and American elm. These trees are often found in lowland areas, close to rivers and marshes. The American elm can live up to 100 years, making it one of the longest-lived trees in the preserve. Go past a nature sign about cherry bark oak, then straight through an intersection where a trail joins on the left. The Lady Bird Trail goes slightly uphill and right as the trail surface changes to grass. The trail surface is now dirt with some lichen and rocks, making for a slippery surface. The trail narrows, with a small creek running on the right. Continue past a trail marker and uphill. Go past a yellow metal marker on the right (an old trail marker) and follow the trail as it goes right and then takes a big bend left. The vegetation has lessened considerably, indicating that this area retains water part of the year. Go past another yellow marker on the right and continue through trees to a Bayou Overlook sign. For a view of Armand Bayou, turn right on a spur trail to reach the overlook. Now retrace the spur to the previous junction and bear right to regain the Lady Bird Trail.

Soon the trail swings right, providing a view of Armand Bayou on your right. Head left at the next yellow marker and back into the forest. Go past another yellow marker on the right and follow the trail as it goes right. The trail becomes grassy and then goes back to dirt just past another trail marker. Once past the next trail marker, the forest vegetation gets much denser, indicating higher elevation. Continue along the trail as it changes from dirt to grass. A nature sign about marshes explains that they form a boundary between water and land.

Cross a bridge and continue on the grass trail. Pass a nature sign about ecotones, the boundary between two adjacent ecological communities such as prairie and forest. Continue past another nature sign explaining that less than 4% of the original prairie in the United States remains. Go straight on the grassy trail, with forest on your left and prairie grasses on your right. Go past a marker on the left and continue straight through an intersection, where a trail joins on the right. Continue past nature signs about prairie invaders and prairie management. Head right, toward a large viewing platform that is part of the prairie home demonstration garden. Go up the stairs and along the platform to view the prairie from above. There is a nature sign about local birds of prey, including barred owl, osprey, red-tailed hawk, red-shouldered hawk, and white-tailed kite.

At the end of the platform are benches. Go left of the benches and down the ramp. Once off the platform, go left to get back on the grassy trail. Just past a garden on your right, turn right to head back to the interpretative center and end the hike.

NEARBY ACTIVITIES

The Martyn Farm is to the right of the interpretive center and includes a garden, barn, windmill, and pond; there are also picnic tables, benches, and a discovery garden for children. NASA Space Center, Clear Lake, Kemah Boardwalk, University of Houston Clear Lake, Lunar Planetary Institute, Challenger Seven Memorial Park are also nearby.

59 CHALLENGER SEVEN MEMORIAL PARK: Boardwalk Trail

KEY AT-A-GLANCE INFORMATION

LENGTH: 2.2 miles

CONFIGURATION: Loop

DIFFICULTY: Easy

SCENERY: Creek beds, woodlands, wetlands, boardwalk, lake, marsh

EXPOSURE: Shady

TRAIL TRAFFIC: Light

TRAIL SURFACE: Asphalt and dirt

HIKING TIME: 1 hour

DRIVING DISTANCE: 9.5 miles from the intersection of Beltway 8 and I-45

ACCESS: Free; summer hours, 7 a.m.–9 p.m.; winter hours, 7 a.m.–7 p.m.

MAPS: USGS Friendswood; trail maps available

WHEELCHAIR ACCESS: None

FACILITIES: Restrooms, picnic tables, learning center, fishing, tours, canoe camp, barbeque pavilion, bird sanctuary, boardwalk, Challenger Seven Memorial, trail signs

SPECIAL COMMENTS: Boardwalks are for nature observation only: bikes and skates are not allowed. Pets on leash are permitted. Overnight camping by Scout groups is permitted by reservation only, (713) 440-1587.

GPS TRAILHEAD COORDINATES

LATITUDE: N 29° 30.504'
LONGITUDE: W 95° 7.987'

IN BRIEF

This hike takes you from the campgrounds around the Challenger Learning Center to a part of the park that has very few people. You pass a fishing lake, hike on a boardwalk, and visit wetlands next to Clear Creek, a natural tributary that empties into Clear Lake, which is adjacent to Galveston Bay. Challenger Seven Memorial Park honors the astronauts who were aboard Space Shuttle *Challenger* when it exploded January 28, 1986, 73 seconds after liftoff. The Challenger Memorial is a replica of the logo the crew members themselves designed for the mission.

DESCRIPTION

To begin the hike, park in the lot across from the Challenger Learning Center and go toward the trail and boardwalk sign. The learning center provides educational opportunities to area school, Scout, and children's groups. These include programs on insects, snakes, turtles, raptors, bats, alligators, crustaceans, and marine life. The center's hours are Monday–Friday, 8 a.m.–5 p.m.; phone (281) 332-5157.

Continue down the asphalt trail, past picnic tables on the left and a restroom on the right. Wind past a large open field on the

----

Directions ⟶

From Beltway 8 and I-45 head south 7 miles on I-45 and exit at NASA Road 1. Turn right and then, at the first light, turn left to remain on NASA Road 1. The entrance to the park is 2 miles ahead on the left. Continue through the park for about a mile, past the fishing lake, to reach the trailhead. Parking for the trail is next to the Challenger Learning Center.

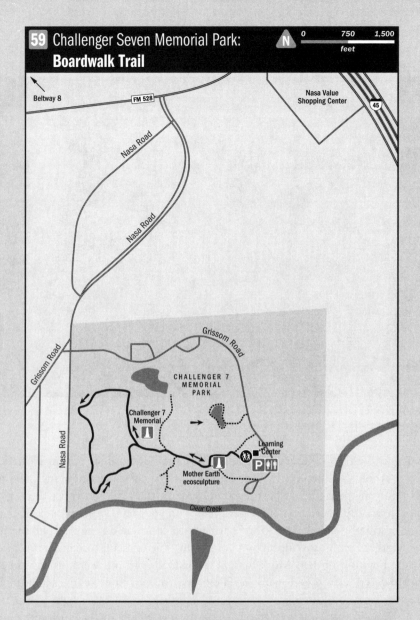

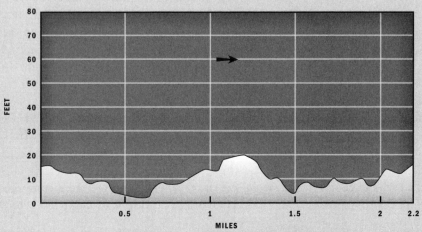

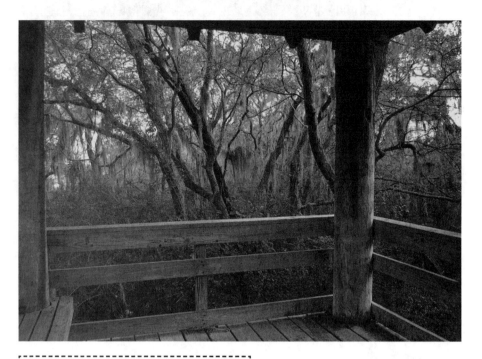

A viewing platform at the end of the boardwalk

right. At the bird sanctuary and boardwalk sign, go straight past a sidewalk to the restrooms. Although the vegetation on the left is thick and dense, the forest floor on the right has been cleared. Stay on the trail and resist the urge to take shortcuts. There is another parking lot on your left, with an open field and swings straight ahead. At a fork, bear right to continue on the trail, hiking past the Mother Earth ecosculpture on your right. The ecosculpture is a large, grass-covered mound of dirt. More than 60 truckloads of sand were brought in and then covered with low-growing buffalo grass. You can climb on the sculpture but bicycles are not allowed.

Head slightly left to get on a boardwalk, which includes three elevated observation platforms for viewing wildlife in the wetlands along Clear Creek. Note that bicycles are not allowed on the boardwalk but are permitted on the park's other trails. On the boardwalk, bear right at a fork to reach the first viewing platform; there are two more ahead—all are covered for sun and rain protection and offer expansive views of the wetlands. There is Spanish moss growing in the trees, creating a very Southern look and feel. When you have finished enjoying the wildlife viewing opportunities, turn around and retrace the entire boardwalk. Once off the boardwalk, turn left to get on a dirt trail. The trail here, partially grass covered, is approximately 7 feet wide. It heads slightly downhill and then right. Go through an intersection, where a trail joins on the left, and go uphill and right. At a clearing where multiple trails converge, take the trail farthest to your right. Hike briefly toward a fishing pond before turning left. Now the trail forks, with both branches running parallel: take the mowed trail on the left. The artificial fishing pond, which is open to the public, is stocked yearly with largemouth bass and catfish. Once through the mowed swath, you reach a large open field with one lone tree. Go left of the tree and to the far side of the open field. Look right for the entrance to Challenger Seven Memorial Park across the field. Find the dirt trail at the far side of the open field and bear left.

At a fork, bear right to hike by a creek. Soon you return to the clearing you visited earlier in the hike. Bear right to retrace your route. Continue past the boardwalk and back onto the asphalt trail until you reach the end of the hike.

Note: Be cautious of poisonous snakes and stay on the trail at all times. There is very little shade on parts of the trail, so be sure to bring sunscreen and a hat.

NEARBY ACTIVITIES

NASA Space Center, Clear Lake, Kemah Boardwalk, University of Houston Clear Lake, Lunar Planetary Institute.

60 GALVESTON ISLAND STATE PARK TRAILS

KEY AT-A-GLANCE INFORMATION

LENGTH: 4.3 miles

CONFIGURATION: Loops

DIFFICULTY: Easy

SCENERY: Bay marshes, bayous, coastal prairie, tidal wetlands, ponds

EXPOSURE: Sunny

TRAIL TRAFFIC: Light

TRAIL SURFACE: Sand and grass

HIKING TIME: 2 hours

DRIVING DISTANCE: 33 miles from the intersection of Beltway 8 and I-45

ACCESS: $5 per person age 13 and older; open 8 a.m.–10 p.m.

MAPS: USGS Lake Como; trail maps available

WHEELCHAIR ACCESS: None

FACILITIES: Restrooms at park headquarters, parking, campsites, nature center, picnic tables

SPECIAL COMMENTS: There are alligators and poisonous snakes in the park, so stay on the trail at all times: the coastal grasses found beside the trail are dense and provide good protection for these snakes. You must pay an entrance fee before starting your hike at park headquarters on the other side of FM 3005.

GPS TRAILHEAD COORDINATES

LATITUDE: N 29° 12.041'
LONGITUDE: W 94° 57.727'

IN BRIEF

Galveston Island State Park is on the west end of Galveston Island and encompasses slightly more than 2,000 acres. The site was acquired by the state in 1969 from private owners under the State Parks Bond Program and was opened to the public in 1975. The park offers camping, bird-watching, nature study, hiking, cycling, fishing, beach access, and swimming.

DESCRIPTION

To start the hike, head toward white posts to get on a grass trail and go north toward an observation tower. The trail is about 6 feet wide, with low coastal grasses and shrubs growing on both sides. It's best to hike Galveston Island State Park in the late fall through early spring, as mosquitoes and the heat can be a deterrent the rest of the year. Continue toward the observation platform and head up the steps for a great view of the bay, marshes, and wetlands of Galveston. Once off the platform, head left (west) of the platform and pass a sign about the Galveston Bay Marsh. Go left at the sign to get back on the grass trail. At a fork, bear right on a sandy trail.

Galveston Island State Park is home to hundreds of species of birds, including

Directions ⟶

From the intersection of Beltway 8 and I-45, head south 32.26 miles on I-45, exit at 61st Street, and turn right. Go 1.65 miles to Seawall Boulevard (FM 3005) and turn right. Go 9 miles to the entrance of the state park, on the left. After paying the entrance fee, turn around and go back to FM 3005. Cross FM 3005 to enter the park on the north side. Take the first left and park in the first parking lot on the right.

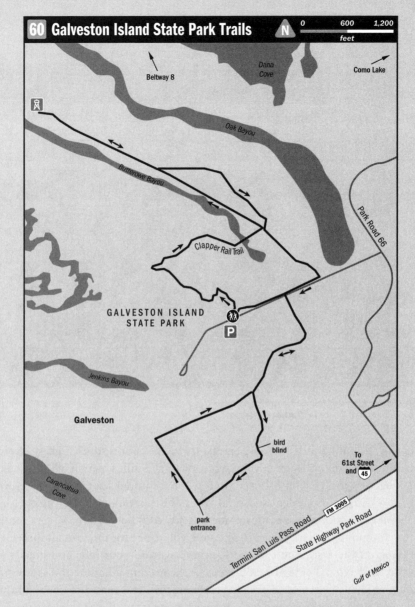

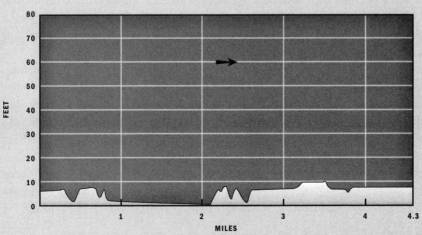

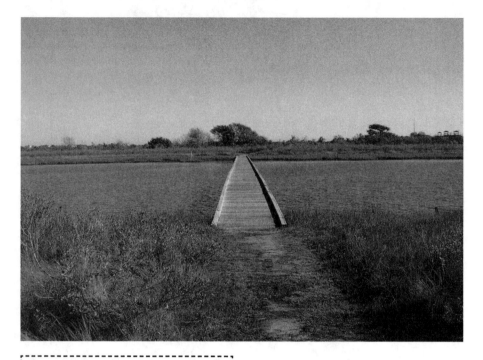

The Clapper Rail Trail over Butterowe Bayou

pelicans, hummingbirds, herons, egrets, owls, spoonbills, ducks, geese, hawks, and eagles. You may also see coyotes, raccoons, armadillos, marsh rabbits, snakes, and alligators. And if you fish, try your luck for spotted sea trout, croaker, redfish, black drum, flounder, and sand trout. The elevation of Galveston Island State Park is 1 foot above sea level, making for very flat terrain. Vegetation less than 1 foot high borders the trail, allowing you to see for miles in all directions. Standing on the trail, you can see Jenkins Bayou to your left, and houses just beyond the bayou. There are crab holes in the ground all along the sandy trail, indicating that this is a good area for crabbing blue crab, calico crab, and fiddler crab. At a fork, bear right and get on a much wider trail. Go to the next intersection, where a trail joins on the right, and follow the trail as it curves right. As you leave the marsh, the trail narrows and trailside grasses increase. Look left for Carancahua Cove in the distance.

Continue as the trail heads slightly uphill and changes to a grassy surface. Vegetation beside the trail here includes prickly pear cactus, mesquite and other shrubs, and coastal grasses. At the next intersection, go left on the Clapper Rail Trail, a long bridge over the Butterowe Bayou. Once off the rail trail, the trail surface changes to shells and sand. At the next intersection, bear left and get back on a grass trail. Butterowe Bayou is now on your left. Where the trail heads downhill, it may be slippery when wet, so watch your footing. Look right for houses around Como Lake. Go through the next intersection, where a trail joins on the right. Now head past a bench and toward another observation tower.

Stay left of the bayou and go past two benches on the left. Sand and low vegetation may make the trail difficult to see: continue to head toward the observation tower. Once at the observation tower, turn around and retrace your route to the first double path you come to. Look left for Texas City and the Galveston Causeway Bridge on a clear day.

Continue retracing the trail until you come to a double path. Take the path on the left, as the one on the right is the trail you were on earlier. The trail surface changes back to grass as you leave the marsh, and vegetation increases on both sides. Go by two benches on the right before the trail curves right. Continue through the next intersection, with the trail you hiked earlier on your right. At the next intersection, bear right, toward the Clapper Rail Trail. Just before the rail trail, bear left on a grass-covered trail. As you head toward the park road, Oak Bayou is now on your left, along with camping and picnic facilities. At the park road, turn right and hike to a trailhead on the left. At the trailhead, go left to get back on a wide, grassy trail. At a fork, bear left, toward FM 3005, which is south (left) of the trail.

Continue past a fishing pond on your left as the trail heads uphill. Go straight through an intersection, past an observation blind on the right. At a stand of trees, head right as the trail curves and continue through the next intersection. FM 3005 is now on your left and a small pond is on the right. At a fork, go left. Continue through the next intersection and past another observation blind, on the right. At the next intersection, turn right to get on a park road that leads past a grassy parking lot. A pond is on your right, and the parking lot is on your left. Go through the next intersection, where a trail joins on the right, and pass a fenced area on your left. At the next intersection, turn right and pass a cattail pond. Continue through the next intersection, where a trail joins on the right, and retrace your route to get on the last loop. At the park road, turn left to return to the parking lot.

Note: Try to hike these trails during the cooler months, as there is no protection from the sun. Pets must be on leash at all times. Fishing is allowed in the bayou but you must have a valid fishing license and observe all state park fishing rules. Check with park headquarters for a list of the rules.

NEARBY ACTIVITIES

Moody Gardens, which has an aquarium, IMAX theater, rainforest pyramid, and private beach; Lone Star Flight Museum; Schlitterbahn (a water park); the Strand Historic District; Seawolf Park; nine historic homes and buildings; and the Railroad Museum.

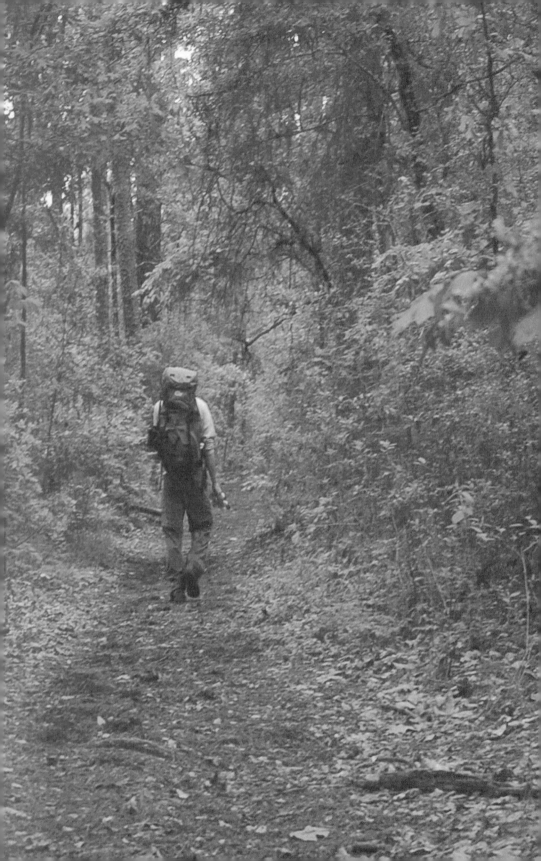

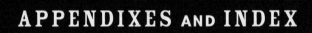

APPENDIXES AND INDEX

APPENDIX A:
OUTDOOR SHOPS

BASS PRO SHOPS OUTDOOR WORLD
5000 Katy Mills Circle, Suite 415
Katy, TX 77494
(281) 644-2200

BASS PRO SHOPS OUTDOOR WORLD
1000 Basspro Drive
Pearland, TX 77047
(713) 770-5100

GANDER MOUNTAIN, locations:
gandermountain.com
Houston/Northwest
19820 Hempstead Highway
Houston, TX 77065
(832) 237-7900

Houston/Spring
19302 Interstate 45
Spring, TX 77373
(281) 288-2620

Houston/Sugar Land
19890 Southwest Freeway
Sugar Land, TX 77479
(281) 239-6720

Beaumont
5855 Eastex Freeway
Beaumont, TX 77706
(409) 347-3055

REI, locations:
rei.com
REI WILLOWBROOK
17717 Tomball Parkway
Houston, TX 77064
(832) 237-8833

REI HOUSTON
7538 Westheimer Road
Houston, TX 77063
(713) 353-2582

ACADEMY SPORTS & OUTDOORS,
locations:
academy.com
290 at 34th
11077 Northwest Freeway
Houston, TX 77092
(713) 613-6300

Crossroads
19720 Northwest Freeway
Houston, TX 77065
(713) 517-3800

Edgebrook
10414 Gulf Freeway
Houston, TX 77034
(713) 948-4100

Gessner
8236 South Gessner
Houston, TX 77036
(713) 219-3500

Houston
7600 Westheimer Road
Houston, TX 77063
(713) 268-4300

Humble
9805 FM 1960 East Bypass
Humble, TX 77338
(281) 964-4760

Katy Freeway
8723 Katy Freeway
Houston, TX 77024
(713) 827-6520

Kirby
2404 Southwest Freeway
Houston, TX 77098
(713) 874-6020

Uvalde
13400 East Freeway
Houston, TX 77015
(713) 445-4400

West Oaks
14500 Westheimer Road
Houston, TX 77077
(281) 556-3200

West Road
10375 North Freeway
Houston, TX 77037
(281) 405-4300

Willowbrook
13150 Breton Ridge Street
Houston, TX 77070
(281) 894-3700

SPORTS AUTHORITY, locations:
2131 South Post Oak Boulevard
Houston, TX 77056
(713) 622-4940

10225 Katy Freeway
Houston, TX 77024
(713) 468-4870

Westgate Marketplace
1210 Fry Road
Houston, TX 77084
(281) 599-1944

11940-A Westheimer Road
Houston, TX 77077
(281) 493-9190

20416 Highway 59 North
Humble, TX 77338
(281) 446-7519

SUN & SKI SPORTS, locations:
sunandski.com
6100 Westheimer Road
Houston, TX 77057
(713) 783-8180

900 Gessner at Interstate 10
Houston, TX 77024
(713) 464-6363

5503 FM 1960 West
Houston, TX 77069
(281) 537-0928

1355 West Bay Area Boulevard
Webster, TX 77598
(281) 823-5154

5000 Katy Mills Circle
Katy, TX 77494
(281) 994-5291

THE WALKING COMPANY
5015 Westheimer Road
Houston, TX 77056
(713) 355-6616

WHOLE EARTH PROVISION CO.
2934 South Shepherd Drive
Houston, TX 77098
(713) 526-5440

APPENDIX B:
MAP SOURCES

DELORME
delorme.com

MAPQUEST
mapquest.com

MAPTECH, INC.
maptech.com

MICROSOFT MAPBLAST
mapblast.com

NATIONAL GEOGRAPHIC MAPMACHINE
nationalgeographic.com/mapmachine

NATIONAL GEOGRAPHIC MAPS
nationalgeographic.com/maps

OFFROUTE
offroute.com

REI
rei.com

TRAILS.COM
trails.com

U.S. FOREST SERVICE
www.fs.fed.us

U.S. GEOLOGIC SURVEY
usgs.gov

USGS MAP STORE
store.usgs.gov

GPS Manufacturers:
BRUNTON
brunton.com

GARMIN
garmin.com

MAGELLAN
magellangps.com

SUUNTO
suunto.com

APPENDIX C:
HIKING CLUBS

AMERICAN HIKING SOCIETY
americanhiking.org

BAYOU CITY OUTDOORS
bayoucityoutdoors.com

HOUSTON SIERRA CLUB
houston.sierraclub.org

HOUSTON HAPPY HIKERS
houstonhappyhikers.org

MOSAIC OUTDOOR CLUB OF HOUSTON
mosaics.org/houston

LONE STAR HIKING TRAIL CLUB
lshtclub.com

SEEING MOUNTAINS IN HOUSTON
bigtent.com/groups/seeingmounts

TEXAS OUTDOOR WOMEN'S NETWORK
townhoustontx.com

THE WOODLANDS HIKING CLUB
woodlandshikingclub.com

INDEX

W

W. C. Britton Park, 263
W. Goodrich Jones State Forest, Middle
    Lake Trail, 136–139
water, drinking, 5, 6, 7
Waugh Drive Bat Colony, 21
weather, temperature, 4–5
West Houston Airport, 113
West Nile virus, 9–10
West of Houston, xii
    featured hikes, 87–121
    map, 85
West Trails, Jesse H. Jones Park, 149–153
West Trails, Mercer Arboretum & Botanic
    Gardens, 132–135

Wheelchair Access (hike descriptions), 3
wheelchair-accessible hikes, xxii–xxiii
White Oak Bayou Hike & Bike Trail, 34–36
White Oak Trail, Big Creek Scenic
    Recreation Area, 172
Whole Earth Provision Co., 291
Wilderness Golf Course, The, 54
wildflowers, best hikes for, xxiii
wildlife, best hikes for, xxiii
Winters Bayou Trail, Sam Houston National
    Forest, 177–180
wooded urban hikes, xxiv
Woodlands, The, 124
Woodlands Hiking Club, 292
Wortham Center opera house, 48, 49

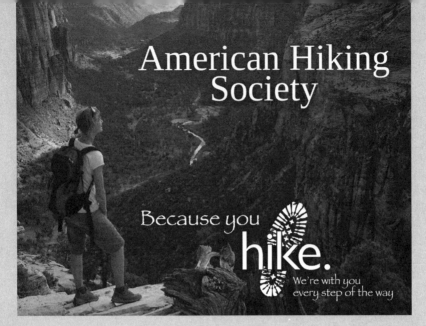

Since its founding in 1976, **American Hiking Society** has been the only national voice for hikers—dedicated to promoting and protecting America's hiking trails, their surrounding natural areas and the hiking experience. **American Hiking Society** works every day:

- Speaking for hikers in the halls of Congress and with federal land managers
- Building and maintaining hiking trails
- Educating and supporting hikers by providing information and resources
- Supporting hiking and trail organizations nationwide

Whether you're a casual hiker or a seasoned backpacker, become a member of **American Hiking Society** and join the national hiking community! You'll not only enjoy great members-only benefits but you will help ensure the hiking trails you love will remain protected and will be waiting for you the next time you lace up your boots and hit the trail.

American Hiking Society

We invite you to join us today!

972-8608
g.org

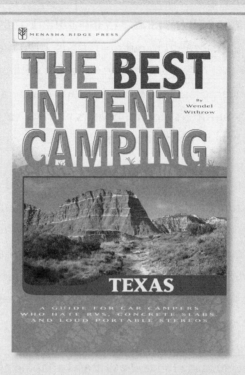
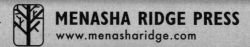

DEAR CUSTOMERS AND FRIENDS,

SUPPORTING YOUR INTEREST IN OUTDOOR ADVENTURE, travel, and an active lifestyle is central to our operations, from the authors we choose to the locations we detail to the way we design our books. Menasha Ridge Press was incorporated in 1982 by a group of veteran outdoorsmen and professional outfitters. For many years now, we've specialized in creating books that benefit the outdoors enthusiast.

Almost immediately, Menasha Ridge Press earned a reputation for revolutionizing outdoors- and travel-guidebook publishing. For such activities as canoeing, kayaking, hiking, backpacking, and mountain biking, we established new standards of quality that transformed the whole genre, resulting in outdoor-recreation guides of great sophistication and solid content. Menasha Ridge continues to be outdoor publishing's greatest innovator.

The folks at Menasha Ridge Press are as at home on a white-water river or mountain trail as they are editing a manuscript. The books we build for you are the best they can be, because we're responding to your needs. Plus, we use and depend on them ourselves.

We look forward to seeing you on the river or the trail. If you'd like to contact us directly, join in at www.trekalong.com or visit us at www.menasharidge.com. We thank you for your interest in our books and the natural world around us all.

SAFE TRAVELS,

BOB SEHLINGER
PUBLISHER